RENEGADE
BEAUTY

RENEGADE BEAUTY

REVEAL AND REVIVE YOUR NATURAL RADIANCE

Nadine Artemis

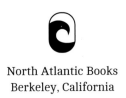

North Atlantic Books
Berkeley, California

Published by
North Atlantic Books
Berkeley, California

Cover art © Andrii Muzyka/Shutterstock.com
Cover design by Jasmine Hromjak
Interior design by Happenstance Type-O-Rama

Printed in the United States of America

Renegade Beauty: Reveal and Revive Your Natural Radiance is sponsored and published by the Society for the Study of Native Arts and Sciences (dba North Atlantic Books), an educational nonprofit based in Berkeley, California, that collaborates with partners to develop cross-cultural perspectives, nurture holistic views of art, science, the humanities, and healing, and seed personal and global transformation by publishing work on the relationship of body, spirit, and nature.

North Atlantic Books' publications are available through most bookstores. For further information, visit our website at www.northatlanticbooks.com or call 800-733-3000.

Library of Congress Cataloging-in-Publication Data

Names: Artemis, Nadine, 1971- author.
Title: Renegade beauty : reveal and revive your natural radiance—beauty
   secrets, solutions, and preparations / Nadine Artemis.
Description: Berkeley, California : North Atlantic Books, [2017] | Includes
   bibliographical references and index.
Identifiers: LCCN 2017037998 | ISBN 9781583949696 (trade paper)
Subjects: LCSH: Women—Health and hygiene. | Beauty, Personal. | Self-care,
   Health. | BISAC: BODY, MIND & SPIRIT / Inspiration & Personal Growth. |
   HEALTH & FITNESS / Beauty & Grooming.
Classification: LCC RA778 .A79 2017 | DDC 646.7/042—dc23
LC record available at https://lccn.loc.gov/2017037998

2 3 4 5 6 7 8 9 Versa 22 21 20 19 18 17

To My Sisters

To my ancestral sisters. To my sister. To my sisters-in-law. To my kin sisters. To my school sisters. To my camp sisters. To my elemental sisters. To my forest sisters. To my Libations sisters. To my friend sisters. To my flower sisters. To my distilling sisters. To my earth sister. To my teen sisters. To my soul sisters. To my future sisters. To all sisters.

Have you ever gotten breathless before from a beautiful face,
for I see you there, my dear.

RUMI[1]

Beauty is not something put together by man. Beauty is when there is
complete self-abandonment, a total relinquishing of the self, the "me,"
with all its aches and loneliness, with all its despairs, anxieties, and fears.
Then you will live in this world as a human being.

KRISHNAMURTI[2]

Beauty! Wasn't that what mattered? Beauty was hardly a popular ideal at
that jumpy moment in history. The masses had been desensitized to it, the
intelligentsia regarded it with suspicion. To most of her peers, "beauty"
smacked of the rarefied, the indulgent, the superfluous, the effete . . . In
a sense, beauty was the ultimate protest, and, in that it generally lasted
longer than an orgasm, the ultimate refuge. The Venus de Milo screamed
"No!" at evil, whereas the Spandex stretch pant, the macramé plant
holder were compliant with it . . . Of course, it wasn't required of beauty
that it perform a social function. That was what was valuable about it.

TOM ROBBINS[3]

All women are beautiful in the ways that we are beautiful. We all have
our unique ways of our own beauty.

ALICIA KEYS[4]

A lily or a rose never pretends, and its beauty is that it is what it is.

KRISHNAMURTI[5]

Beauty is life when life unveils her holy face.
But you are life and you are the veil.

KAHLIL GIBRAN[6]

Contents

Foreword

I first met Nadine through her products—glass bottles filled with heaven. I was transformed by the beauty she created, and soon I fell in love with her as a person.

We met at a hotel one winter evening in Toronto. I was shooting a television show, and she was flying home from speaking at a health symposium. By chance, we aligned in this brief moment and were able to spend some time together. We sat for hours drinking green juice and talking endlessly. I wanted to know everything about Nadine. Her beauty is intoxicating, yes, but when she speaks, it is very clear that she is a leader in the health and wellness movement.

We spoke until the wee hours of the morning, and a deep friendship formed instantly. It was evident within minutes that I had so much to learn from her.

Nadine is one of the warmest, smartest women I have ever met. Her knowledge of health and her care for the natural world are a much-needed feminine pillar in the times we are living in.

When so many businesses are aligned with only profit instead of values, I see Nadine as not only a maverick in the health/holistic movement but also a leader in what a truly conscious business looks like.

She is a steward of nature and of self-initiated wholeness, steeped in the practice and flow of connecting to one's own innate and natural wisdom.

I use every product Nadine makes. Through my friendship with her, I have begun to see my life in metaphor with plant wisdom. When I feel lost and need grounding, I reach for my frankincense. When the world feels heavy and my heart is aching, I pour rose geranium on my chest. This awareness has come as a direct result of knowing Nadine and using her products as a way to support my health and the health of my family. As I reconnect with this knowledge, I bow in gratitude to Nadine. When people stop me and ask, "What is that oil you're wearing?," I share Nadine, and in doing so I know they are headed toward a soulful connection to nature and to themselves.

This book is a gift to humanity. Nadine's beauty emanates through the written word and pierces directly into the heart. The world needs this. I need this. We all need this.

Carrie-Anne Moss

Mother, Actor, Founder of Annapurna Living

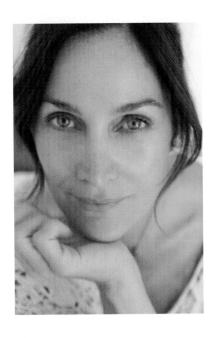

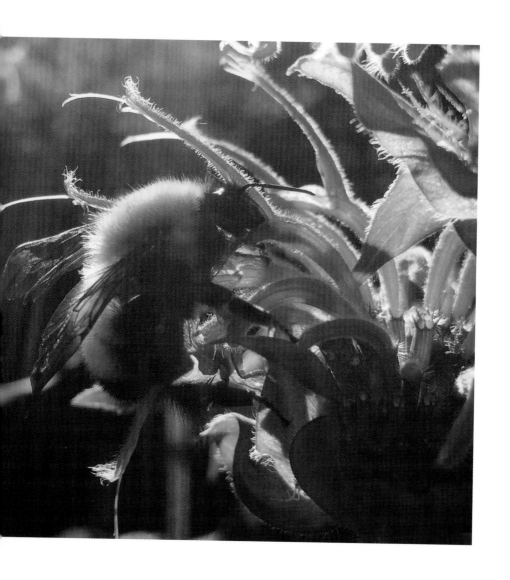

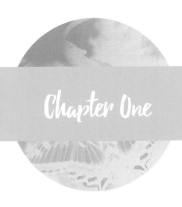

Chapter One

AN UNIMAGINED BEAUTY FLOWS THROUGH YOU

The current culture of beauty is industrialized. Flaws are highlighted and criticized while supermodels' cheekbones get mythologized. The fantasy of female is advertised, leading our thoughts to compare and analyze.

In the pursuit of beauty, we have sprayed on the Obsessions, filled our mind with flawless Photoshop impressions, and laid bare our skin to serious synthetic aggressions. We have Botoxed our expressions, shared sisterly confessions, and endured serious surgical sessions. We dress, on occasion with duress, and fear to digress from beauty regimes appointed by glossy magazines. We have plucked, polymerized, plasticized, plumped with fillers, preened with Listerine, perfumed with Poison, peeled with chemicals, and preserved with parabens. We have poured on, picked upon, and thought we were wrong, so we over-stripped, oversqueezed, and tried to appease the skin we are in.

Dizzying arrays of industrial tricks advertise assurances of self-esteem applied with acne-bleaching cream. We attempt to scrub clean with danger-ous daily routines of douches, deodorants, wipes, puffs of powder, foaming cleansers, and creams to glorify someone else's scheme of being poreless and pristine. Meanwhile, the majority of modern cosmetics cause our skin cells to atrophy, shrivel, and shrink, leading us to think we need to do more and more as bottles amass around our bathroom sink.

Our present day perception of beauty is parched. The focus is on the exter-nal. This vanity of the veneer has created an intense atmosphere that interferes with our body's innate intelligence. Through the haze of this critical gaze, we chase unrealistic perfection and prop up these excessive ideals even though we know the standards are unreal. And boy have we been buying into it at $244 billion a year globally![1] Devouring the Fantasy, the Allure of the perfect contour; creating CoverGirl Complexions; lambasting in Lancôme lotions; dousing ourselves with the fumes of Shalimar, Opium, and Envy perfumes; frescoing our face with perilous paint; and attempting to Keep Up with the Kardashians' surgical fashions.

Over the last twenty years, thousands of women have come to me with their beauty questions. These women are distraught with dilemmas, and the nature of their questions is complex. "Beauty" has led us astray into dangerous terrain. It is time to declare a permanent fast from this pressing paradigm and reconsider the cultural creeds that cause us harm. It is time for a renegade vision of beauty.

Renegade Beauty is not about skincare regimes, and it is not about twelve-step programs for washing your face. It arouses a new set of questions: Is beauty in the eye of the beholder, or are we beholden to live in a state of comparison to the chimera airbrushed images of plasticine-like skin? Is beauty flawless skin or a feeling from within? Is it an emerging inner glow, or something we don't know?

Inspired by the philosophy of vitalism, *Renegade Beauty* surrenders to the seduction of doing less and allows the elements and the life force of nature to revive the body, skin, and spirit. True beauty, healthy and lasting beauty, is expressed from within when we are nurtured by nature. When everything artificial, contrived, and synthetic falls away, the breathability and the beauty of our own nature can shine through.

Yet, we seem to have lost our connection with the natural elements that sustain our body's self-renewing systems. We begin our journey in the not-too-distant past when our lives were integrated with nature, and it furnished our health and beauty. I reveal the philosophy that caused our shift out of nature and briefly examine why and when we withdrew from the natural world around us, and the devastating health, emotional, and cultural problems that resulted. We will also briefly review the historical definitions of beauty from ancient Egypt to Plato, the Renaissance and Enlightenment periods, and the golden mean.

The quest continues with an introduction to the energizing elements that support health and beauty, including the sun, fresh air, water, the earth, and the bountiful gifts of the earth, plants. Prepare to get personal, all the way down to your cells and bacteria. Beauty culminates in the millions of tiny cells and bacteria in our bodies. I invite you on a joyful journey of cellular rejuvenation. Along this journey, we get curious about common beauty complaints, and I explain what is occurring on the cellular level. I offer practical suggestions to rejuvenate the cells and reenergize health. Drawing from food science, I translate current nutrition research on what foods are health sustaining and what foods are best left uneaten.

The sun, the moon, the wind, the rivers, the rain, the soil, the trees and leaves are all here to bathe in, on, and around us. They are the source of our beauty. These elements of nature replenish us because our bodies—our skin— are in relationship to the whole cosmos. This is the creed of Renegade Beauty.

I think we must stop treating beauty as a thing or quality, and see it instead as a kind of communion.[2]

Drink in the dew of perfumed petals, allow innate intelligence to inspire your life, and let nature attend to your Renegade Beauty.

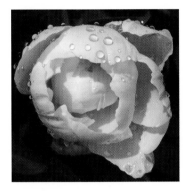 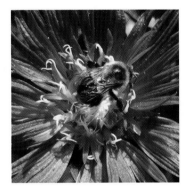

Communing with the world-cosmos-earth grants us grace, strength, and vitality. Nature is the "Is" of what is real. The elements of earth, sun, water, and air and the botanical blessings of plants are here to help us care for our being. Sungazing, sunbathing, forest bathing, moon bathing, cold clear lake water bathing, lying-on-the-earth bathing, and fresh-air bathing nourish and revivify. It is my desire to rouse your inner-beauty compass, to lead you to your guidance, not be your guidance. May this book be a seed along the way.

Where shall you seek beauty, and how shall you find her unless she herself be your way and your guide?

Kahlil Gibran[3]

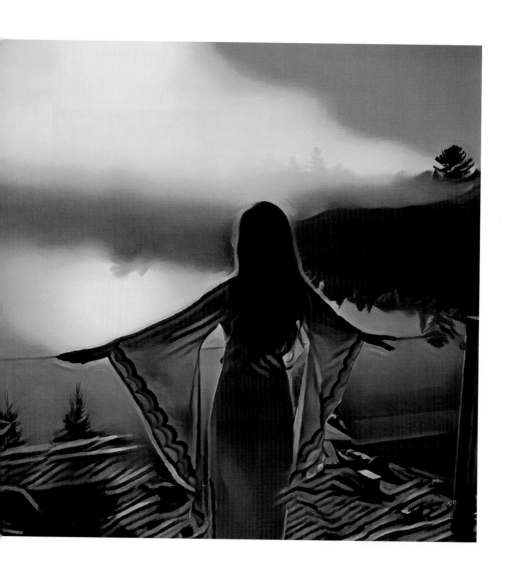

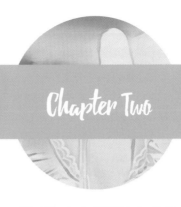

Chapter Two

BEAUTY IS
A PATHLESS LAND

Do you know how beautiful you are?
I think not, my dear.

Hafiz[1]

This book is an invitation, an illumination to dive into your being, to be the beauty and the beautician, the music and the musician, the desire and the desired. Beauty is a pathless land. There is no arrival. There is an is-ness. It's a living thing, a light inside that is revealed. Beauty ripens as your relationship between you and your thoughts, between you and you, becomes unabridged.

When we fear the unknown zones of our body, we swim in a sea of uncertainty that secedes us from our inner compass. Cultural concentration on the external has distanced us from the eternal engine of desire that calls forth life force into our beings. We focus on the smoke of the symptoms instead of the roots of solutions and simple ablutions that can care for and attend to feelings full of beauty.

Beauty is caught in consumerism's spin of acquiring and applying attractiveness with a cash-cow quagmire of chemicals that cannot see the beauty of the forest through the trees. The prompts to primp, polish, and perfect widen the wedge of self-doubt. These insecurities can stifle hormonal secretions of glands and can brittle bones by drying up marrow. Feelings of strife stagnate the blood. Anxious complaints taint the liquids of the liver and tighten the heart's natural desire to expand.

We are always comparing what we are with what we should be. This measuring ourselves all the time against something or someone is one of the primary causes of conflict. Now why is there any comparison at all? If you do not compare yourself with another, you will be what you really are.[2]

When we compare, the world seems unfair. Comparing ourselves to ourselves causes us to condemn parts of our actions and appearance. We compare ourselves to the "more" of friends and to images in movies and magazines, constantly measuring ourselves against someone or something. Caught in a daily dialogue of inner conflict, comparison creates a rift that erodes confidence and breeds fear. Attempting to discover who we are through this divided thinking leads us to perceive ourselves through a fragmented reality. This inner schism between what is and what should be is a siphon that drains away our vital energy.

Engaging with life without the lens of comparison creates vast clarity as the mind is immersed in life's totality.

In this sense, "Beauty is when you are not."[3] When we get out of the way, we observe without processing the perceptions of self-identification and without the clutter of comparison. There is freedom in our furrowed brow as limited thinking gets liberated. This brings equanimity to both the insult and the compliment. If you are looking in the mirror and scrutinizing your skin for the next place to scour or the next pore to pick, you are having fissured thoughts that can be fraught with doubt and judgment. Is it possible to lift the needle off the record spinning in our minds and get out of habitual grooves of thinking? Is it possible to stop a negative thought? Yes! By tuning in to our feelings, we can catch a ride on the compass of our internal guide.

Find daily moments of time to divine awareness into the momentum of your mind's mental chatter, the brain's backlog of banter, and become aware of the contents of the river of your thoughts meandering in your mental spheres all day every day. By slipping into the stream of thinking, we can tune in to the feelings that go with these thoughts. If it doesn't feel good, it does your body no good to keep on playing the song of the thought. Feelings are signals, our inner-compass clues, that a thought is out of alignment with our true tune, which is worthiness: complete and absolute worthiness.

Focus on what makes you feel good. Think: what do I enjoy about my skin, hair, hands, my body, being, and senses? Start with general gratitude for being alive and having hundreds of body systems flow without you having to make it happen. This clears a space for the etheric grace of cosmic companionship.[4]

The invisible mist of our thoughts has a relationship to the element of ether. Ether is the unseen fifth element, the substratum of space, the omnipresent emptiness, the void that impels source substance into being. Ether is intangible, whereas the other elements are tangible; ether is immaterial, whereas water, earth, wind, and fire are material. Ether is the ethereal catalyst that coalesces with vapors of thought. The mind is composed of ether: thoughts and emotions ride on waves of cerebral space; spirals of DNA store the ether of unseen cellular memory. Tuning in to the energy of all that is, merging with the wholeness of existence, fusing to the fulsome frequency of who we are, allow a full flowering of our worthiness. The "rose opens because she is the fragrance she loves"; the flowers' fragrance arises "above all for their own sake, for what we enjoy of its sweetness as something external can surely be no more than a faint reflection of what is enjoyed by the living flower itself."[5]

The source that sprouts seeds into a kaleidoscope of colorful blossoms, into chalices of sweet-scented nectar, is the same source that breathes life into us human beings. Your worthiness is without an opposite; it is innate. A "feeling of unworthiness runs rampant on our planet, and much of human thought is directed toward lack, which only promotes more disallowance of alignment"[6] to the stream of well-being that flows through our bodies. Grow the garden of your mind to commune to the tune of good-feeling thoughts, and discover an emotional invincibility that is a true reflection of your intrinsic worthy nature.

> Consider that you radiate. At all times. Consider that what you're feeling right now is rippling outward into a field of is-ness that anyone can dip their oar into. You are felt. You are heard. You are seen. If you were not here, the world would be different. Because of your presence, the universe is expanding.
>
> Danielle LaPorte[7]

THE BENEDICTION OF BEAUTY

Inhale. Exhale. Wherever you are at with your body, it's all right . . . always, as the "benediction is where you are."[8] The benediction of beauty begins by surrendering the how and blossoming into the expanse of now. Unconditional acceptance of who you are, what you are, and where you are aligns heart and mind. Appreciation is the exquisite all-accepting song that attunes your body to you. Appreciation is the elixir of the adrenals, soothing the source substance of the kidneys. In appreciation we live in gratitude of the gift of our body, an elegant instrument to live in. In meeting life, we turn to face the sun as flowers do, and experience the eternal dew that everlastingly renews.

> *I want to feel the divine pouring through me in every moment . . . Watch bees sipping juice from flowers. Do that with the mystery of presence. Let your body become honey made from that sipping. We are the unlimited wine you dream of, the reviving light. As you restore that in yourself, you will find fulfillment in every pleasure you pursue.*[9]

AN INVITATION TO ILLUMINATION

Charge your inner fountain of felicity with this invocation of body illumination that is a tonic to tone, an elixir of appreciation to feel good, and a cordial of communion to flourish the deepest wilderness of your being: from the visceral mixing of elements to the stellar constellation of your spirit. Gamble your life on living, and let the calibration begin.

> *Enter in*
> *To your skin*
> *Enter into the formless wisdom of your heart and mind.*
> *Inhaling, exhaling*
>
> *I appreciate my spirit that brings beauty into my being.*
> *I appreciate my heart that lifts to the pulse of loving, bringing beaming radiance to my face.*
> *I appreciate my mind's creativity, clarity, and innocence.*
> *I appreciate my lungs and chest that fill with breath, energizing my body.*
> *I appreciate my thyroid that balances my being.*
> *I appreciate my bones' strength and mineral-rich marrow.*
> *I appreciate my liver's fuel and all the substances it filters.*
> *I appreciate my blood and lymph's ceaseless circulating flow.*
> *I appreciate my mitochondria and the wilderness of cells that light my body's ways.*
> *I appreciate my microbiome's design of diversity that is the terrain of my immunity.*

I appreciate my billions of beneficial bacteria that take care of me so beautifully.

I appreciate my kidneys' essential offerings of vital energy.

I appreciate my stomach and intestines that deliver zest for life.

I appreciate my playful flexibility and moving muscles.

I appreciate my spine that is a scepter of my sovereignty.

I appreciate my nerves nestled in their tranquil sensory web.

I appreciate my veins' verve and vigor.

I appreciate my eyes' clear luminosity and my ears that hear melody.

I appreciate my nose and its ability to delight in a rose.

I appreciate my mouth that expresses the beauty of my heart and mind.

I appreciate my molecules of bliss that rain from the hypothalamus of my brain.

I appreciate my endocrine glands and hormones that harmoniously secrete vital essences.

Embraced by the fragrance of grace, my health flourishes in the wisdom of security and uncertainty. With each breath, I inhale the unknown and welcome it as a source of strength and nourishment. I revel in the infinite intelligence expressed by the deity of spontaneity in every cell and organ. I am thankful for all of my relationships and my relationship to creation, to the elements, and to the cosmos of all living things. I am thankful for the infinite stream of well-being that flows to me and through me. With my heart enraptured and spirit enthralled, I invite beauty to be my guide, to be the weaver of my thoughts and speech. My day-to-day play with providence is a revelrous reception and banquet of beauty that infuse me with the joy juice of love.

Thank you.

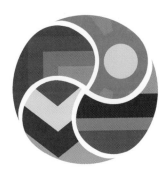

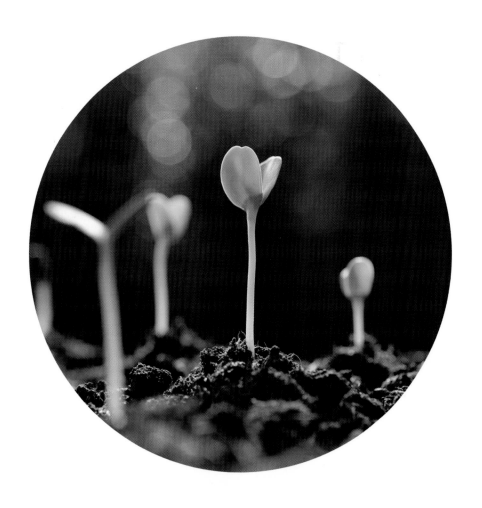

Chapter Three

IN THE BEGINNING

Be the detective of your own life. Attentively discover your own mysteries and early whisperings that will lead you on the pathless path to where you want to be. Teach yourself your relationship to your inner system. Live life from this inner cosmos, and you will blossom in the world around you.

These are thoughts that I share with my son, Leif. I know that these are simply words and that it will be his life experiences that foster his being. We talk about these things as I am hopeful that as he grows and flows with life, he may stay tuned toward self-knowledge and self-discovery. And then, as he sifts and sorts his way through life, he will understand his unique path that has been developing within since his earliest inspirations. As I gain hindsight, I am in deep appreciation of all the breadcrumbs along the way that led me to where I am now. Listening to the early whisperings, my being is imprinted by pindrops of moments creating a collage of confluence in present time.

There once was a girl with a wild look in her eye and a smile that reached to the tip of her cheek. She cleaned up nice, yet her dress was often a mess with pockets full of acorns and findings from the forest, and there was always a curl that longed to unfurl. One day she sat—hands in lap—at the dining room table tuning in and out of the murmuring grown-up din. The raspberries gathered earlier that day had stained the fingers of her imagination. With a rosy glow she gazed out the window and saw friends of branches and birds sway, beckoning her foray. So without a sound, she slipped off her shoes, and her little feet whisked her away to the woods to play. Entranced by the galaxy in a patch of grass, she started to daydream and wondered if every flower was a flask of fun? If petals were spoons for pouring forth perfume? If there is a great pantry filled with ladles of moonbeams and goblets of sun? If bark is the bottle of a tree that holds the secret sap for a scraped knee? And so she asked on into infinity.

She swished bottles and mixed brews, and wished to adorn everyone with garlands of nature. This is the story of how nature found her and how she found you with this book in your hands.

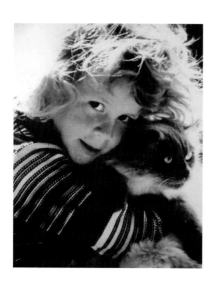

If the sun was out, so was I, and I was happy. Like most parents at the time, mine simply required me home by dark. I would stay outside as long as the sun did. We had a cottage on a lake by the forest, and I could play outside for hours examining closely the patterns of nature. Even when I was very young, I could spend hours on a patch of earth with an array of leaves, mushing mud, flowers, and bark from trees, or hang out in our tree fort in the middle of the forest. We often visited friends in Nova Scotia during the summer. There, the forest was replaced by the beach. The intersection of sea and land offered an array of entirely new elements—wind, waves, sand, shells of all colors, and big, bright-purple starfish. Enamored by these purple creatures, I thought I could take one home. I tried. Upon my return, I was carefully unpacking the bright-purple starfish I had wrapped in my clothes. My mother walked in and asked, "What is that smell?" It was the rotting purple starfish that hadn't survived in my luggage.

When I wasn't outside, I explored the house. I loved to mix liquids, mostly from my mother's bathroom cabinets, and I sometimes found bottles with the skull and crossbones symbol. I discovered that those particular bottles frothed and foamed when mixed. I often poured samples of my perfumed mixtures into shells for safekeeping until my mother would sniff them out and find them among my drawer full of pressed petals, acorns, stones, and dried leaves. I yearned to bottle nature so I could have it at home with me.

School interested me when it intersected with nature. I attended St. Mildred's School, an all-girls school in Ontario set by a small forest with a creek. I would stare out the window and yearn to go out for recess and lunch hours. We swept the forest floor for all we could find. We ran back and forth from the edge of the forest to the creek. We organized logs, leaves, and rocks in the forest and built a small community of forts to play in. We were constantly entertained and creating with the gifts of nature.

As I got older, I still wanted to be outside, yet with different aspirations. St. Mildred's was serious about order, and they were strict about the uniform. I was always trying to alter the uniform somehow, even slightly, to see what I could get away with—wearing penny loafers instead of oxfords or a cashmere sweater instead of the itchy polyester navy-blue sweater they required us to wear. Recess and lunch became an opportunity to sneak in sun and to test the boundaries of the uniform guidelines. We pursued sun as if it were forbidden fruit. One spring we began bringing books to lunch and recess. It must have puzzled a few teachers. Luckily, none of them asked questions or watched us long enough to realize that we were not turning pages. We positioned ourselves just right, backs to the school, facing the sun, opened our books, unfolded our aluminum foil bookmarks, and basked for glorious minutes in the reflected rays of the sun.

I was a schoolgirl in the 1980s, and I had bottles and bottles of makeup. I was the youngest in my family and I accumulated hand-me-down bottles of lotion and makeup from my mother and sister. I had several palettes of eye shadows—one had thirty vivid colors, including electric ultramarine blue and Elizabeth Taylor violet. I would often bring my collection of makeup to school, and we would have so much fun applying Egyptian-style eyeliner accompanied with dragonfly-green mascara.

Pop culture soon propelled me a step further into my preteen cosmetic creations. On the TV show *Square Pegs*, I heard a teenage Sarah Jessica Parker and Jami Gertz talking about their potential career paths. One asked the other, "What do you want to do when you're older?" The other replied (imagine this in a full Valley Girl accent), "I want to name lipsticks—like Very Red, Very Very Red, and Very Very Very Red." It was comical, yet that tiny moment struck me; the idea of a career of naming potions intrigued me. At the same time, I was enjoying a novel series called *Sweet Dreams*, which I am sure the faculty of St. Mildred's would not have approved of. One of the characters was a high school girl who made her own makeup, and I found that fascinating. My potion-making past was revived, and I began making my own makeup concoctions. I loved the sheer-white lip gloss look from the 1960s, so I made some myself by taking white eye shadow and melting it with pots of lip balm. It was my first "product," and I adored wearing it. I called it Moon Swoon. I am still making it, yet with much, much better ingredients.

My creative evolution continued when we took a family trip to Europe the summer after my eighth-grade year. I discovered the pharmacies, especially in France and Italy, lined with bright bottles of exotic European designer ablutions. In Paris we went to Le Printemps, a grand department store, and they had hundreds of perfume samples in tiny replica bottles instead of little vials. I collected them all, took them home, and mixed them to make my own scents to wear. For better or worse, no one in my hometown smelled like me. My mother, Deirdre, was an art historian and award-winning interior designer, so she was keen on us visiting every architectural wonder and what felt like every church in Europe. The highlight of Paris was stumbling upon the quaint Fragonard Museum. Here glass cabinets glimmered with vintage bottles, apothecary jars, and perfume instruments. Imprinted on my mind was the history of olfactory arts and ancient aroma artifacts.

The next school year, I began to find ways to integrate my perfume passion with my education. While trying to decide what to create for a science fair project, I found a book in the library on cosmetics making. The chapter on perfume included formulations and was fascinating. I was enthralled to read more about perfume's true roots in nature and that these substances were available in present time, as something called essential oils. Now everything was connecting to the aroma artifacts at the museum; now I could gather my own substances, rather than mixing from bottled perfume. I determined that I would re-create Nina Ricci's *L'Air du Temps* for the school science fair. My mom, always encouraging creativity, drove us to the health food store in Toronto. Here I inhaled my first oils of ylang, jasmine, neroli, lemon, and orange and I was hooked. It was a whole new world of fragrance; the aromas had a depth and a regal reality that I had not known in the 1980s aromascape of saccharine fruity fantasies of watermelon and strawberry bubblegum, powdery florals, fluffy candy-floss fragrances, and musky men's colognes. I didn't quite understand the discernment between natural and synthetics at this stage, yet these new plant aromas awoke an olfactory lightbulb of possibilities in my mind.

My creative energy continued to develop, along with my energy to challenge convention. Limited by our uniform, my friends and I unconsciously became cosmetic activists at St. Mildred's. I was in high school, obsessed with perfumes, mixing makeup, doing hair for my friends, and having nail-polish parties at lunch where we would experiment with French manicures and hues of Schiaparelli pink and lilac purple. The faculty at St. Mildred's did not approve, and soon there was a no-color nail-polish policy. We continued to push boundaries with hair. One day we would show up with wild hair spiked up with gel. The next day a no-gel policy was introduced. As new loopholes in the Golden Rule Book were found, we would test them only to find new rules put in place.

It was the 1980s. We were unaware that the wave of consumer culture was reaching its zenith—at least I was. I was wearing electric-blue mascara. There was no large-scale awareness of the danger of plastics or dangerous chemicals in cosmetics. There was little talk in the West of consumerism, except what to consume. It was time to explore, and there was so much to adorn! My grandmother gave me a subscription to *Vogue* magazine. I was intrigued by the scents in the pages and the *avant garde* ads. I was introduced to all the baubles you could buy and apply in pursuit of idealized femininity. It all seemed very playful and fun.

Intentionally or not, the womenfolk at St. Mildred's were shaping my destiny. Some teachers were simply boundaries I could bounce myself off of, though others inspired my young spirit and guided my growth. My sixth-grade teacher, Mrs. Murray, was one of these. I spent much energy generating giggles and laughter, which she (understandably) saw as disruption. Some teachers would pull me aside to lecture; others sent me to visit the principal. Mrs. Murray chose a different route. She kept me inside one day for recess. "You're a leader," she said. "How would it be if you used your leadership strength for good, as opposed to being the class clown?" She gave me a book called *I Dare You!* I vividly remember this little hardcover book inspiring and inviting me. Mrs. Murray was direct: "I dare you," she said. "I dare you to be a leader."

I didn't realize until years later that the book was a classic, and I give the writer, William H. Danforth, thanks for his shared wisdom, though I am still more struck by Mrs. Murray's willingness to thoughtfully inspire and suggest that I take the innate energy that I had been using for fun and turn it into something that could benefit myself *and others*.

I accepted Mrs. Murray's challenge. I made attempts to use my powers for good, yet the improvement process was veiled by aluminum-foil tans, makeup, makeovers, and fun with friends. The next year, another feminine figure stepped into our school life. Ms. Palazzi replaced Mrs. Bull as principal. Mrs.

Bull had been a classic girls' school principal—stern at times, yet grandmotherly and sweet. She retired, and in strode Ms. Palazzi—a former model, over six feet tall, highly educated, and from New York. She was perfectly coiffed and styled. She wore pastel-pink linen suits and cream cashmere sweaters. "Stunning and unforgettable. Ubiquitous and inexhaustible. A force in education. Tall and imposing. Awe-inspiring. Action packed. Undaunted. That is Linda Palazzi."[1] She was forward-thinking and would talk to us about career paths and leadership. My frequent forays into fashion activism and class clownism provided me with several opportunities to sort things out in Ms. Palazzi's office. Through all of these, she remained composed and exhibited leadership and grace.

Then I was off to university. I focused my degree on philosophy and women's studies, and I became the Women's Issues Commissioner for the university. Leading a dynamic group of young women as the Women's Issues Commissioner at the university was the beginning of a new season for me. Our primary goal was to raise awareness. We researched reports about the presence of dioxins that made tampons full of chemicals. At the time our province was talking about changing the laws so that women could have the same rights as men regarding being shirtless in public, and we brought in speakers to inform the community about this topless topic. I heard about a model, Marla Hanson, who had been the victim of a knife attack and was left with scars on her face. Her case had been a big news item, and we brought her in to speak about the modeling industry, deconstructing the media, and reading the undercurrent messages in ads.

Finally, I found myself as interested in what was happening in the classroom and in my books as I was in the sun and flowers outside. I was challenged to develop skills in critical thinking, critical analysis, and writing. We wrote essays in high school, of course, yet I was more entranced by daydreaming about fun in the sun or the forest floor and what my friends and I would do after school. However, in university I had some intelligent and intriguing teachers, and I began to dig deep.

Women's studies was cross-disciplinary, so we learned about women's lives through many cultural lenses—Women in Film, Women in Africa, Women in Judaism, Women in Literature, Women in African American Literature. We read Toni Morrison and Zora Neale Hurston, and we listened to jazz. We were introduced to and explored an array of new concepts—the male gaze, mimicry, the vagina *dentata*, Freud's dark continent of the female body.

The *Beauty Myth* by Naomi Wolf was one of our textbooks! I wrote a paper on the masterful masquerading of Madonna and her ability to flip the script of classic female objectification. I explored how her crafted image intertwined with disrupting the perceived excesses of the female body. This was my introduction to thinking about the health of the vagina, breasts, breast milk, menstruation, and how women's bodies are perceived to be fluid and without boundaries. I was amazed and thoroughly engaged that we could learn about this in an "institute of higher learning."

We read *Our Bodies, Ourselves,* and learned about the horrors of IUDs and other forms of birth control. Interviewing midwives for a project helped me begin to understand the business of birth. I wrote about women in Taoist China and the Taoist sex practices. I wrote my thesis paper on the female orgasm, "Oscillating Orgasms: Beyond the Pleasure Principles of Female Orgasms." We read about female circumcision in Uganda and studied the relationship between traditional culture, colonialism, poverty, and international aid. We debated whether or not it was a healthy concept to refer to the earth as Mother Earth, considering our historical treatment of women and nature. I remember coining the term "eco-misogyny" for a paper. For one class I researched and wrote about the role of female animals in farming. Of course, all factory-farmed animals are getting a raw deal, yet it is even more of a sad situation for the females, as they are the ones reproducing and being overmilked. I analyzed the relationship between hormones in cow's milk and the pumping of hormones into women from the birth control pill to hormone replacement therapy (HRT).

Along with the growing awareness in my academic work of all things female and natural, I was learning to be on my own. Instead of living in residence, I found a quaint cottage with a little woodstove in the backyard of a house. It was on a picturesque street with a humble health food store called *Grains and Beans and Things* that operated out of a barely transformed house. I dropped in every day after class and eventually bought every bean and book in the store.

As I continued my school studies, I furthered new frontiers in food preparation. I read many health books, including *How to Get Well* and *Swedish Beauty Secrets* by European naturopath Dr. Paavo Airola and *The Goldbecks' Guide to Good Food* by Nikki and David Goldbeck. This educational book took readers around the entire supermarket and deciphered the fine print on labels. It was revolutionary. I learned among other things that an ingredient on a label can be a placeholder for an exponential amount of hidden ingredients and that all-bran cereal was a health food farce because of all the strange, unnatural fibers and other elements that were added to the mix.

These simple experiences in new ways of thinking and new foods were stirring my inner alchemy. The unadorned nourishment of my first flaxseed and rosehips porridge was a type of homecoming. Tasting this honey-infused flax breakfast warmed my heart, and it was the beginning of never eating processed food again. Soon I discovered the farmers' market and the delights of freshly baked sourdough bread and shiitake lentil stews. A whole world of nourishment opened up as I discovered this portal to new palettes of possibility. It may seem to create a bottleneck in food choices, yet it really expanded my gourmet reality as it introduced me to edible herbs, unusual varieties of greens, new soups and stews to brew, making milk from oats, fermented cultures, farm fresh eggs, and an array of authentic fats and oils. I was in a whole new food heaven.

One morning I came across *The Phil Donahue Show* on TV. He was talking about a book called *Diet for a New America*. The guests that day were John Robbins, Raul Julia, and Lisa Bonet. They spoke about not eating animal products and that there was a primary connection between food production, our health, and the health of the planet. In a sweet circle-of-life moment, years later, I was at a friend's birthday party and a lovely woman approached me to say thank you. She had recently heard a talk I had given on breast health. As we talked, I realized it was Lisa Bonet, and it wasn't until she walked away that I remembered how seeing her talk about the quality of food and factory farming all those years ago had been a pivotal moment, an encouraging game-changer for me to question the production of food and self-care products and then venture into making my own skincare creations.

This encouraged me to decipher the cosmetic codes of all my bath products, which led me to my fuller understanding of the beauty industry. This compelled me into a product purge. I had been excited about The Body Shop, because their products seemed more natural than the classic beauty-counter brands. I had their pineapple face wash, body oil, and dewberry perfume. Yet when I started researching the nitty-gritty of ingredients, I realized how unnatural these items were and that there was no such thing as a dewberry in nature! It was understanding that the "cleaner" beauty brands were of the same ilk as the classic ones that brought me back to the wonderful world of essential oils.

Determined to exclude processed bodycare from my life, I collected every book on essential oils and making cosmetics I could find. I was totally intrigued by ancient formulations and European alchemy of the eighteenth century just prior to the advent of synthetics. Among my favorite books were *Perfumes and Their Preparation*[2] and *Perfumery and Kindred Arts: A Comprehensive Treatise on Perfumery,* which included a history of perfumes, a complete and detailed description of the raw materials and apparatus used in the perfumer's art, with practical instructions, careful formulas, and advice on the fabrications of all the best preparations of the day, including essences, tinctures, pomades, powders, oils, emulsions, cosmetics, tooth powders, sachets, and essential oils.[3]

The books described aromas I had never heard of, and my nose would not rest until it could inhale every pure ingredient on the planet. I dove into research and recipes; I wrote to consulates, distillers, and raw-material suppliers in foreign lands. I found exceptionally pure and artisanally crafted essential oils, oils that were distilled slowly and at lower temperatures that protect the oils from being oxidized and produce oils brimming with botanical constituents. I pursued the highest-quality raw materials and never settled. I found the best of the best. I was aware that I had been living in the synthetic world and could now discern the really real from the pseudo-real. Once I discovered the bright palette of pure, clean essences, I could not fathom using anything else.

I started receiving samples of oils: neroli from orange groves in Tanzania, luminous ylang ylang from Madagascar, beloved bergamot from the Jasmine Coast of Italy, and very velvety lemongrass from Zanzibar right from the distiller. These were organic, artisanally distilled oils that were a whole new level of purity. This was when I olfactorily understood that most of the available essential oils on the market, including the ones at the health food stores, were using highly adulterated "essential oils" sourced from companies that were mainly based out of warehouse-laboratories that make "nature-identicals." I learned by smelling. The scent trail led me to the purest oils and the fascinating realm of research and sniffing and whiffing essences from all over the world—and they all smelled leaps and bounds more beautiful than what was available on the shelves of a store. I sourced oils that were not even mentioned in aromatherapy books at the time, such as ravensara, manuka, and boronia, and I started importing quantities of quality oils.

I fitted my cottage kitchen with beakers and blenders, bottles and jars. And I began to mix and melt, to brew and make balms, to pour and perfume my way to making skincare creations. Some of my first products were solid perfumes with jasmine and linden blossoms, lip balms, body massage oils in recycled wine bottles, chest balms with eucalyptus, and therapeutic blends like Waitress Legs for clearing up spider veins. From this I formed my first company, *Artemis*

Essentials. Family and friends enjoyed my creations, and it was so fun to see my efforts bloom, encouraging me to dive in more fully.

During those university years, elements of my early passions and current education merged into one. My desire to push past established boundaries developed into questioning established norms regarding what we put in and on our bodies. My love of nature guided me into identifying the healthiest path that values the vitalism of beauty and the cosmos.

In my final year of university, I was so eager to graduate, because I knew exactly what I had to do. Within months of graduation, I opened my first store, *Osmosis,* on Queen Street in Toronto. It was North America's first full-concept aromatherapy store. It was such a special place from the moment the doors opened. There was a striking mural on the back wall of Van Gogh's *Irises* and a draped fabric ceiling that was welcoming. There was an exquisite blending bar with a menu that offered essential oils by the drop and personalized perfume creations. People would drop in to this scent salon just to relax in the aromatic ambience and to converge in conversations with people who had similar passions. I cherished those conversations—it was a beautiful place and a beautiful time. There was lots of media interest, and I found myself on television and in national newspapers and magazines sharing the vision. I began speaking at aromatherapy conferences, where it was delightful to meet pioneers in the field, Dr. Kurt Schnaubelt, John Steele, Robert Tisserand, Valerie Ann Worwood, Jeanne Rose, Dr. Daniel Pénoël, and Dr. Pierre Franchomme. I traveled to meet my essential oil distillers, and I taught workshops on making incense and medicinal blends and on skincare and crafting perfume. I lectured on smelling without thought, and on essential oils for family health care, for pregnancy, and for perfumery.

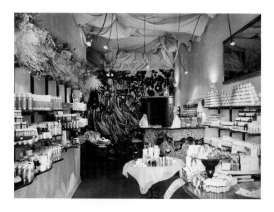

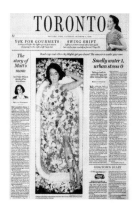

Another full-circle moment that percolated with the providence one discovers while being the detective in one's life was the first time I met aromacologist John Steele. He was talking about aromatics in ancient Egypt and the Temple of Luxor. My great-grandfather, Marcus Worsley Blackden, had been the president of the London Egyptology Society and a member of The Hermetic Order of the Golden Dawn. He was a gifted artist and intellectual. He worked on translations of the Egyptian *Book of the Dead* and worked as an illustrator on archaeological digs with Howard Carter, who later discovered King Tut's tomb. I had grown up with these paintings of his of the goddess Isis and of the Temple of Luxor. So John was talking, and I was listening intently. As John talked about hypnotic blue lotus flowers and the design of the Temple of Luxor, I didn't need to see his photographs—I knew it from the painting. Yet I had not known about the inside of the temple. John explained how the interior was architecturally designed with chambers to reflect the interior of a nose—the entire olfactory system. I was learning—absorbing new information—and I was also being fulfilled. It was an ancestral affirmation on my scent trail.

Clients and friends I met at *Osmosis* created serendipitous occasions to make meaningful connections. One of these happened in the early days of *Osmosis*. At the end of every day, I would turn up the volume and mop the floor. Alanis Morissette's album *Jagged Little Pill* had just been released, and it became my mopping music. Alanis was on tour and came to town for a concert. She had expressed to a mutual friend that she wanted to visit a store called *Osmosis*. Her friend called me and 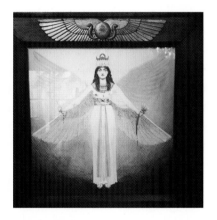 we set up a midnight rendezvous after the concert at the store. It was so much fun! She was like a connoisseur kid in a candy store, delighting in every smell at the scent bar and picking up on the many subtle nuances of the essences. To this day in her scent library she still has bottles of *Osmosis* blends smelling as lovely as the day they were poured.

The store could have continued to bloom, and there were offers to franchise, yet I longed to live in nature; I had to focus on finding a forest to live in.

It was a difficult decision, yet I closed the store. That had been quite a run—studying, importing, and creating a store. So I lived like I was retired for a year, yet it was really just a pause . . . to think and to re-create. Although I still had a handful of private clients and worked on some perfume projects, I wanted to recalibrate for a moment. I composed a special project: making unguent perfumes in one-of-a-kind vintage compacts. These compacts were little gems, each one and each perfume unique in its shape, color, and texture. I called them Moisture in an Oyster, and they were featured in *The Hollywood Reporter*.

During this semi-retirement, I had time and space to simply be. I went on many camping trips and immersed in nature. I camped in the deserts of Arizona and California to experience the skin's relationship to the sun through applying infusions of jojoba and essences of tamanu, myrrh, frankincense, and seabuckthorn berry. A few years later, these botanicals became the ingredients that are in Everybody Loves the Sunshine. In the summer I would travel to the forests of Algonquin and Killarney, where I had canoed often in my youth. Then I met Ron.

Upon our meeting, I was compelled by Ron's life force and the crazy wisdom of his playfulness. Soon after we met, I was scheduled to travel to Arizona again for another conference. I told him I was ready to go, and he said, "I am coming with you." It was a beautiful moment. It was the first month in our relationship and things were fresh and new, so I was a little nervous too. We went to Arizona together and while I was doing conference things, Ron gathered orange blossoms. He asked the hotel concierge for a needle and thread and then proceeded to sew orange blossoms into garlands for a necklace for me. I was blown away. It was such a loving, enchanting gesture. The next day we invited people from the conference to our room for a hydrosol cocktail party. We had rare distillations of blue lotus, pink lotus, rose, and frankincense hydrosols. It was a whimsical word-of-mouth invitation, and we had a crowd. One attendee was Horst Rechelbacher, the founder of Aveda, who had just sold his company to Estée Lauder. We talked briefly and he said, "This is fun! Let's go out for dinner." We left our party and went to dinner with an industry giant.

Horst was a lovely man, and we had a great evening. He was starting to explore creating a new product line. He loved the innovations of my creations, and we engaged in lively discussions about natural beauty care. At one point he said, "You're the real deal. It would be so much fun to work together." Alas, there was no professional collaboration between us, yet it was sweet to be appreciated by somebody who had such a dynamic career. It was a great moment for Ron and me to be involved in that weekend together. We had joined forces in the Canadian winter when there wasn't much nature budding to explore and appreciate. So we ventured over to camp in Joshua Tree. We made sun teas with chaparral and sage, we slept under the stars, and we hiked. He was absorbing and loving all the smells as we went. At one point he put sage up his nose as we hiked so he could really take in its aroma. I loved that he would do this, and I thought, "He finds a needle and thread and sews fragrant garlands. He just shoved sage up his nose in Joshua Tree. He is so the one for me."

Some nights we would stay up till dawn, imbibing essential oils, drinking exotic elixirs, and sinking into a world of luscious libations. It was on a night like this that Ron became impassioned about working together. So we did. We started making yoga truffles and chocolate bars, and co-created new perfumes and blends together. And the beginning of Living Libations bloomed.

Then we took to the woods together.

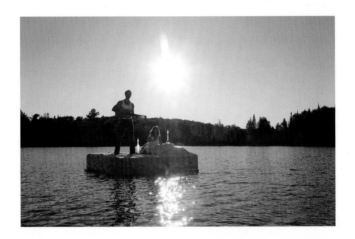

With freedom, books, flowers, and the moon, who could not be happy?

Oscar Wilde[4]

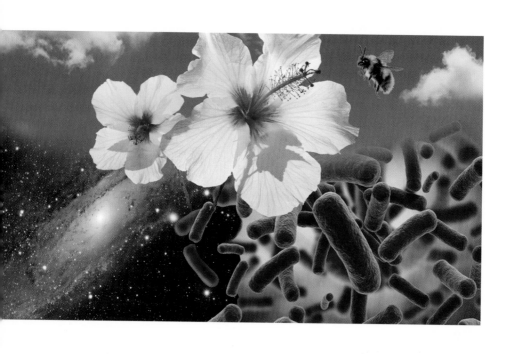

Chapter Four

THE MYSTERY AND HISTORY OF BEAUTY

From Milky Way to Microbiome

When we contemplate the whole globe as one great dewdrop, striped and dotted with continents and islands, flying through space with other stars all singing and shining together as one, the whole universe appears as an infinite storm of beauty.

John Muir[1]

Suggesting visions of ripe fruit, Euripides, an ancient Greek philosopher, defined beauty as "being of one's hour." He believed that even something or someone usually considered ugly can transform into a thing of beauty when that person steps into one's own fullness of being by dwelling in the present.

Greek society was very interested in the notion of beauty, and an influential ethic of beauty in ancient Greek culture relied on mathematics. There are three elements of beauty: proportion, symmetry, and coherence. This notion of beauty was more than an ideal; it was to be implemented, imitated, and revered in how they lived their lives and how they formed culture. *Eudaimonia*, often translated as "happiness through flourishing," adheres closer to the spirit of the word, and is an expression of beauty well-lived. Aristotle proposed that virtue is fundamental for human flourishing and offered the golden mean as the sweet spot of virtue that exists between extreme character traits. The classic example highlights courage as the virtue, with recklessness and cowardice as the extremes. To the ancient Greeks, the golden mean was an ideal of beauty because it encouraged human flourishing via symmetrical virtue.

Leonardo Fibonacci, a thirteenth-century monk, noticed a particular pattern that was repeated in nature: branches on trees, petals on flowers, and sunflower seeds. This pattern, now called the Fibonacci sequence, is "Nature's numbering system"[2] and it still awes and inspires mathematicians and scientists today. From this sequence the "golden ratio" (1.618), otherwise known as phi, was computed, and this ratio is often called the perfection of beauty and design. (We can also thank Fibonacci for displacing the Roman numeral system and popularizing our current numerical system and symbols.) There is more on the mystery and beauty of Fibonacci later in this chapter.

THE GREAT DIVIDE

Early seventeenth-century ethicists have a lot of explaining to do. Until that point in history, life energy was a mystery of nature that commanded respect. Life was mostly agrarian, and the culture was organized to *live with* the land, and from that land people gained all that was needed for life. Humans still regarded themselves as human animals as part of nature.

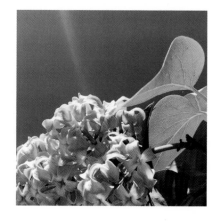

All this began to change with the arrival of two powerful philosophies in the late Renaissance period (fourteenth to seventeenth centuries): rationalism and materialism. These philosophies reduced the created world, including our bodies, to autonomous machines. Humans were allowed the privilege of souls and minds, though the rest of nature, plants and animals, was devalued to simple material substance: a series of pumps, joints, and levers devoid of a conscience, soul, or any divine energy. In this way, humanity was removed from the created order and elevated above it. This ethic slowly seeped into the beliefs of the cultural key-bearers—the church, the arts, and education—thus, it eventually seeped into the social conscience, and today it dominates public life and private sentiment.

The Industrial Revolution began in the mid-1700s with the advent of machines, new standards of efficiency, mass manufacturing, and urbanization. As agrarian life shrank and the new mechanical view of nature infiltrated our basic assumptions, a wedge was driven between humans and the rest of creation. We became agrarian-agnostics unaware. For this, both humans and nature have paid the price.

Along with these changes, the philosophy of beauty changed. Beauty no longer was considered an inherent characteristic of things—flowers, fields, people, animals. It lost its place as a cultural ideal or truth and became subjective, an opinion, a passing sensory experience: "Beauty is in the eye of the beholder."

Immanuel Kant and Edmund Burke, eighteenth-century philosophers, extended a difference between the classical or philosophical meaning of beauty and of the "Sublime". The sublime was recognized as a powerful, astonishing, almost fearful, physiological response to a vision or experience. For example, sublime is the emotional experience of viewing Gothic architecture, extreme mountain peaks, and powerful storms on the ocean. The experience of beauty, on the other hand, is pleasant and inspiring, such as viewing a field of wildflowers, a cozy library, and children at play.

The ideal of beauty was not fully lost, yet. Beauty was a central concern of Friedrich Nietzsche, who argued that beauty is a personal ideal, an illusion that veils reality, and almost a lie. Even though, or perhaps because, beauty is an illusion, Nietzsche argues that it can save us in tragedy, in darkness, and from the suffering that all of us experience in life. Beauty is the dream-beacon on the hill on a dark night that produces hopeful, inspiring light to guide the way, even if it is all make-believe.

The contemporary era, the twentieth and new twenty-first centuries, saw an increasing rejection of the pursuit of beauty by artists and philosophers alike. This has culminated in postmodernism's antiaesthetics, where art across all aesthetic fields is produced for the sake of pure art in lieu of beauty. The notion of beauty was demoted to "pedestrian."

The ideal of beauty was usurped by consumerism, and suddenly beauty got gooey. Beauty in our current cultural landscape is dictated to us by glossy magazines, celebrities, commercials, and the critique of mass media. Beauty was degraded from an ideal, a mathematical ethic, and even a dream-beacon to a common act of commerce.

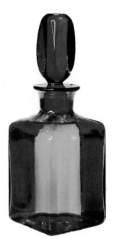

On average, women use nine personal care products every day, and 25% use as many as fifteen products daily.

The passageways of womanhood (and manhood) are wallpapered with beauty ads that point to products that promise to shape our destiny. Beauty is purchased as a fashion that is applied to the body or worn as the newest cut of jeans. It is sold as glittery bottles of antiaging serums, body-shaping surgeries, and eye-color-enhancing eye shadow. Beauty is for sale if you are willing to pay the price.

"Beauty is not caused, it is."[3] Beauty is resilient.

The materialist and rationalist divide is beginning to crumble as we learn anew how vital to our well-being a relationship with nature is. Some contemporary philosophers, artists, and even some scientists are beginning to reengage and reconnect with the concepts of beauty, nature, and human flourishing.

Dr. Elaine Scarry, the author of several lovely books, including *On Beauty and Being Just*, invites an academic and public revival of the appreciation of the beautiful. Her thoughts on beauty elevate the everyday natural beauty around us, things such as flowers and sunsets. As an obsessive gardener and flower aficionado, Scarry admits to often losing herself in the beauty of the natural world.[4]

Our world has become dehumanized. Man feels himself isolated in the cosmos, because he is no longer involved in nature.

Carl Jung[5]

The human need and longing to reconnect to the sustaining energy of the natural world are real. In 2005, Richard Louv hypothesized that limited exposure to nature contributes to health and behavioral problems, citing increases in ADD/ADHD, depression, obesity, and myopia as a "nature deficit disorder."[6] In *The Nature Principle,* Louv reasons that "reconnection to the natural world is fundamental to human health, well-being, spirit, and survival."[7] We see it in science with the hygiene hypothesis and various microbiome projects and in agriculture with the swell of organic farming, homesteading, and permaculture farming. It is also on the rise in the field of natural aesthetics, such as horticultural design shifts toward natural gardens and native plant preservation.

VITALISM

Vitalism, a late nineteenth-century philosophy, is garnering renewed support as a viable bridge between our nature-deprived society and its shallow beauty and a life-affirming, holistic way of being and of being beautiful. Arising from the natural sciences, vitalism asserts that we honor the complexity of life, every living thing's innate spirit, and the necessity of its connection and interconnection in its own environment. Innately linking science, ethics, and aesthetics, vitalism is rejuvenating

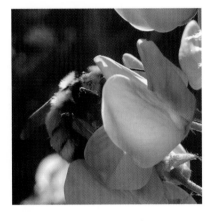

new research in both hard and social sciences, and it may just change the way we think about ourselves and beauty.

One vein of vitalism in particular speaks to the interconnectedness of human beauty and nature. In 1846, English art critic John Ruskin conceived of Vital Beauty in volume II of his book series *Modern Painters.*[8] Ruskin was an outsider to academia, and his broad ideas are more cosmology than philosophy. In an argument that is strikingly familiar today, Ruskin decried the "loss of fellowship with nature"[9] in the urbanism of his post–Industrial Revolution era, and he wanted to draw humanity back into relationship with creation.

Ruskin defines Vital Beauty as the energetic beauty of thriving, living things. It is "the expression of the happiness and energy of life, and . . . with the representation of moral truths by living things. These beautiful truths exist as part of a divinely ordained great chain of being in which each living creature plays a role as agent and as living emblem of divine intention."[10] Vitality springs from the joyful fulfillment of each living thing's function and engagement with its lived experience.[11] This living energy is governed by laws of growth that Ruskin named "circles of vitality," and these life-laws provide order and organization to life that we can investigate and step into.[12]

Ruskin's theory embraces direct personal experience and relationship with and among all living things: plants, the cosmos, animals, humans, and ecologies. These dynamic, intimate interactions are "an attunement with life and its processes." With this, he transforms beauty from a purely intellectual pursuit and a remote admiration to a "living-with" and "a sympathy" with our coinhabitants of the planet.[13]

> Man is a microcosm in whose flesh resonates and reverberates the whole of creation, in whose mind creation comes to consciousness. . . .
>
> Vigen Guroian[14]

Delving deeper into Ruskin's theories that link nature, beauty, and health, he takes cues from Aristotle by relating beauty to flourishing; plants, animals, ecologies, and humans (as well as every natural element in Ruskin's theory) embody beauty when they are flourishing with health. However, Ruskin does widen the ancient Greek concept of flourishing by stating that flourishing can occur only while in intimate relationship with nature. An integral part of Ruskin's vitalism is the human symbiotic dependence on natural things to flourish; he believes that "much human strength and health of spirit comes from nature."[15]

Looking at iron, one of the most common chemical elements on earth, Ruskin demonstrates how deeply humans dwell within the circles of vitality operating in nature. Iron tends to rust, and the iron oxide produces gems, which everyone admires and enjoys, as well as offers up the essential nutrient that nourishes nature and sustains life. He inquires, "Is it not strange to find this stern and strong metal mingled so delicately in our human life that we cannot even blush without its help?"[16]

Learning to see these circles and the intrinsic value of all the elements of nature, not just iron, is more than an important skill. It is a tender way of being in the world, a way of truly seeing nature in relationship. Ruskin implores us to use our imaginations to see things anew and to develop in ourselves "natural piety."[17]

Ruskin's cosmology of Vital Beauty births a garden of healthy, radiant beauty by embracing our embodiment as earthly creatures living in a symbiotic relationship with nature. *Renegade Beauty* embraces this new epoch that regards beauty as a living, self-organizing system embedded in healthy ecology and nature. This is a beauty that can be stepped into by interacting intimately with nature.

Vital beauty is not just about the careful observation of landscape and natural phenomena but about a sympathetic immersion in shared being.[18]

Is it really as simple as spending more time outside? more time in our gardens? Perhaps beauty graces us by intentionally cultivating the garden that grows in us.

Let's now take a step closer to nature to examine a detailed look at what nature herself can teach us about beauty.

Wilderness is not a luxury but a necessity of the human spirit.

Edward Abbey[19]

SACRED GEOMETRY: NATURE'S GRAND DESIGN

Beauty is a manifestation of secret natural laws, which otherwise would have been hidden from us forever.

Johann Wolfgang von Goethe[20]

There is wholeness in creation: a unity in design, pattern, ratio, and energy. And this wholeness and unity occur at all scales, from microparticles to the cosmos. This unity in form is often called "sacred geometry." By studying the meta-form of nature we learn about the physical properties of each thing and recognize that they are metaphysical symbols of the interconnectedness, the relationship, of all

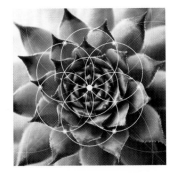

things to the whole. These geometric designs and patterns inform our ideas of *beauty*.

One such mystery found in nature is the fractal repetition of numbers represented in forms and patterns; the same statistical character and harmonic intervals repeat on the micro and macro scales.

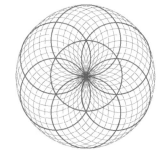

Beyond beautiful, sacred geometry is also nature's design principle, as it is an efficient and purposeful means of organization and growth. It is a cosmos-wide functioning system displayed in both living beings and inanimate objects. Nikhat Parveen, a mathematician, elegantly described the Fibonacci numbers as "Nature's numbering system . . . and applicable to the growth of every living thing, including a single cell, a grain of wheat, a hive of bees, and even all of mankind."[21]

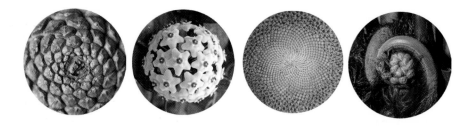

The Fibonacci sequence shows up in the golden ratio (or phi) as the ratio representation that reflects the perfection of proportion in beauty and design. The actual value of phi is approximately 1.618, and this value is divined by dividing a Fibonacci number by the number before it: 34 divided by 21 = 1.619. When this ratio is used to draw the proportions of rectangles, triangles, spirals, and so on, the figures will be pleasing to the human eye.

This sequence of numbers is nature's formula for growth, so not only is it beautiful, it is also evolutionarily and mathematically efficient and effective. It mysteriously occurs all around us; we live in the midst of Fibonacci sequences, and it is even at work inside of us. Hurricanes, spiderwebs, pinecones, pineapple fruits, and seashells are all Fibonacci patterns with phi ratios. A honeybee colony's reproduction patterns also fall along the Fibonacci sequence.

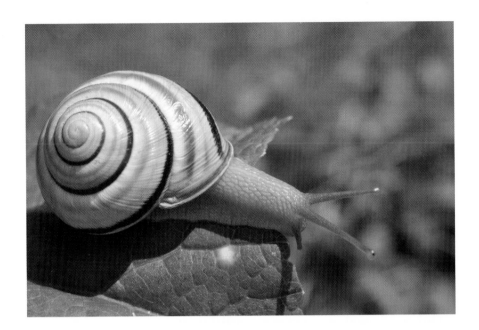

In normal, healthy plants, the cells are self-organizing and grow in a symmetrical pattern that is a Fibonacci sequence spiral pattern. The number of petals on a flower is usually a Fibonacci number. Scientists have discovered that this growth pattern allows the plant to use the least amount of energy needed for growth, and the geometric patterns of the cells and leaves are perfectly arranged so that the plant can absorb the maximum sun rays and efficiently collect and channel rain. This sequence is so reliable in nature that deviations from it are often used as indicators of genetic damage.

A DNA molecule's double-helix spiral measures 34 angstroms by 21 angstroms wide; both 34 and 21 are Fibonacci numbers, and the ratio is 1.6190476. The golden ratio is 1.618. The perfect golden ratio, otherwise known as phi, the perfection of beauty and design.

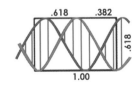

The dimensions and ratios of the human face and body, and even the uterus, are organized in Fibonacci sequences and ratios. For example, the ratio of the forearm to the hand is phi. The proportions of the whole face as well as the length of the nose and chin, the position of the eyes, and the size of the mouth are phi: mathematical beauty. Dr. Jasper Verguts, a gynecologist, measured the ratio of length to width of his patients' uteruses, and the ratio of fertile, healthy uteruses was 1.6. In infant girls the ratio was 2 and by postmenopausal age the uterus shrinks to about 1.46. During the most fertile years it is 1.6.[22]

TOTALLY TUBULAR: TOROIDS

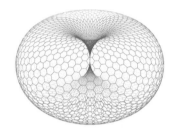

Another self-organizing pattern found in nature is the toroid, or torus, which is the mathematical term for a doughnut-shaped figure. Toroidal energetic models are found extensively in nature across that scale, from the cosmological down to the quantum. When gases or liquids close into a doughnut-shaped loop that spins multidimensionally, inward and around, it is called a toroidal vortex. (Think tornadoes and smoke rings.) These toroidal systems are an elegantly efficient means of stable energy flow and information sharing.

Galaxies are toroidal energy systems. Our sun is enclosed in a large toroidal field. The sun's field exists inside an even larger toroidal field that encompasses our entire galaxy, the Milky Way. Earth resides inside the sun's toroidal field, and earth's atmosphere and ocean waves are toroidal, influenced by earth's magnetic field that protects us from the sun's electromagnetic radiation.[23]

Our body is also a toroidal tube. The alimentary canal that runs from mouth to anus serves as the hole through our doughnut tube. Most of the energy that we need comes from the nutrients pulled out of our food and drink via our digestive tract, with all the lively magic that happens there in the alimentary canal.

The red blood cells that carry oxygen and nutrients to our cells are toroidal. As a red blood cell matures, its nucleus is pushed out of the cell, changing the shape of the cell from round disk to biconcave or closed torus. The toroidal shape provides more surface area on the cell to bind oxygen and carbon dioxide during gas exchange. The shape also helps to ensure the survival of red blood cells as they flow through the rough waters of the bloodstream, because the torus shape provides more flexibility than a perfect sphere.

Sperm cells and viruses contain toroidal loops of DNA, and it is also common among DNA-binding enzymes. Many of the proteins involved in DNA metabolism adopted the ring shape, and they may assume this shape because of some yet unknown advantages in interacting with DNA. The structures and formations of these tiny toroids are yet to be comprehended by science.

The divine design of toroidal shapes, the golden ratio, and the Fibonacci sequence confirms coherence with the order of the universe, with the elements, and with the precise patterns of life. When we resonate with the coherence of the cosmos, we dissolve the illusion of separateness and we connect to the source of all things. Connecting to this infinite intelligence attunes us to our inherent perfection and our inherent worthiness, and we discern that we receive resources from Source as we allow the beauty of nature to continually revive our being.

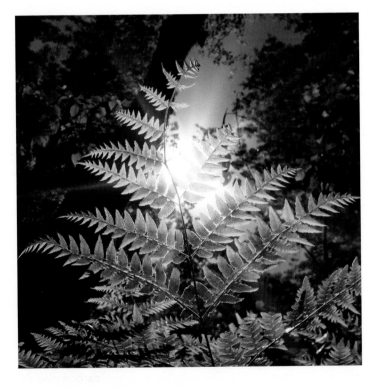

Every particular in nature, a leaf, a drop, a crystal, a moment of time is related to the whole, and partakes of the perfection of the whole.

Ralph Waldo Emerson[24]

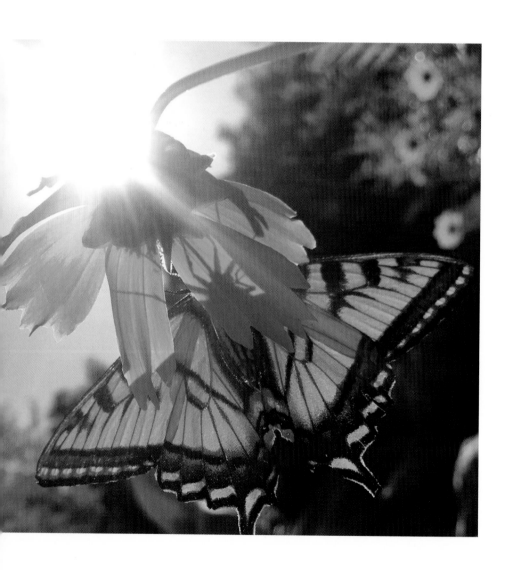

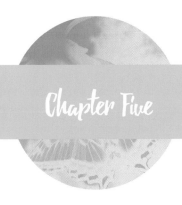

Chapter Five

NATURE IN RELATION

Introduction to the Elements

*Forget not that the earth delights to feel your bare feet
and the winds long to play with your hair.*

Kahlil Gibran[1]

When we think of beauty and self-care, we need to look beyond the bottles at the cosmetic counter and bring in the confluence of the cosmos. In many ways, our skin is starving for a reunion with the elements. Our skin is sequestered from the celestial spheres, the sun, soil, water, and airy atmospheres that sustain our body's self-renewing systems. The recipe for wrinkles and rashes is our current lifestyle that shuns the sun and consumes food grown in the shadows of factory farming and pesticides: rancid, bleached, refined carbohydrates, along with corn syrup and artificial sweeteners, all mix in our bodies with the residues of caustic cosmetics and tainted tap water.

Our beings, our bodies, our skin are inseparable from nature and are intertwined with particles that have passed through the vast reaches of time and space. We are bacterial blasts from the past, and it is our current task to allow the elements, the life force of flowers and air, to revive our skin's self-repair. Let's dive into our divine skin and nourish our pores that are parched for a real-to-the-feel reunion with the gorgeous garden of our being.

Each element exists in intimate relationship with our bodies: our cells and bodies are vessels of water's liquid life, the spirit of air enters our nostrils and lungs, sun shines divine into our pores, plumps our receptors, and stirs our circadian rhythms. The essence of earth sustains us with living, giving gifts from the soil.

The elements of nature—the sun, the moon, the wind, the waters, the rain, the soil, the trees and leaves—they are the source of our beauty. They replenish us because our bodies are in relationship with these cosmic collaborators.

 ## SUN ELEMENT

The sun has been my faithful lover
For millions of years.
Whenever I offer my body to him
Brilliant light pours from his heart.

Hafiz[2]

Every morning the revelrous reveille of the rising sun makes the sky grow lighter, the stars become dimmer, and the dew on silvered fields lift into the air. Flowers open, reptiles bask in warmth, green leaves renew their daily task of churning carbon dioxide into oxygen. The sun rises every day, yet it goes in and out of fashion. We have been lobbied into a loss of sunlight. Sun-

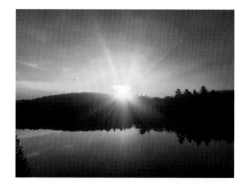

damage debates make us shun the sun and fear exposure from simple jaunts, like walking from the parking lot to the mall. Media and magazines have us so convinced, we have winced at these life-giving rays; with sunscreen applied and sunglasses over our eyes, this is advised to prepare our bodies to engage with the sun.

The sun needs a new PR agent.

In fear of this blaze, we have had a few decades of fun under an air-conditioned sun, fluorescent rays have lit our days, and light from computer screens has affected the expression of our genes. On every tropical trip, sunscreen's grip has stifled serotonin, while waterproof PABA has blocked the brain's good-feeling GABA. We have sunbathed in Bain de Soleil's carcinogenic oxybenzone glaze, choked our vitamin D receptors on Banana Boat. All the while, we think we are doing our part in being SunSmart.

As we got used to alarm clocks, we forgot about the sun, which awakens our circadian rhythms and stirs crickets into song. We forgot about our innate need for cosmic pollination; that our blood, hormones, and skin are aroused by the warm wavelengths of creation. Since ancient times, this molten mass of our mythology, this mysterious companion of the earth, has been revered. Deprived of the sun's divinity, we speculate the sun's danger and make imitations and synthetic suns of our own. As far as we have come from Apollo and his chariot moving the sun across the sky, we still need the sun. No matter our inventions, from lightbulbs to vitamin D supplements, the sun is the maker of our mornings and ruler of our days.

In our ancient odes to the sun, we have Egyptians raising babies to greet the sun's rays and Greeks praising the benefits of *heliosis,* which they defined as therapeutic sun exposure via sunbathing and sungazing. The original Olympic athletes were required to sunbathe to let the sun strengthen their muscles and nerves. Ancient architecture was optimized to interact with the sun. Pliny the Elder of Rome declared, "The sun is the best of all self-administered remedies." Ancient physicians affirmed the sun to be "the best food and medicine" in the world. Even today's microbiologists advocate that the sun is the best disinfectant.

> *I am not surprised that ancient people worshiped the sun, the only thing we know that gives without expectation or even possibility of return. The sun is generosity manifest.*
>
> Charles Eisenstein[3]

> *Even after all this time,*
> *The sun never says to the earth*
> *"You owe me."*
>
> Hafiz[4]

Doctors in the 1800s thought that "invalids should seek the sunlight as do flowers."[5] Our ancestors spent most of their waking hours outside without being afflicted by epidemics of skin diseases. At the turn of the century, as life became industrialized and many people moved from the countryside to towns and cities and worked more indoors, the white plague of tuberculosis wiped out hundreds of thousands of people, and an epidemic of rickets warped the bones of children. This plague of illnesses led to the medical study and application of heliotherapy, sun therapy, as a successful treatment for various sicknesses and wounds. At the time, complete cures by sunlight of tuberculosis and many other diseases made headlines around the world.[6]

Sunlight ripens fruit, guides the growth of trees, prompts petals to close at dusk and awake at dawn. Sustaining solar rays penetrate the deep layers of our planet. And although we try to deny, the sun ignites the deep layers of our skin, our hormonal secretions, and our cells.

As we court the sun and recognize it as a cosmic catalyst, a bestower of beneficial nutrients, we can begin to understand that our skin is designed to be exposed to the sun's rays, that there is an energy exchange with solar ethers that only happens in our skin. This relationship, this union between our bodies and the sun, offers revitalizing nourishment. When our bodies sunbathe and bind with the seminal strength of the sun, the effect of this union is an energy that animates our vitality, our innate immunity, and the very marrow of our bones.

This may sound like a lot to digest: suns are waiting to emanate from your pores.

Hafiz[7]

Chapter Seven delves further into considering what our bodies are currently offering to the sun's rays, if there is such a thing as a healthy tan, or if we can just wear sunscreen, take vitamin D supplements, and forget about it.

The earth has received the embrace of the sun and we shall see the results of that love.

Tatanka Iyotake[8]

WATER ELEMENT

In one drop of water are found all the secrets of all the oceans; in one aspect of You are found all the aspects of existence.

Kahlil Gibran[9]

Waves of water wash over our existence from springs and seas to lakes and the water in leaves; all life sips these aquatic secretions. We are bodies of water that thrive on hydration, right down to our bacterial and cellular nation.

Clouds emit rain and our eyes do the same as inner emotional currents ebb, flow, and form tears. Water quenches the deep thirst of our longing to live, to be both drunk and drank. Waters wash through our being, continually rejuvenating our blood, lymph, nervous system, cells, and cerebrospinal fluids. There is a tidal pull to water intake, and it is vital to know what your body of water prefers. There is a fine composition between damp roots and dried branches. Spring water sings to your cells, and juiced plants nourish deep cellular layers. Drink flowers, sip trees, wet your whistle with leaves. Raise a cup to give cheer; know the element of water is near and dear. Be the moist air, soil, and seed that opens to receive.

Not only the thirsty seek the water, the water as well seeks the thirsty.

Rumi[10]

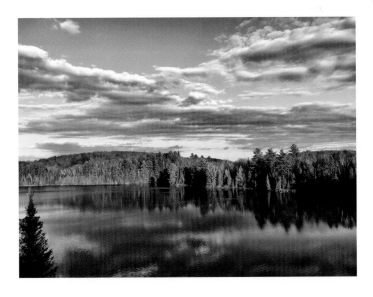

Water is life, yet when stagnant, polluted, and sterilized it can be a harbinger of disease. Water is a living energy that needs care. Although chlorine chemical treatment bleaches out harmful bacteria, it destroys the beneficial bacteria too, while bleaching our blood supply and thus weakening our immune system.

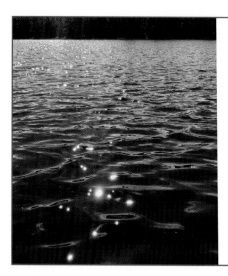

We are thoroughly watery:

• Brain and heart are 73% water.
• Lungs are 83% water.
• Skin is 64% water.
• Muscles and kidneys are 79% water.
• Bones are 31% water.

When we are born, we are about 78% water, and this drops as we age to closer to 50% in the elderly.

Lean tissue holds more water than fatty tissue, and reductions in lean body mass equal less total body water.

Drink pure spring water, which is always naturally cool and clean. Tap water is a fountain of fluoride, chlorine, and dozens of other chemicals. More energy is encapsulated in every drop of good spring water than an average-sized power station is presently able to produce.[11] The Associated Press conducted an investigation into the pharmaceuticals found in U.S. tap water that found traces of drugs in twenty-four major metropolitan areas, with several cities not testing or not reporting.[12] The U.S. government does not regulate levels of prescription drugs in the water, even bottled water. If access to spring water is challenging,[13] a filter that can clear contaminants from tap water is highly recommended.

Actually, the mysteries of water are similar to those of the blood in the human body. In Nature, normal functions are fulfilled by water just as blood provides many important functions for mankind.

Viktor Schauberger[14]

Rumor has it that we need eight glasses of water a day; however, there is no scientific claim to this theory. Your ever-wise body will tell you when it is

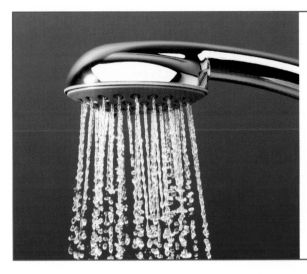

Some of the 300 chemicals in tested tap water.

Fluoride
Chlorine
Antibiotics
Synthetic Hormones
Bronchodilators
Antidepressants
Sunscreen Ingredients
Beta-Blockers
Pesticides
X-ray Contrast Agents
Cleaning Solvents
Fragrances
Nicotine
Veterinary Meds

time for a drink. Thirst sets in once you have lost about 2 percent of its needed water. If you drink to satisfy your thirst and if your urine is clear to pale yellow, then you are well hydrated.

Heed your thirst and sip all day. If you drink too much water, or too much too quickly, the delicate balance of electrolytes in the blood can drop dangerously, causing the cells to absorb too much water and essentially drown. And if you are really dehydrated, downing lots of plain water can flash flood your system and stress the kidneys. It is best to sip slowly and steadily to replenish your fluids.

Our bodies are the boundaries and banks as rivers of capillaries guide the flow of water through our being. Our cells float in a sea of water. Water is the fluid of life. The unique, invaluable properties of water make it a wellspring for health.

Human Photosynthesis: Water and Sunlight

Water in a cup and water in your cells are not the same thing. In *Water, Cells, and Life,* Dr. Gerald Pollack, a professor of bioengineering, explains the role of water in the functioning of cells. We all learn as kids that water can carry an electrical charge, which is why we do not use a hair dryer while in the bathtub. Pollack describes water that is structured in our cells as a battery that can hold and deliver energy. Our cells are exposed to energy as near-infrared light, a.k.a. ultraviolet sunlight. As light hits the water in the cell, water is split into positive (H+) and negative (OH-) ions. (This is the same first step as plant photosynthesis.) This separation of charge is potential energy stored in a cellular battery.

Critical nutrients dissolve in our body water so that they are in a form that can feed our cells. The stickiness of water (it is the property of water that makes one raindrop stick to another as they run down the windowpane) allows our body to transport the nutrients through the body. Precious water in our body also allows our bodies to flush out waste. Water is beautiful.

Consider the significance of solar-powered humans and human photosynthesis. Seek the sun! And consider that perhaps we are more like the plants than we thought. (And eating green leafy plants and drinking chlorophyll provide nutrients for our cells.)

> *Water is the blood of creation. Our own bodies are eighty percent water*
> *. . . We tend not only the garden that we call nature but also the garden*
> *that is ourselves insofar as we are constituted with water and are born*
> *anew by it.*
>
> Vigen Guroian[15]

Water and Moist Skin

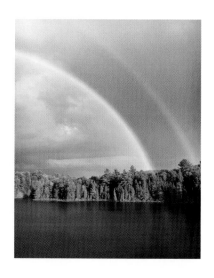

Instead of water hydrating our bacterial hive, a chlorine-clean bathing routine can harm our skin's hygiene. Cleaning our body in chlorine kills the friendly flora that helps skin stay supple, resulting in drying dysbioses from dandruff to dermatitis. Furthermore, the plethora of products applied to our skin creates additional loss of water content from our cells. This happens through a process called osmosis after applying glycerin and humectant products that temporarily plump skin, yet ultimately cause cells to shrivel and shrink.

The water content of our skin cells determines how moist and supple our skin is. Water contains minerals that inform the skin's cells. Intrinsically entwined, mineral content in the cell dictates the water content within it, and the mineral content dictates how receptive the skin is to water. Water provides for cell function and efficiency of cell-to-cell communication. The skin is a great giver to the rest of the body, and even if other organs need water, water goes to the skin first. Early wrinkles are dehydration asking for more water. Dehydration can accumulate over the years, and result in lack of cell flexibility, leading to dry, sagging skin and dark circles under the eyes. Water is a beauty fluid. Drink up!

Drinking water is essential, and feeling water on your skin and moving in water is wonderful! Immersing yourself in water's fluid embrace allows the body to feel grace. Our ancestors knew the value of water's wholesome ways, and spa-like bath houses became a prevalent part of water's waves through history. Cross-culturally, bathing practices shaped society: the Great Bath of the Indus Valley Civilization, the *gymnasia* of ancient Greece complete with aromatic-oil massages, the *thermae* of the Roman Empire, the Byzantine baths, the Turkish *hamam,* Indonesian stone bathing pools, the *banya* of Russia, Finnish saunas, Native American sweat lodges, Japan's natural hot spring *onsens,* and the *jimjil-bang* of Korea—these cultures knew the fine art of being ensorcelled by water's rejuvenating liquid life. See the bathing section in Chapter Thirteen for tips on boosting your baths with botanicals, minerals, and the elements. So get caught in the rain, dance in misty drizzle, dive into cool lakes, hop into hot springs, steam your skin in the sauna, float in the sea, jump in the ocean waves, and steep in a hot bath to feel water's wellness ways wash over you.

The upholder of the cycles which sustain all Life is water. In every drop of water dwells a deity whom indeed we all serve.

Heart, "Dreamboat Annie"[17]

Viktor Schauberger[16]

AIR ELEMENT

Warm winds caress her
Her lover it seems

Heart, "Dreamboat Annie"[17]

Life breathes us. The world breathes in me. "Spirit" comes from the Latin word *spiritus,* meaning "to breathe." Every spirited thing in the cosmos has a respiration rhythm. So many sunrises and sunsets have infused the air with infinite intelligence and our ancient ancestors' breaths. The atmosphere is an exhalation of the earth. Trees exhale and we live!

I am all breathing.[18]

We all breathe the same air. We exist in a vital ocean of air, we breathe each other's breaths, and we inhale the exhalations of plants. We inhale oxygen, nitrogen, and argon. Argon is an inert gas; inert means this gas does not interact with other elements, which also means that ancestral argon molecules, millions of years old, are still being inhaled and exhaled as part of the earth's rapturous respiration cycle. "I imagine the earth with its circle of vapors like a great living being which inhales and exhales eternally."[19]

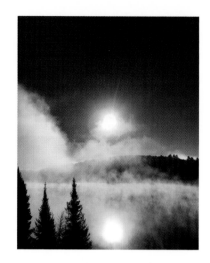

Fresh breath? Our breath is not our own. Every breath connects us to ancient plants and beasts and our own ancient ancestors:

How about air? Also vital. A single breathful draws in more air molecules than there are breathfuls of air in the entire Earth's atmosphere. That means some of the air you just breathed passed through the lungs of Napoleon, Beethoven, Lincoln, and Billy the Kid.

Neil deGrasse Tyson[20]

Air constantly renews our cosmic health, and the air we breathe connects us with the cosmos; "each time you inhale, you are drawing into yourself an average of about one atom from each of the breaths contained in the whole sky . . . and each breath you breathe must contain a quadrillion atoms breathed by the rest of mankind within the past few weeks and more than a million atoms breathed personally sometime by each and any person on Earth."[21]

Contrary to the essentiality of air, many of the products and practices we employ in our modern era block the breath of our skin and our skin's microbiome. Petrochemical-based beauty products act like Saran Wrap, and our clothing alters the pH of skin by encouraging a buildup of secretions that throw off the skin's respiration system and the biome's balance. Because we will most likely not start walking around naked anytime soon, we need to correct our concept of skincare by not clogging our skin with chemicals that leave an invisible yet respiration-robbing residue. Additionally, we can refine our fashion for a little more freshness; feet with fungal infections should not be in synthetic socks and shoes all day. A diaper rash needs fresh air, and our genitals rebel at polyester underwear.

Air bathing is a bath in cool, fresh air. It has since fallen from fashion, yet at the turn of the century, air bathing was elevated to an atmospheric cure that led to vigorous health. Contrary to his contemporaries, who thought that cold air produced colds, Benjamin Franklin, a believer in air bathing, thought that illness came from being inside without ventilation and with airborne germs. He found that the practice opened the pores and refreshed the body by drawing toxins from the skin. Famously, he would sit buff in front of the open windows of his home to get the full effects of the increased airflow. Wise doctors today recommend air baths for soothing sleep and stronger immunity. Hopefully you can find a secluded area to luxuriate in aerating air baths outdoors, and in cooler months simply sit in the cross-breeze of open windows, breathe, and enjoy some herbal tea.

> For my panacea . . . let me have a draught of undiluted morning air. Morning air! If men will not drink of this at the fountain-head of the day, why, then, we must even bottle up some and sell it in the shops, for the benefit of those who have lost their subscription ticket to morning time in this world.
>
> Henry David Thoreau[22]

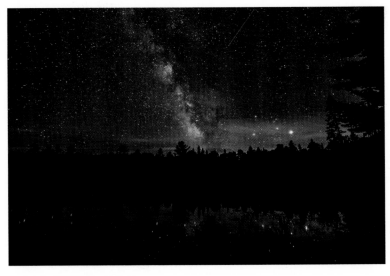

John Lehmann

Night Air

I caught the happy virus when I was out last night singing beneath the stars. It is remarkably contagious, so kiss me.

Hafiz[23]

There was a time when people were afraid of the dark. The eras of the epidemic diseases of cholera and the plague were ruled by the miasma theory. This theory states that a poisonous, smelly vapor spread disease through night air. Come nightfall, people hurried home and shut their doors and windows tight in an attempt to protect themselves from illness. Granted, poor sanitation caused stinky air that would grow more rancid as humidity rose at night. The miasma theory was, of course, discredited with the nineteenth-century discovery of the germ. Even so, much like our predecessors, we tend to go inside at night, when really we ought to be embracing the fresh night air.

Almost every element on Earth was formed at the heart of a star.[24]

We Are Stardust

Your beauty comes from the same source that bursts stars into the night sky. Humans have a natural affinity for and curiosity about the stars, and perhaps this is because these heavenly bodies are our kin. From the meteorites that plant microbes on our planet to the carbon content of our bodies, we are linked to the atoms of comets that fell to the earth and the elements of exploding stars. Physicists tell us that 93 percent of the mass of our body is stardust. This may be a revelation to us, but Paracelsus, the sixteenth-century alchemist, instinctively understood our intimacy with the galaxy when he wrote that we are an "extract from all the stars and planets."[25] We want to soothe the stardust that is us and bathe our bacteria in a bevy of life-affirming elements.

Think back to chemistry class. Every element in the periodic table other than hydrogen was created by an exploding star. These elements are all stardust. The human body is composed of about 7×10^{27} atoms, and 4.2×10^{27} of those atoms are hydrogen. Most of the hydrogen in our body is the H in our H_2O. The human body is about 60 percent water, and hydrogen doesn't have much mass. Physicists tell us that 93 percent of the mass of our body is stardust![26]

Embrace the night. On a clear night, go outside and find a dark place away from city lights, which steal the show of the stars. Lie down under the night sky and attune to your wonder. Be in awe of the vastness of space. Find your North Star, moon bathe, and become aware of the interconnectedness of your life with the stars, the cosmos, and deep space.

> *So she sat on the porch and watched the moon rise. Soon its amber fluid was drenching the earth, and quenching the thirst of the day.*
>
> Zora Neale Hurston[27]

Moon bathing is a different type of cosmoetic (a cosmetic creation of the cosmos) than sunbathing. Moonlight is the absorbed and reflected rays of the sun shining divinely upon the earth. Its luminescence has a cooling, refreshing yin energy, whereas the sun has a warming yang energy. To moon bathe, familiarize yourself with the lunar cycles and venture outside when the moon is in its waxing gibbous, waning gibbous, and full-moon phases. If possible, connect your bare feet to the earth and keep your eyes open to receive the moon's illuminating cosmic wavelengths. Moon gazing is a serene dream that vespers to our internal rhythms and sublime spirit.

> *Well, it's a marvelous night for a moondance*
> *With the stars up above in your eyes . . .*
> *And all the night's magic seems to whisper and hush*
> *And all the soft moonlight seems to shine in your blush . . .*
>
> Van Morrison, "Moondance"[28]

Summer night air is especially sweet, once the sun sets and the air cools, and if you are lucky, the air is filled with the heady, intoxicating fragrance of night-blooming flowers releasing their essences into the dark. Many of the components of these night-flower aromas are aphrodisiacs that can reduce stress and lower blood pressure. You can plant your own moon-bathing garden as a peaceful prelude to sleep by including a few of these sweet night-bloomers.

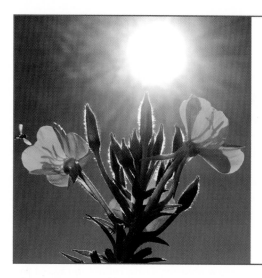

Glorious Night-Blooming Flowers

Evening Primrose
(*Oenothera biennis*)
pictured

Vining Moonflower
(*Ipomoea alba*)

Night Phlox
(*Zaluzianskya capensis*)

Evening Stock
(*Matthiola longipetala*)

Flowering Tobacco
(*Nicotiana alata*)

Night-Blooming Jasmine
(*Cestrum nocturnum*)

EARTH ELEMENT

Dirt is the fountain of all cleanliness.

In the children's book written by Frances Hodgson Burnett entitled *The Secret Garden,* the daily chores of tending to a forgotten garden engage and enliven a young orphaned and forgotten girl. As she spends her days outside digging, pulling weeds, planting seeds, and rebuilding the old garden, the pink returns to her cheeks, the light returns to her eyes, she forgets her sorrows, and she learns to live and play as a little girl ought. There is something lovely and mystical in that story, and it bears witness to a truth understood by devoted gardeners: there is something about getting our hands dirty that makes us happy.

We have never been taught what it means for us to commune with trees, to treat other species as peers with rights, to relate to mountains as animate, to live in balance with the air, to feel the pulse of the ocean in our own blood. We have never experienced a sense of give-and-take with the soil and the rocks.

Jim Nollman[29]

Soil organisms live in the soil, and we play temporary host to some of them as friendly gut microorganisms that are part of our gut health and equilibrium. Our sterile society that shuns soil, and the distance our food travels from farm to table, have reduced our interaction with these soil organisms.

A strain of bacteria that lives in the soil, *Mycobacterium vaccae,* decreases anxiety, boosts moods, and improves cognition. Dr. Christopher Lowry, a neuroscientist at the University of Bristol in England, discovered that the soil-borne bacterium stimulates the immune system and encourages balance in brain chemistry resulting in improved mood. He speculates that *M. vaccae* may be used in the future to treat inflammatory diseases.[30]

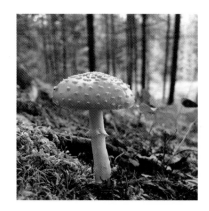

The impact of soil organisms on our health was the subject of a 2005 double-blind research study. The study tested the efficacy of a pre- and probiotic supplement composed of soil organisms on irritable bowel syndrome and the symptoms of general ill feelings, nausea, indigestion, flatulence, and colitis. The results of the study found that the soil organism in the supplement caused "significant reduction" in nausea, indigestion, flatulence, and colitis.[31]

We can benefit from *M. vaccae* as well as other soil organisms by taking a walk in the woods or digging in the dirt and inhaling the bacteria. Or consider eating unwashed homegrown, organic fruit and vegetables.

Distraught Dirt

Synthetic soil additives used widely in commercial agricultural fields, home gardens, and landscapes have devastated the soil microbiome. Most food crops and annual flowering plants rely on bacteria (in lieu of fungi) to digest nutrients and to deliver crucial nutrients from the soil to plant roots. Perennials, shrubs, and trees rely on fungi in the soil for their nutrients. The heavy use of fertilizers, pesticides, fungicides, and herbicides as well as poor soil and water management have created a bacteria and fungi drought and left behind depleted soil, which is less than ideal for a long-term plan for sustainable farming in a world with an ever-growing population.

Aside from stepping away from synthetic products and processed food, we can reintroduce life and health to our land by adding organic matter to our gardens via composts, mulch, leaf mold, and permaculture practices that feed and boost microbial life. We can encourage food-producing farms to follow suit by purchasing fruits and vegetables from organic growers.

Rehabilitating depleted soil is slow work, though. The good news is that microbiologists are using the technology developed to map the human microbiome to identify and isolate healthy soil microbes. If suitable microbes are reintroduced to the soil, it will speed up restoration and sustain the crops we rely on for food and the plants and flowers that we love to nurture in our home gardens.[32]

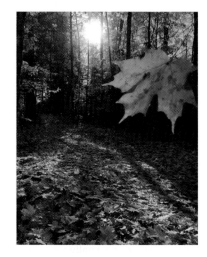

> *There is something so holy deep inside of you, so ardent and awake that needs to lay down in the soil.*
>
> Hafiz[33]

To lie on the earth, for me a quintessential delight. And for all humans, an essential health habit is to get to feel the ground and get grounded. Earth bathing by connecting skin to soil creates an electrically charged conduit that makes our bodies feel good.

Our skin needs the earth element as it continually rebuilds itself with nutrients captured from the cosmos, using the food and water that flows through us as fuel and microbial material. What is applied to the skin goes in, circulating with our cells and mingling with our microbes. When we apply the right things, the skin's ability to absorb is a gift of life. To do this, we need ingredients grown in healthy soil, not in pesticides and petroleum oil.

A nation that destroys its soils destroys itself.

Franklin D. Roosevelt[34]

The plundering of earth with pesticides leads to a loss of the labyrinth of life forms that sustain our skin. Glyphosate pesticides disturb the home of our microbiome to a devastating degree as the added surfactants bring this brew to a new level of toxic residue. Manufacturers maintain that glyphosates are harmless to humans because the action they use to kill weeds, called the shikimate pathway, is absent in all mammals. However, the shikimate pathway *is* present in the billions of bacteria in our skin and guts, and that is how glyphosates cause widespread systemic harm.

There are hundreds of ways to kneel and kiss the ground.

Rumi[35]

Because we are in a deep relationship, inextricably linked, to the earth element, what we do to our bodies we also do to the earth; and what we do to the earth we do to our bodies. In *Sacred Economics*, Charles Eisenstein draws the parallel between our heavy reliance on fossil fuels and our willingness to plunder the earth to get the energy we need and the "violent" methods we use to jolt more energy from our bodies: coffee, stimulants, threats, motivational techniques, money. "The personal and planetary mirror each other," he writes. "We don't really want to do it to our bodies; we don't really want to do it to the world."[36]

Nature's peace will flow into you as sunshine flows into trees. The winds will blow their own freshness into you, and the storms their energy, while cares will drop away from you like the leaves of Autumn.

John Muir[37]

Gifts of the Earth Element: Plants, Flowers, and Trees

When I am among the trees,
especially the willows and honey locusts,
equally the beeches, the oaks and the pines,
they give off such hints of gladness.
I would almost say that they save me, and daily . . .

Mary Oliver[38]

The Land of Is, my homeland, nestles among evergreen forests, wildflower fields, and cool, spring-filled lakes. Our sun-filled days are spent outdoors. Nature is our playground. Between my soul and the landscape, between my soul and our horizon line, there is a constant and eternal conversation, a secret correspondence that fluffs the filaments of my being. When we arrived on this land to live, joy gushed from my heart as I realized that I would now live where I had been already living inside my chest.

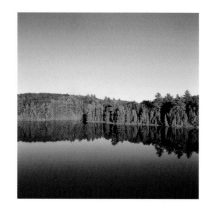

We also revere nature as our medicine chest; after a day outdoors, our hearts are expanded and we feel healthier.

> For the most part they quenched their thirst with deep draughts of mingled dew and rain, flavored with forest flowers and the airy taste of the thinnest clouds.

C. S. Lewis[39]

COSMOETICS: BRING ON THE BOTANICALS

Flowers stretch to touch sunlight from a star light-years away, and by swirling their yearning photons together with the elemental alchemy of water and carbon dioxide, cells are patterned into metamorphoses of colorful, fragrant blossoms. Plants are cosmic chemists, endlessly assembling the molecules of the world, and we live by the grace of this assembly. Plants mix elemental matter into the manna that continually rebuilds our body throughout our lifetime. This is the nature of "cosmoetics": a cosmetic creation of the cosmos. The etymology of "cosmetic" is the art and preparation of beautifying, and cosmoetic is the art and preparation of beautifying with natural creations from the cosmos.

It is the life force of this plant perfection that we want to mix and meld with our microbiome. Plant tissues are made up of cells that produce lipids and aromatic essences. These secretions are pressed and steamed from cells within the plant's epidermis to produce botanical extracts, and these oily

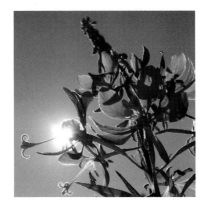

secretions work synergistically with our cells. Plants ally with our bodies, turning on electrons, protective genes, and anti-inflammatory proteins; stimulating circulation; feeding immunity; and disrupting the destruction of collagen.

Light becomes plant by being transformed into color, nectar and scent. Inside the plant is brewing; everything begins to boil—bathed in light, it erupts into an "enlightened" state of feeling and being in which it becomes conscious of the work of a higher power.[40]

FOREST BATHING

Shinrin-yoku, the Japanese practice of forest bathing, harnesses the medicinal power of botany to harmonize our health. Since 1982, the Japanese government has designated forty-eight official forest therapy trails to encourage citizens to spend more time in the woods to bolster their health.[41]

> *Thousands of tired, nerve-shaken, over-civilized people are beginning to find out that going to the mountains is going home; that wildness is a necessity.*
>
> John Muir[42]

Yoshifumi Miyazaki, a physiological anthropologist, studied the physiological and psychological benefits of forest bathing and concluded that humans feel most comfortable and are most healthy while in nature, *even those who dislike outdoor endeavors.* We evolved with and in the natural world, so our cells, systems, and rhythms recognize the cells, systems, and rhythms of nature. Miyazaki suggested that close contact with nature restores our minds and also our bodies.[43]

Qing Li, another Japanese scientist, needed quantifiable evidence of the health benefits of forest bathing so he designed an experiment where twelve businessmen went on a three-day hiking trip in the forest. Blood and urine samples were collected and tested from all the men before and after the trip. Their hormone levels, blood pressure, and levels of natural killer cells were tracked. Miyazaki's hypothesis was confirmed: in all twelve men, blood pressure and cortisol levels dropped, and most notably, the men's natural killer cells increased by 40 percent. A month later, the NK cells were still elevated. NK cells are a type of lymphocyte vital for immune health. They stealthily kill off stressed and infected cells and tumor-forming cells.[44]

It's the Trees!

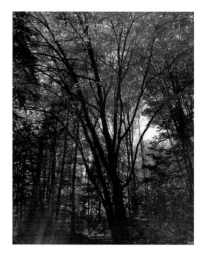

Li suspected that not just a psychological cause, but a biological process, was influencing these changes, and he thought it had something to do with the aromatic molecules of the trees. The scent molecules of trees, called phytoncides, are volatile organic compounds, and terpenes are the main component. Coined in 1928 by Russian biochemist Boris P. Tokin, "phytoncide" means "exterminated by the plant." Dr. Tokin established that these substances are part of the botanical self-defense system;[45] they deter insects, animals, and microbes from eating the plant. The concentration of phytoncides in the air in the forest is temperature dependent. It is higher in the summer than the winter, and it peaks around 30 degrees Celsius (about 86 degrees Fahrenheit).[46]

To test the phytoncide theory, Li sequestered twelve subjects in hotel rooms. In some rooms, he vaporized hinoki cypress essential oil, and the other rooms received nothing. The cypress oil breathers had a 20 percent increase in NK cells and reported feeling less fatigued. The control group reported almost no changes. (Li saw the same increase in NK cells in a subsequent petri-dish test.) Li remarked, "This is big. Pharmaceutical drugs makers can only wish that their pills would have such an impact."[47]

A study from China focused on *Cryptomeria japonica* tree oil (which contains limonene, another type of terpene), and the participants reported improved sleep quality, lower anxiety, and less pain.[48]

Pines and conifers release large amounts of phytoncides into the air to suppress surrounding microorganisms, bacteria, and fungi from invading them.[49] Other plants, including spices, onion, garlic, many varieties of flowers, tea tree, oak, and countless others, release these compounds as well.

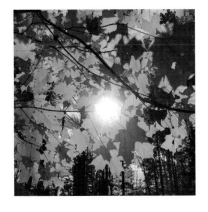

Trees are poems the earth writes upon the sky.

Kahlil Gibran[50]

Our health is deeply influenced by these little plant-powerhouse molecules. When the molecules are inhaled or absorbed through the mouth and skin, they travel in the bloodstream, are pulsed through the body, and instruct the brain. Ongoing research demonstrates that phytoncides increase NK-cell levels as well as increase anticancer proteins and proteases (granulysin, granzymes A and B, and perforin) that cause tumor cells to self-destruct. They also relax our parasympathetic nervous system, thus reducing stress hormones, which are widely understood to inhibit NK-cell activity.[51]

I wonder if clear-cutting and deforestation correspond to increases in disease in those areas and in the world.

Terra viriditatem sudat.
The earth exudes freshness.

Saint Hildegard of Bingen[52]

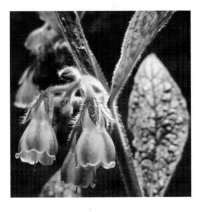

MILIEU OF MICROORGANISMS:
MORE THAN MEETS THE EYE

Our planet is inhabitable due to the busy lives of microbes. Microbial species vary in size, shape, biochemical activities, chemical composition, and nutritional needs, and there is a multitude of species. And they are *everywhere*.

Each living creature must be looked at as a microcosm—a little universe, formed of a host of self-propagating organisms, inconceivably minute and as numerous as the stars in heaven.[53]

The Challenger Deep in the Marianas Trench off the coast of Guam is the deepest place on earth at 36,070 feet (10,994 meters) below sea level. In March 2013, researchers discovered that the deep darkness of this trench supports a thriving microbial community.[54] Up high in the atmosphere, tossed about by the winds and living in the clouds, abundant colonies of microbes eat airborne pollutants and may possibly influence weather patterns.

The world flourishes with tiny lives that are an integral part of the complex system of life. In the universe, there are billions of galaxies. Our galaxy, the Milky Way, has somewhere between 200 billion and 400 billion stars. Your body contains upward of 130 trillion cells. You are like a galaxy of stars, as beautiful, mysterious, and complex.

The philosophy of vitalism affirms that an environment that propels life and health can be cultivated when we recognize our body's inherent complexity and wisdom and its inextricable connection to the world it inhabits. Our most intimate connection with the world is through our own body ecology.

A tiny world flourishes in you. Of the 130 trillion cells in your body, only about 30 trillion of them are human cells. You play hospitable host to more than 100 trillion bacterial and fungal cells that have coevolved with us and in us. Up to 3 percent of a human's weight is microbial mass. That means that if you weigh 120 pounds (54.4 kg), then up to 3.6 pounds (1.6 kg) of that is your microbiome. A microbiome is the microbes and their relationship with their host and with other microbes in a specific location or habitat. Your microbiome includes all the various microbes that thrive in your gut, vagina, anus, nose, mouth, and skin.

If we examine one person's oral microbes and gut microbes, there is an incredible diversity. The difference between those two communities, according to biologist Rob Knight, is "bigger than the difference between the microbes in this reef and the microbes in this prairie . . . a few feet of difference in the human body makes more of a difference to your microbial ecology than hundreds of miles on Earth."[55]

Researchers at the Human Microbiome Project have identified the boundaries of our human microbes in the Western world. (Well, they *think* they have. . . .) They collected samples from the skin, nose, mouth, lower intestines, and vaginas of 242 people and "calculated that more than 10,000 microbial species occupy the human ecosystem."[56]

The microbial garden of our body has untold and yet unknown capabilities.

The plethora of microbes in us contributes more genes responsible for our survival than we contribute. The Human Microbiome Project researchers estimate that the human microbiome contributes some eight million genes to our health and survival—that is 360 times more bacterial genes than human genes.[57] These microbes account for the majority of our production of nutrients, including methylated folate, fatty acids, fat-soluble vitamins, detoxification, and immune signaling.[58]

These bacteria build colonies that act as "virtual organs."[59] Some species communicate with the body via lymphocytes through the epithelial cells, and others communicate via nerve endings in the intestinal walls. Some bacteria signal to our native cells that unfriendly microbes are invading and that the immune system should be activated.

The late Dr. Eshel Ben-Jacob of Tel Aviv University photographed stunning images of the growth patterns of colonies of bacteria.[60] These images, such as Vortex Blue, highlight the power of sacred geometry. Bacterial colonies grow in a Fibonacci pattern that is beautiful, efficient, and effective; the growth pattern mathematically minimizes the bacteria colony's exposure to outside toxins.[61]

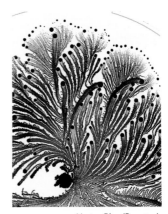

Vortex Blue (P. vortex),
by Eshel Ben-Jacob

Quorum Call

Bacteria cells and colonies have a few means of communicating with each other. The cells produce a lubricating substance called surfactin that carries messages between bacteria, and this lubricant can also create currents to push toxic substances into external areas of the colony to provide the best survival rate for the colony.

Bacteria cells also talk to each other via chemical messengers, and the bacteria don't even need to touch. They can communicate at a distance using chemical messages.

Using special signaling molecules, bacteria talk to each other and share information about their population numbers. The number of signaling molecules in the environment increases as the population grows. This cell-to-cell communication is called "quorum sensing." Quorum sensing turns on the genes to direct normal bacterial activities that only make sense when the group of bacteria is large enough to produce an effect and allows them to synchronize their processes, such as antibiotic production, toxin secretions, and biofilm formation.

Think of biofilm as a hotel for microbes (bacteria and fungi). These biofilms protect microbes and allow colonies to thrive in extreme environments, such as hot hydrothermal vents, miles deep in Arctic ice, and powerful acidic solutions. Biofilms are composed of hard, rigid layers of proteins that form strong bonds to a surface and are hard to penetrate from the outside. Microbial residents in biofilm are by nature pathogenic, medically dangerous, and difficult to dissolve. Oral plaque, buildup on medical implants, catheters, and stents, and lung-clogging mucus in cystic fibrosis are all examples of biofilms. They are also associated with colon and rectal cancers. The presence of a biofilm in the colon before evidence of cancer can indicate precancerous tissue changes related to the invasion of bacteria and increased cell proliferation.[62]

Beyond Probiotics: The Microbiome in Your Guts

Microvilli are small hairs that line the intestines to increase surface area for greater nutrient absorption. The tiny spaces between the microvilli provide the perfect environment for bacteria to thrive. These microbes in our guts secrete enzymes that we rely on for efficient digestion and make the nutrients in the food that we eat more available to us. They help us break down fats, carbohydrates, plant material, and proteins that we couldn't digest on our own. They extract energy from undigested carbohydrates that ferment in the gut, and some bacteria produce vitamins and anti-inflammation compounds that mediate our immune response to swelling, pain, and other disease issues.[63] On the flip side, reductions in gut bacteria colonization contribute to malnutrition and obesity and increased intestinal permeability and inflammation.[64]

More than 100 million neurons weave between the muscle layers of the gastrointestinal tract. This is roughly the same number of neurons in the brain. Almost 80 percent of the neurotransmitter serotonin, which is involved in learning, memory, mood, and sleep and a million other tiny interactions, is made by the neurons in the gut and is transported to the brain. The GI neurons both send and receive messages from the brain via the vagus nerve, which is sort of like the telecommunication system in the body that wanders through the body from the brain to all internal organs. The communication that travels between the brain and gut is called the gut–brain axis.

Gut–Brain Axis

The gut–brain axis is a two-way street connecting the gut and the brain. Communication between the gut and the brain travels via nerves and body fluids along the vagus nerve, and they communicate a *lot*. Over 90 percent of the nerve pulses in the vagus nerve are communication from the gut to the brain.[65]

Gut bacteria use the vagus nerve to communicate with the brain, too. Gut bacteria and gut neurons actively interact, and their interactions are vital for our health. Gut bacteria are experts in molecular mimicry. They produce copies of important peptides that travel via the bloodstream to the brain. These peptides alter emotions and behavior.[66] They make large amounts of molecular copies of serotonin, gamma-aminobutyric acid (GABA), and other neurotransmitters, and our bodies rely on these bacteria and their secretions for homeostasis.[67]

Low levels of prefrontal cortex GABA can mean anxious feelings, poor concentration, and issues with long-term memory. Being severely short of GABA may contribute to ADD and autism.[68] Gut bacteria help a baby's brain develop in utero. The bacteria modulate an important factor for new synapses to grow and communicate with each other.[69] Gut bacteria help to organize the human nervous system. A deficit in this can mean increases in stress hormones, which in turn contribute to addictive behaviors, seizures, and the onset of depression.[70]

From Symbiosis to Dysbiosis

Medical researchers are convinced that our bodies thrive when these micro-mutualist partners live on and in us, and that without them our bodies tend to go awry. They have elaborate interactions with our immune system, our skin, our mouth, our guts, brains, eyes, and even our DNA—we inherit our mitochondrial microbes from our mothers. When our microbiome is in symbiosis, all is well.

Symbiosis is a mutually beneficial relationship between two organisms sharing an environment. The word actually means to "live in harmony." Microbial symbiosis occurs when there is healthy microbial diversity living harmoniously with the host. The opposite, microbial imbalance, is called dysbiosis. Microbial disharmony may underlie increases in allergies, asthma, autoimmune disorders, obesity, diabetes, and mental, emotional, and behavioral issues.[71]

A dysbiotic gut opens the body to opportunistic pathogens—bacteria, yeasts, and fungi—that are normally suppressed by a healthy microbiome. These opportunistic species result in leaky gut, and the yeasts and fungi can sneak through the gut perforations and cause skin rashes, acne, and eczema.[72]

Having the wrong kind of gut bacteria can lead to chronic inflammation, which can lead to bone-mineral loss and osteoporosis, and that includes loss of tooth and jaw bones, too. Vitamin D, also important in bone formation as well as a myriad of health functions, is contingent on gut bacteria to be absorbed from food. A vitamin D deficiency may indicate a gut imbalance.[73] Gut bacterial imbalance results in chronic inflammation that can lead to damage to collagen and the skin bacteria, which contributes to rapid aging.[74]

Early findings point to problematic areas of the Western lifestyle as disruptive to our precious microbial balance. The findings include processed foods in the diet, ever-increasing exposure to antibiotics, and the growing trend toward cesarean-section births, depriving the baby of the vaginal microorganisms that "seed" its gut. Some over-the-counter drugs, such as proton-pump-inhibitor heartburn drugs, are also disruptive.

OTHER THAN HYGIENIC: THE DIRTY TRUTH ABOUT ANTIBACTERIAL PRODUCTS

Hygiene Hypothesis

Before the first antibiotic (which translates as "against life") was introduced, unfriendly, invasive microbes were a serious concern; we were plagued by the plague as well as tuberculosis, syphilis, and pneumonia. Back then, scientists tended to believe that bacteria-free living was healthy and safe, and exterminating our bacteria was their new goal.

We are beginning to see the error of this way of thinking. Immunologists and epidemiologists are increasingly supporting the hygiene hypothesis, which states that many of the advances of modernization, such as good sanitation, antibiotic exposure, excessive cleanliness, and urban or indoor living, interrupt the normal development of the immune system. Living in an ultraclean, sterile, and synthetic-soap-cleaned environment may inhibit proper immune development in children. Decreasing occurrences of childhood infections and exposures to diverse microbes and helminths in the developed world resulting from better hygiene may be the origin of skyrocketing levels of allergies, asthma, and autoimmune disease. Our immune systems may need these exposures to develop balanced regulation of the body. Without proper exposure to "dirt," our immune systems fail to mature.[75]

Antibiotics are a blessing to people in medical crises with an infection. However, the overuse of antibiotics today has led to bacteria that are not killed by antibiotics because they have mutated to be resistant to them. By age forty, the average Westerner will have been prescribed thirty courses of antibiotics![76]

You take antibiotics even if you do not swallow the pills. Even if you have diligently avoided antibiotic prescriptions, they still seep in by consuming supermarket food. All antibiotics have their allowable limits in the food and water supply. They are on our food, in our drinks, coating our vegetables, and fed to animals raised for meat and dairy. Milk can have up to 100 micrograms of tetracycline per kilogram. Antibiotics are indiscriminate assassins. Antibiotics are in our hand soaps, dish soaps, lotions, and cleansers. Until recently, not much thought was given to the effect of all of this on our friendly bacteria, even as our bodies felt their absence. Any surviving resistant bacteria mutate fast and bask in the empty niches the antibiotics made. Soon pathogenic biofilms bloom, and we no longer have protection from infection.

Let's turn our attention to the hype about antibacterial soaps and sanitizers. Kline & Company market researchers state that there is a $350 million annual market for antibacterial soaps in the United States.[77]

Introducing Monster Bugs

Antibacterial soaps have the potential to create antibiotic-resistant bacteria. Drug or antibiotic resistance results when a small number of a bacteria population are genetically mutated in a way that the drug or chemical doesn't kill it—but it will kill the other bacteria, opening the door to proliferation. If this happens over and over, worldwide, there will be no drug or chemical to kill that strain of bacteria. Some bacteria species have developed resistance to several different drugs and chemicals. The World Health Organization calls bacterial resistance a "threat to global health security."[78]

In the autumn of 2016, the FDA banned the use of consumer antibacterial products, declaring that antibacterial soaps and gels are not more effective in preventing illness than standard soap and water, and that some of the chemicals used in those products are even harmful. Nineteen antibacterial chemicals[79] were included in the ban, and producers were given a year to phase out these products.[80]

We hear about the current health scares and the "flu of the day," and we may wonder how we can stay safe. What can we use to wash away the bugs? Nature has provided for us a clear alternative for keeping us healthy while boosting our mood and immune system, and there is no evidence that bacteria develop resistance to botanical oils. Our best defense against illness is our own immune system. So, while we want to be diligent in protecting our health, we can refrain from worry and obsessive degerming for the future health of our children.

WELCOME TO THE POST-PATHOGEN BIOME ERA

Obsolete, or soon to be, is the medical directive to scrub ourselves, inside and out, from the microbes that share our bodies; whereas once they were a source of fear, now our microbiota are founts of wonder for medical researchers.

The Western diet and lifestyle do not support a diverse, robust symbiont population.

Immunity

Our native bacteria are better at keeping us healthy and our immune system in top shape than the best medical technology and drugs. A group of microbiologists examined what happened to salmonella, a potentially deadly foodborne pathogen, in a healthy gastrointestinal system. When they exposed salmonella to fecal bacteria collected from people with healthy GI tracts, the bacteria inactivated the salmonella.[81]

One contributor to an altered gut microbiome is vitamin A deficiency. Retinoic acid produced alongside the bacteria from vitamin A activates T_h17, an immune-system helper cell. Too much T_h17 can stimulate autoimmune conditions; and with too little, we are susceptible to infections. This all-important balance—not too much or too little—is why keeping a healthy microbial population is key, and it is something that drugs can't fix.[82] Our bacteria teach our immune systems what and how to attack when viruses and pathogenic bacteria invade.[83]

The Human Microbiome Project is developing a pharmacopoeia of our microbes and their chemical secretions. When we know which microorganisms and which secretions are important to keeping our health in balance, it could be that medicine in the future may focus on treating or preventing microbiome disorders in lieu of treating disease. Down the road, our drugs may be targeted probiotics and their prebiotic food.[84]

Rewilding: Body as Ecosystem[85]

In this fresh new field in microbiology, there is still plenty of room for clarity and nuance. Yet one conclusion is clear: we are healthiest when our bodies are thriving ecosystems, and to get there we may need to reintroduce or "rewild" ancient microbes into our lives. Dr. Rob

> Bacteria
> "Never doubt that a small group of thoughtful, committed citizens can change the world. Indeed it is the only thing that ever has."
> —Margaret Mead

Dunn succinctly states that for our health and our children's health "we need to come up with a new way of restoring elements of what once was."[86]

Trailblazing the way to "rewilding" the human body, some sufferers of Crohn's disease, multiple sclerosis, irritable bowel syndrome, asthma, and allergies are intentionally acquiring anew some of our old body microbial wildlife that we lost due to Western living. Some of these daring people have walked barefoot through the pit latrines of nonurbanized, non-Westernized people groups. Others have intentionally consumed helminths, with the goal of repopulating their bodies. Some of these people have experienced miraculous healing.[87]

> After all, perhaps dirt isn't really so unhealthy
> as one is brought up to believe.
>
> Agatha Christie[88]

Does Koala Bear Poop Smell Like Cough Drops?[89]

On the medical front, a cutting-edge therapy called fecal microbiota transplantation (FMT) transfers healthy, microbiota-rich feces from a healthy person to a person with a dysbiotic gut. So far, the treatment's greatest success is in treating severe diarrhea from an infection of antibiotic-resistant *C. difficile* linked to 14,000 deaths in the United States every year.[90] In one study, FMT cured 15 of 16 people, whereas antibiotics cured only 3 of 13 people.[91] Consider how nature does not let the smallest piece of excrement go to waste: there are always three to four creatures fighting over it.[92]

We will revisit this concept of rewilding later, albeit on a less drastic level, as we consider how our body ecology, our microbiota, makes us beautiful.

VITAL RELATIONSHIPS

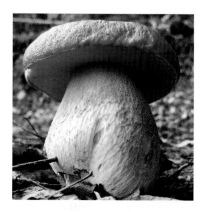

*And each one there, has one thing
  shared
They have sweated beneath the
  same sun
Looked up and wondered at the
  same moon*

Neil Diamond[93]

We have been caught up in the pursuit of beauty, the pursuit of purchases for acquiring beauty, rather than revealing beauty and basking in our relationship to the elements. We exist in a vital relationship, a vital interplay, with the elements. Yet our current consumer culture attempts to deftly defy and deny this relationship with warnings of the sun's danger, promoting polluted water bottled in plastic, and pushing pesticides to deplete the soil as we douse our houses with chemical "air fresheners." All this in lieu of wisely soaking in

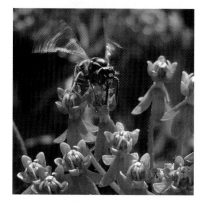

the sun, drinking pure water, eating and gardening naturally, and freshening our homes with spring-scented breezes blowing in through open windows.

For millennia, humans sought to live beyond survival, making more permanent shelters, storing foods, and easing access to water, and we have indeed succeeded with plumbing, electricity, and housing. Now that survival, for many, has been removed from our daily equation, we can enjoy the elements in such a sweet way. Now more than ever, we can engage with the elements rather than being overexposed.

Currently, we create lifestyles that quarantine us from the elements, and what is pouring out of our beauty-care bottles is without vital fluids, without life force. It is without the essential matter that has interplayed with the elements, emerged from the soil, drank in delicious dew, been refreshed by rains, been strengthened by the sun, absorbed air, and basked in breezes.

If there is a remnant of plant matter in modern skincare solutions, as with our supermarket food supply, then it has been bleached, deodorized, refractionated, isolated, mixed with synthetics, and stripped of its vital gifts to remain stable on store shelves for decades. What feeds our skin and bodies now is lifeless, yet we get caught up in the game because we are sold on the advertised acclaim, convenience, and fantasy of it all.

So we have sequestered ourselves from this dynamic interplay of sensations, the vital élan that nourishes and renews in ways that synthetics never can. Every plant has engaged with the elements, the luminous life cycle, and this is at the heart of capturing the quintessence of plants, the purpose of distilling, extracting, and decanting the sap, the elixir, the essence so we may partake of and commune with these botanical blessings from the earth's heirlooms.

We are in a vital relationship with everything that goes on, in, and around our bodies. I prefer to perfume with the aromas of creation, sluiced from sap, pressed from petals, tinctured from trees, so that I may adorn with and inhale molecules that message to my senses, cells, and endocrine system sensual indications of the earth's regenerative floral forces.

The elements are essential to animate our lives. Immersion in these vital interactions animates our beauty and engages us with the fulsome power of the universe.

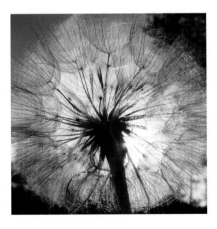

The sun itself cannot enlighten the world
without receptive souls experiencing its radiance.[94]

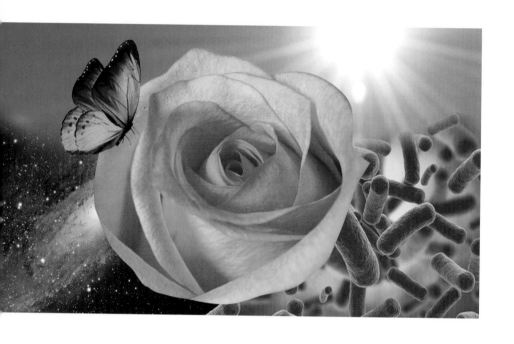

Chapter Six

THE MOIST ENVELOPE OF THE SOUL

Loving the Skin You're In

My childhood was steeped in summer's light rays and days of endless play in nature. Then in my teens, my bathroom blossomed with bottles upon bottles of beauty products that came with a whole new set of rules of what to do to my body. Beauty magazines with their still scenes of everlasting glamour enamored me and my friends with their promises of perfection and luxurious beauty. I loved dabbling in lotions and potions and mixing makeup. On long school road trips, I would pull out my palettes of eye shadows, blushes, and hairbrushes and would glam up my girlfriends as we sat in the back of the bus.

Luckily, by the time I was eighteen, I had sifted and sorted my way through synthetic skincare and I understood that all these products were just chemicals dressed in false finery; even my Cucumber Face Toner from The Body Shop had never encountered a cucumber and was just scented rubbing alcohol. Realizing that every bottle was really hollow, I purged this petroleum promised land of products, and this was when my approach to beauty got *renegade* and I began to care for my body in a whole new, wholesome way.

If I could offer advice to that teenage self, I would say:

Age awakens your inner sage, yet it's never too soon to comprehend,
Your body is your best friend.

Enjoy the sun but forget the sunscreen and pools of chlorine.
Bask in those rays, just not with baby oil and tinfoil.
Ignore beauty magazines. They set you up to compare.
And living in comparison makes the world seem unfair.
Let loose hair strands relax.
Floss, but not with petroleum wax.
Exfoliation is overrated.
Six steps to wash your face is too complicated.
The ancient beauty secrets you crave are in the forest, not the mall.
Play hooky with flowers and tune in to your intuition, above all.

Differing from my teen self, I like to do as little as possible by way of beauty maintenance and avoid perpetual loops of products and appointments. I would rather make a date dipping in a lake. Effortlessness is my guiding light when it comes to skincare; let's delve in to activating our skin's self-regenerating systems and engaging nature's elements as our finest skincare.

Maybelline was right—she *is* born with it. Our greatest beauty secret, our microbiome, was woven into us in our mother's womb. The flora of our fabric gets its initial inoculation going through the birth canal. Our first sips of life are in these secretions. Baby's skin, fresh from its nine-month nap in amniotic fluid, is covered in a waxy, white vernix sheath that is home to the maternal microbiome's genome and is a gift to our future skin's glow.

In today's rush to rinse the baby, this waxy sheath, this probiotic patina, is removed. Babies born by cesarean section are more vulnerable as ambient bacteria, instead of their mother's, colonize their skin. Maternal flora, our soul-starter culture, is activated by the 200 prebiotic oligosaccharides found in breast milk. Formula feeding impairs microbial diversity, as formula lacks the innate matter to nourish microbes. For many, these missing microbes increase their risk of infections, allergies, and an array of skin disorders.

Our health, and thus our beauty, comes down to the millions of microbes and minute cells in our bodies. Healthy cells are alive. They are filled with vitality. They are filled with order, and they are reflecting the order and vitality of nature. The total health of our cells is reflected in the health of our skin.

The glow and energy of the healthy woman is the
ultimate beauty, the only beauty that will last.

Jane Fonda[1]

OUR SKIN CELLVES

Millions of illuminating light cells dance in our being as starry galaxies within our galaxy: cell by cell, thought by thought, life. Let each cell reflect a star. The care of creation sets the cells afloat in a swirling sea of illuminated ether. Inhalation births millions of new cells, and with exhalation, millions expire. Entirely fresh blood, skin, and organ cells are renewed every moon cycle. Infuse your cells with the holiest of telluric tones, and trust the precision work of the body. This is the rhythm of nature; these are the four seasons in a day. The death and life of breath: the green leaves exhale, and we live.

Healthy cells are essential to resplendent skin. We want to ennoble the cell with the right environment. That means on a core, primal level we need a good balance of water, oxygen, and nutrients. Cells have a breathing cycle, an inhalation and an exhalation. Respiration equals resplendence. Oxygen is fundamental for the metabolic function of the cells. Imbue your being with fresh air, movement, and everything that gets oxygen going to the cells. Skin needs and feeds upon the elements.

This moist envelope of our soul is a living, breathing, communicating, and regenerating tissue. It is our largest organ of elimination, secreting out sweat and sebum while keeping out infectious invaders. This miraculous medium is the real estate coveted by every cosmetic that aims to penetrate pores, solve insecurities, and systematize skin types. Dry, oily in the T-zone, combination skin—these are not types but symptoms! Symptoms vary from subtle to severe, yet they all point toward skin microbiome imbalance.

Only a few millimeters of skin separate our bodies from the outside world. Yet its multilayered microbial design provides us with the perfect protection. There are four main levels in the very thin, top layer of our skin called the epidermis. The outermost protective layer, the stratum corneum, keeps skin elastic and prevents water evaporation. The stratum lucidum, found only in naturally thickened skin, is a translucent layer of flat, dead skin cells that is only three to five cells thick that protect the skin from friction and force. The hydro-lipid barrier, the stratum granulosum, produces ceramides and phospholipids. The immunologically active stratum spinosum is a net-like layer that provides protection to the basement layer, the stratum basale, which generates keratin and melanin cells and pushes them up to the stratum corneum every fourteen days. This continuous process culminates in the loss of 40,000 cells every minute of our lives!

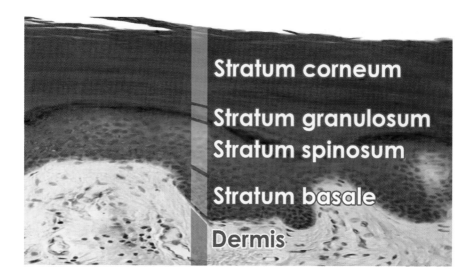

Stratum corneum

Stratum granulosum

Stratum spinosum

Stratum basale

Dermis

The outermost layer, the stratum corneum, is composed mostly of dead cells, which has given rise to the practice of chemical peels and excessive exfoliation. Yet this vital layer is our topsoil that feeds our friendly flora. Cell loss is designed to precisely match cell production. Exfoliating cells away too quickly tips the balance, and cell loss exceeds cell production. This signals stress in the skin. Our epidermal ecosystem requires a healthy stratum corneum because it is our most antiaging and anti-infection layer. When we remove it prematurely, the young cells underneath are left vulnerable.

With this juicy layer jeopardized, toxins and harsh chemicals irritate the new skin, inducing inflammatory issues. If this layer is disturbed regularly, as it is with daily exposure to foaming cleansers, creams, and chlorine, it creates an ongoing health deficit of missing microbes, inflammation, abnormal cells, and easy entrance for toxins.

THE BACTERIAL BANQUET ON YOUR SKIN: MICROBES

We live our lives in perpetual bacterial bloom, our skin a tapestry teeming with microbes. A whole ecosystem resides on the surface and multilayers of our skin. Our cutaneous microbiome is in constant contact with the immune, digestive, nervous, and hormonal systems. Disruption results in dysbiosis. Acne, eczema, psoriasis, dermatitis, keratosis pilaris, rosacea, melasma, hyperpigmentation, fungal infections, *Candida,* skin lesions, dandruff, age spots, blemishes, blackheads, dry, scaly, uneven skin, and more are all manifestations of bacterial imbalance. The unfriendly microbes that cause imbalance live on everyone's skin. Yet, when microbial diversity mutates and plummets, pathogenic bacteria breed and trigger skin issues. Our skin needs bacterial diversity to thrive and to keep all the flora friendly instead of fostering the frenemies that cause disruption and disease.

For decades we have known about the toxicity of modern toiletries and its effect on our skin, cells, and hormones. Now, revolutionary research about the skin's microbiome reveals new levels of damage to our dermis that the daily doping of lotions and soaping is doing to the firmament of flora that supports our skin. There is a balance of bacteria that tends to the soil of our skin, and not one of them is parched for petroleum and paraben.

Skin microbes are pervasive through the layers of the epidermis. When the skin is injured, our native skin microbes invade the area to defend against nonnative pathogens, which prevents infection. (This is a good reason to avoid antibacterial soap!) For example, *Staphylococcus epidermidis,* commonly found on the skin, secretes a substance that improves wound healing, reduces inflammation, and inhibits the pathogenic S. *aureus,* also known as the superbug MRSA.[2] Bacteria also regulate skin collagen and protect the skin from UV damage. Gut bacterial imbalance results in chronic inflammation that can lead to damage to collagen and bacteria, and this contributes to rapid aging.[3]

Any disturbance to the skin microbes can cause the delicate microbial balance to become out of whack and can make us unwell. As Dr. Bruce Agnew of the National Human Genome Research Institute recently said, "If the microbiota is sick, the human host will probably get sick, too."[4] All changes and disturbances to the skin microbiota have contributed to the rising rates of chronic inflammatory and autoimmune diseases seen in wealthier countries that tend toward hypersanitation and the abuse of antibiotics.[5]

Modern skincare routines often suppress the beauty of this symbiotic system. The bacteria domesticating our dermis are altered by what is applied topically. Just as toxic food and chemical irritants induce leaky guts by microscopically perforating the intestines, the rubbing and scrubbing of our skin with a daily diet of chemical cleansers and creams fumigates our friendly flora. This defoliation of our flora-nation mutates microbes and makes them extinct. By removing this protective bacteria and their food source of sebum, cells,

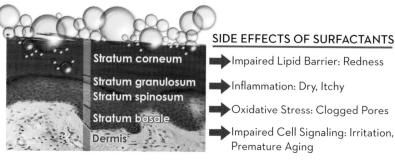

Surfactants Remain in Statum Corneum Layer

SIDE EFFECTS OF SURFACTANTS

Stratum corneum

Stratum granulosum
Stratum spinosum

Stratum basale

Dermis

Impaired Lipid Barrier: Redness

Inflammation: Dry, Itchy

Oxidative Stress: Clogged Pores

Impaired Cell Signaling: Irritation, Premature Aging

and lipids, we disrupt the homeostasis of our skin's oasis. Ancient cultures with highly sophisticated ablutions would oil their skin for cleansing and renewing, lubricating lipid layers with exquisite fresh-pressed fats—now we scrub and surfactant everything.

Studies show that surfactants in cosmetics dissolve our skin's natural ceramides, enzymes, and hydro-lipid barrier. These surfactants that make skin squeaky clean also insert themselves into the stratum corneum and stay there even after rinsing, initiating chronic degradation to this delicate layer.[6] This results in inflammation and microbial elimination, which may manifest as melasma, blemishes, redness, dryness, and irritated skin. Chronic damage to this layer essentially exterminates our skin's "first responders" to injury and infection, and along with it goes our moist envelope of protection. Venturing into the world without the integrity of this top layer and its full-flora intact is like leaving the front door wide open while away on vacation.

The penetration of chemicals we commonly use creates a vicious cycle of dermal dysbiosis and premature skin conditions that are difficult to escape. To this mix we add washing in water that is soaked in pharmaceuticals,[7] fluoride, and chlorine, further eradicating essential bacteria. The resulting skin issues may send us seeking a dermatologist. Dermatologists' prescriptions are steeped in side effects, have low success rates of resolving skin aliments, and often spawn new ones. Among this arsenal are antibiotics, retinoids, and cortisone creams that deplete our bacteria teams. Restoring beneficial bacteria, rather than further depleting it, should be the key to all skin therapy.

Microbe Matrimony: The Union of Skin and Guts

The skin and the guts are inexplicably bound in a relationship with bacteria. Healthy skin and a healthy gut are lined with billions of beneficial microbes. These bacteria boost our immune system and aid in absorbing nutrients.

Research indicates that probiotics and rebalancing the gut microbiome can inhibit hair loss and solve skin issues. A flourishing bodywide microbiome, boosted by probiotics to help regain some of our microbe species and diversity, can help skin be less sensitive to UV rays,[8] along with helping the skin maintain the acid mantle and its moisture, preventing cell abnormality, improving vascularization, regulating collagen, and more!

For beauty's sake, we must befriend our bacteria. Ultimately, this is what unplugs pores perpetually, not an aesthetician's extractor or plastic exfoliating beads, as blackheads begin in a congested colon, rosacea is linked to leaky guts, and acne arises from oxidization. *Bacteria are the best beautician.* By outsourcing our beauty routines to bacteria, we let the microbes micromanage our skincare with their beauty-stimulating secretions that clean pores and keep skin strong and supple. A healthy microbiome is your best friend forever and works like the best beauty cream ever!

Beneficial Bacteria Beauticians

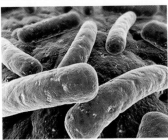

Regulate Collagen
Prevent Infections
Improve Vascularization
Regulate Innate Immunity
Maintain Acid Mantle
Prevent Cell Abnormailty
Regulate Lipids, Peptides, Sebum
Maintain Moisture
Help Heal Burns, Scars & Wounds
Reduce Sensitivity to UV
Upregulate Vitamin D Receptors (VDR)
Communicate with Guts, Brain, Hormones, & Nerves

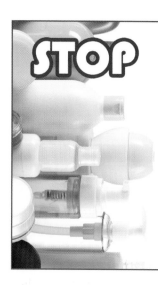

Damaging Skin and Mutating Microbes
with synthetic skincare containing
antibiotics and chemicals

Showering in Chlorine

Washing with Antibacterial Soap

Peeling Away the Epidermis
with chemical peels and over exfoliation

Foaming Face and Body with Surfactants

Irritating Skin Via the Guts
with pesticide-laden processed foods

Cooking with Rancid, Processed Fats
that oxidize, prematurely age, and hyperpigment skin

Applying Questionable Naturals

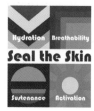

Stop. Seal. Seed.

The best way to achieve flawless skin, besides Photoshop, is to maintain a microbiome of beatific bacteria by
following these three steps: Stop, Seal, and Seed. Stop-
ping is all about arresting the affliction upon our skin's
microbiome. Sealing is about healing the skin. Seeding
is about allowing the infinite intelligence of the body's
microbiome to continually replenish the skin.

Stop

The first step is to give your bathroom a makeover and set free the toxic bottles of
empty promises that claimed to quick-fix or correct skin type and advertised active
ingredients with hype. We need to cease the supersanitized, synthetic routines that
are harming our skin's hygiene. There is no need for chemicals to feel fresh and be
clean. We need to shower, sweat, and stimulate yet not mutate our microbiome.

Stop showering in chlorine. Cleaning in chlorine kills the friendly flora that
helps skin stay supple, resulting in drying dysbioses from dandruff to dermatitis. If municipal tap water is pouring from your faucets, use a shower filter—and
it is handy to have a bottle of spring water for washing the face.

Stop using antibacterial soap, which breeds superbugs and decreases our
protection from pathogens. Seriously, no foaming the face and body with soap,
ever: just pits and bits.

Stop irritating the skin through the guts with processed food, corn by-products, refined carbs, synthetic sugars, soy, and processed vegetable oils that quickly oxidize, prematurely age, and hyperpigment skin.

Stop applying questionable "natural" products. Just because there is an image of lavender fields on the label does not mean the bottle is full of intelligent ingredients. Rancidity, refinement, and hidden ingredients mean that not all naturals nourish the skin.

Here are a few more surprising less-than-natural "all-natural" ingredients: Aloe vera juice usually has hidden preservatives of sodium benzoate and potassium sorbate, which are toxic to microbes. Witch hazel is never one single ingredient, even though it may be listed as such. It is a concoction of harsh alcohols and chemicals. Glycerin is highly processed, and it is a humectant that provides temporary plumping but leads skin cells to shrivel through a process called osmolarity. "Natural fragrance" on a label sounds natural, yet this phrase refers to a group of aromatic ingredients that can be isolates, or fractions of essential oils chemically derived and genetically modified.[9] See Chapter Twelve.

Hyaluronic acid is also best left in the bottle. Scientific evidence has demonstrated that topical HA is unable to penetrate the skin and is rapidly degraded on the skin surface.[10] Its molecule size is far too large to effectively absorb, and that is a blessing considering how it is made. Originally extracted from rooster combs, now it is made by bacteria fermented on tuna-viscera residue and mussel-processing wastewater.

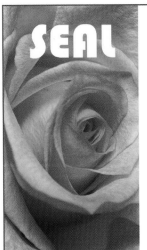

SEAL

Seal Hydro-Lipid Barrier—recover integrity of the stratum corneum with soothing serums

Settle Sebaceaous Glands—with jojoba botanical biotic skin serums

Wash with Oil—gently stimulate; whisk away dirt and makeup

Happy Hands—scrub with natural bar soap and further disinfect with tea tree

Unclog Pores—with stimulation seed masks, cleansing with oil and botanical-biotics; balancing digestion

Inhibit Pathogen Parties—with botanical-biotic serums that inhibit quorum sensing

Heal and Seal Guts—eat for your microbiome

Spot Treat—blemishes, bumps, cuts, scars, melasma, and acne with botanical-biotics

Arm Pits—sandalwood, baking soda, or a sea-salt spray

Shampoo—add baking soda to chemical-free shampoo to detox scalp and hair

Dry Brush—stimulate skin lymph system

Sunbathe—with pigment botanical oils and chlorophyll-infused water

SEAL

When we think of skin solutions to heal and seal our skin, we need to step away from the bottles at the cosmetic counter and bring in the confluence of the cosmos. The next step in healing the skin and recovering the integrity of the epidermis is to repair the hydro-lipid barrier that seals the skin. It is time to stop the spin-cycle of surfactants and begin washing with oils. It may seem strange, washing with oils. People think that oil will leave their skin feeling oily and less than clean, though this isn't the case when organic, authentic, fresh-pressed botanical oils are used to cleanse the face. A lotion is made by combining an oil and water with an emulsifier, so washing with oil makes a fresh lotion on your face. There is a power of nowness to it; it is a fresh aqua oleum.

Indeed, not all oils are created equal. There are many "natural" oils that will never go near my skin! Grapeseed, peach kernel, sunflower, and almond oils are often rancid right off the shelf. Beyond the ick-factor of putting rancid oils on the skin, the rancidity can create free-radical damage. Moreover, they are often contaminated by solvents and additives in the refining process. Other oils, such as argan and olive, have serious issues with production and purity; even in Morocco, where the argan tree is native, it is difficult to find argan oil that has not been mixed with mystery oils.

Yet pure, organic oils, such as gorgeous golden jojoba, are loving lipids that lubricate the skin so that makeup and dirt are gently whisked away and natural skin oils are left intact. In fact, cleansing with these oils also stabilizes

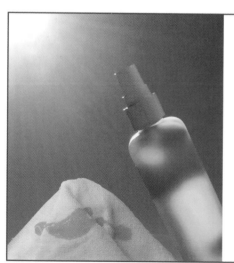

Washing with Oil

1. Wet Cloth, Squirt on Oil
2. Wash Face with Oiled Cloth
3. Massage a Squirt of Oil onto Face

our native, friendly skin bacteria and enhances protection from pathogenic bacteria. Soothing serums of seabuckthorn and jojoba deliver phospholipids and balance the biome, keeping cells perfectly plump. Jojoba is a liquid plant wax that settles overactive sebaceous glands. This liquid wax is perfect for the task because it is symbiotic with our sebum. No more nitpicking pores! Jojoba unplugs pores by dissolving oxidized sebum.

Prevent pathogen parties with essential oil serums that inhibit pathogens without eradicating beneficial bacteria. Dab on botanical-biotics to treat pimples and hyperpigmentation. We can pour frankincense on our flora, rose on rosacea, myrrh on melasma, and cypress on psoriasis. Essential oils protect us in much the same way that they protect the plant against pathogens while helping friendly bacteria. Each oil is made of hundreds of special substances that defy the development of bacterial resistance. The same substances that stop quorum sensing and kill pathogens also boost the skin's beauty by removing toxins, delivering nutrients, and stimulating cells.

It is the life force of this plant perfection that we want to mix and meld with our microbiome. Plant tissues are made of cells that produce lipids and aromatic essences. These oily secretions, pressed and steamed from cells within the plant's epidermis, are excellent for skincare as they work synergistically with our cells. These essences ally with our bodies, turning on electrons, protective genes, and anti-inflammatory proteins, stimulating circulation, feeding immunity, and keeping collagen healthy.

With synthetic skincare devastating the dermis, and with ingredients, like parabens, that are problematic at an infinitesimal amount of 0.01 percent, we can see how each particle matters. Each drop must contain boundless, bioactive, botanical beauty. When nature provides such exquisite and effective elements to graciously attend to our skin, we must see the use of synthetics as the definition of insanity.

Seed

Our skin continually rebuilds itself with the elements captured from the cosmos, using the food and water that flows through us as fuel and microbial material. What is applied to the skin goes in, circulating with our cells and mingling with our microbes. When we apply the right things, the skin's ability to absorb is a gift of life. To do this, we need to seed our skin with wild and organic ingredients grown in healthy soil, not in pesticides and petroleum oil.

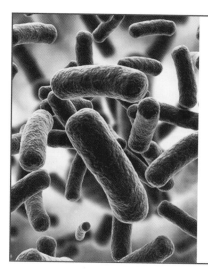

SEED
Studies Show Probiotics Benefit Skin:

Rebuild Microbial Diversity
Boost Skin's Innate Immunity
Strengthen Skin Barrier
Maintain Acid Mantle
Increase Ceramide and Lipid Production
Balance Sebaceous Glands
Help Skin Maintain Moisture
Harmonize Skin to Receive Sun's Rays
Support Collagen Synthesis
Alleviate Rosacea, Eczema, Psoriasis, and Dermatitis
Help Heal Burns, Scars, and Wounds
Prebiotics—fiber-rich oligosaccharides feed probiotics
Probiotics—look for fifty billion CFUs, diverse in Lactobacillus and Bitidus species

Healing and sealing the guts are as foundational to skincare as digestion is a direct door to every pore. A less-than-stellar diet and digestive disorders will manifest in the skin. Even wholesome food can affect the skin if you have an unknown sensitivity to it. Organic foods such as cashews, eggs, and potatoes can cause breakouts for some. If you experience a reoccurring rash or stubborn acne, tune in to your diet and skin cycles and see if there are foods triggering it.

Avoid processed foods, GMO corn and soy, and the abundance of gluten grains that can contribute to chronic inflammation, spikes in blood sugar levels, and digestive upset. Also avoid cooking with rancid, processed fats and oils that oxidize on the grocery-store shelf and contribute to premature aging and hyperpigmented skin. (See Chapter Seventeen, "Renegade Beauty Solutions," for more.)

Build your body's reserve of bacteria by ingesting and applying prebiotics and probiotics through diverse dietary deposits and skincare that thrives with the biome. Researchers are developing ways to deliver probiotics to the dermis, yet we don't have to wait! Currently, commercial topical probiotic treatments are mixed into microbe-mutating petroleum-based ooze. Instead, simply open a probiotic capsule, add to a wholesome skin serum, clay, or honey mask, and apply.

Chapter Fifteen includes a Cosmoetic Materia Medica and Renegade Beauty Recipes. Specific skin solutions can be found in Chapter Sixteen.

The Care and Feeding of Your Microbiome

Trying to get good symbiont bacteria to grow without making improvements in your stress, diet and lifestyle is like trying to grow seeds in the dark or on a parking lot.

Dr. Richard Matthews[11]

The foods you eat mainly determine which types of bacteria live in your gut. For example, *Bacteroides* are more prevalent when the diet is heavy on protein and animal fats, and *Prevotella* are associated with high-carbohydrate diets.

Long-term dietary changes can shift the microbial population.[12] Foods that are bacterial boosters are often referred to as "prebiotics." Digestion-resistant starches are the food preferred by 90 percent of our gut-loving bacteria. These starches pass unchanged all the way through the digestive system to the colon, where the bacteria feed on them. These friendly flora digest them and turn them into a substance that feeds the cells of the colon.[13] Resistant starches also lower inflammation in the colon, which should reduce the risk of colorectal cancer,[14] elevate insulin sensitivity,[15] and balance postmeal blood sugar levels.[16]

A Delightful Diet for Friendly Gut Flora

Fortunately, there are tasty foods that are chock-full of resistant starches. By adding a few of these to your daily diet, you can bless your gut microbiome and

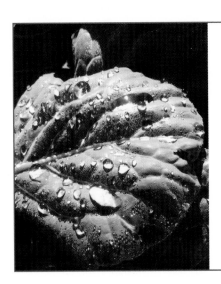

Prebiotic Foods
- Green bananas
- Cooked, cooled potatoes
- Oats
- Chicory
- Dandelion Root and Greens
- Plantain Flour
- Onions, Garlic, Leeks
- Jicama
- Jerusalem Artichoke
- Cassava
- Raw Collards
- Raw Asparagus

your skin. Soluble fiber is broken down and fermented by colon bacteria. Prebiotics, including inulin, oligofructose, and FOS (fructooligosaccharide), cause remarkable changes in the bacterial mix of the colon.

Dietary Adversaries of Healthy Gut Microbes

Processed sugar, carbohydrates, and fats and factory-raised meat and dairy are adversaries to our biome. For more than fifty years, subtherapeutic doses of antibiotics have been added to the daily feed of factory-raised animals to promote weight gain. (The mechanism of action is unknown.) We know that the antibiotics are passed into the meat and dairy, resulting in humans gaining weight and lowering immunity, resulting in a depleted immune resistance to fend off pathogens as these daily doses deplete bacterial diversity and mutate microbes.

Eating for Beauty

Imbibe dewdrops, savor solar rays, taste invocations of twilight, lift your chin to the silvery decantations of moonbeams. Welcome life in. Digestion is the resurrection and the life of the body. Food is for nourishment, delight, and abundance; let goodness be your guide. To eat is to give the body life force. Choose the purest. Digestion is the discernment of the senses. Extract what is sweet and savory; ingest the best water and food possible. Your body works as a whole, continually releasing and renewing; even laughter giggles the heart, sending nutrients everywhere.

Hearty fuel fans the flames of the belly. Tend to this purifying fire that distills inner essences and dissolves waste. This begins with relaxing and relishing, in eating and preparing meals. Invite the reception of food. Welcome minerals and enzymes to the banquet. Each meal is your body. As you are alive, eat living foods. Eat the laughing berries; these are the seeds you need. Provide nourishment to yourself, as the earth provides. Figure out what this means for your body. This is a call to digest life. Digest its beauty, freshness, pulse, and charm. Take it *all* in. The bounty going in illuminates your entire insides.

Dietary fat is vital for whole-body health and beautiful skin, and some fats are better than others. The fabulous fats in rich avocados, pasture-raised dairy, and real, organic olive and coconut oils support our cellular integrity and keep the skin soft and supple from the inside out. Processed omega-6 polyunsaturated fats and trans fats, found in every processed food on the supermarket shelf, impair intercellular communication and suppress immune functions, which are associated with skin aging and hyperpigmentation. These oils are chemically unstable and oxidize readily to form free radicals that prevent flourishing health; free radicals pillage DNA, organs, blood vessels, immunity, and the skin.

Also, avoid wheat and sugar as if your beauty depends on it . . . because it does! Sugar and wheat gluten trigger a cascade of inflammatory responses in the body and skin. It is important to keep blood sugar levels balanced. Spikes in blood sugar levels occur after eating sugar and refined carbs. In response to a rise in blood sugar, the pancreas pumps out insulin, which moves the sugar from the bloodstream to either muscle storage or fat storage. High blood sugar and spikes expose the cells to continual tidal waves of insulin, and they have only one defense against this assault and that is to become resistant to the effects of insulin. This can cause inflammatory skin issues such as hyperpigmentation and premature aging, as well as an increased risk of skin tags and a host of significant health issues.

Glycation occurs in the bloodstream to a small amount of free blood sugar from refined carbohydrates. The glycation process occurs when the sugar attaches to tissue proteins and rearranges their structures. Collagen is a long-lived protein that is susceptible to glycation, which can degrade collagen and impair it from forming healthy structures, which leads to wrinkling, sagging, and creping skin. See "Glycation" in Chapter Seventeen for more information.

Colorful meals of organic, wholesome foods, healthy fats, proteins, fruit, and vegetables are the first step toward properly functioning melanocytes, reducing low-level inflammation and reversing oxidative damage. For nutrient-dense diets, wild, homegrown, and organic foods are optimal. In this day and age, due to a myriad of factors, sometimes we need to supplement to be sure we are sated with the full spectrum of vitamins and minerals. Minerals are a language of earth and light that commune with the wisdom and connectedness in every cell. These secrets of stones and soil secrete frequencies of internal light that inspires ribbons of DNA and cells to play. A radiant terrain brims in our bodies when we are replete with minerals and vitamins that pollinate electrical possibilities into each cellular calyx.

The following vitamins and minerals are special allies for radiant skin:

* Zinc contributes to hormonal balance and repairs the skin.

* Omega-3 EFAs balance hormones, maintain cell-membrane health, and promote youthful skin.[17]

* Vitamin C is a powerhouse antioxidant to reduce oxidative damage.

- Vitamins B3 and B12 may reduce inflammation and clear out the lipofuscin in hyperpigmentation and age spots.

- Essential fat-soluble vitamin E, another powerful antioxidant, has been proven to slow the aging of skin cells and help diminish the appearance of scars. Always ingest natural vitamin E, which is listed on the label as d-alpha-tocopherol, and avoid synthetic vitamin E, which is listed with just one more letter, dl-alpha-tocopherol, yet is vastly different in its molecular makeup.

- Curcuminoids found in turmeric's yellow pigments protect cells from oxidative stress.

- Polyphenols, such as resveratrol in knotweed, grapes, cranberries, and blueberries, help to reverse some DNA damage in the body and skin cells. EGCG in green tea is a good option, too.

- Minerals of magnesium, iodine, sulfur, selenium, and silica are essential to skin and light up the cells within.

- Red clover, chamomile, passionflower, and indole-3-carbinol found in cruciferous veggies help the body clear excess estrogen that contributes to melasma. Avoid foods containing soy, because it contains plant estrogens that simulate human estrogen.

And when you crush an apple with your teeth, say to it in your heart,
"Your seeds shall live in my body,
And the buds of your tomorrow shall blossom in my heart,
And your fragrance shall be my breath,
And together we shall rejoice through all the seasons."

Kahlil Gibran[18]

THE DISH ON SOAP

The Babylonians mastered soap-making between 2800 and 2200 BC, and they wrote the recipe for it on a clay tablet: water, wood ash, and cassia oil.[19] This is the magic formula for soap: water, an alkali, and a fat (lipid). Since its discovery, we have used it to clean ourselves, our homes, our animals, and our transportation. We love our suds!

Chemically, soap is a salt of a fatty acid. Maybe soap chemistry isn't enthralling, yet it is good to understand. One end of the soap molecule attaches to water, and the other end of the soap molecule repels water but attaches to oil. When you lather up with soap, one end of the soap molecule attaches to the oil on your body and all the dirt and bacteria that are trapped in that drop of oil. The water end of the soap molecule attaches to the water from the faucet. It is the mechanical action of rubbing the skin that removes the most germs. The friction breaks up and removes the biofilms that house pathogenic bacteria, and rinsing well washes the oil and its germy cohorts off the skin.

But there's more: the fatty acids in the lipid used to make the soap are antibacterial, so soap kills some bacteria instead of just rinsing it off. Different lipids contain different fatty acids, and different fatty acids kill different kinds of bacteria. This antimicrobial action of fatty acids is why healthy skin is self-disinfecting; the natural oils in our skin contain antimicrobial fatty acids. Isn't our skin amazing?[20]

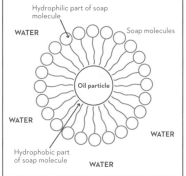

There are parts of our bodies that are exposed to a heavy load of bacteria, dirt, environmental toxins, and waste, and these areas of the body could use a little help from soap to stay clean. These parts are our pits, private bits, and hands. Our warm, damp armpits offer an irresistible invitation to bacteria. Although many are not hosts to bacteria that promote an unpleasant body odor, a quick wash with a pure bar of soap and warm water every few days will keep populations of bacteria at a healthy level and prevent biofilms from forming.

Proper hygiene requires washing our derrieres. Although practicing good post-bowel movement cleanup (wiping from front to back) is great, it isn't enough. Our private bits are a rich environment for bacteria—warmth, dampness, darkness, and food. A gentle soap-and-water washup is all you need for cleanliness. Our yonis (Sanskrit for the female genitalia) are self-cleaning and do not need to be thoroughly washed, so be sure that any soapsuds that flow to yoni-land are fully rinsed off.

Hand-Washing: Health Is in Your Hands

When it is cold and flu season, hand-washing signs such as "Clean Hands Save Lives" pop up everywhere. The Centers for Disease Control estimates that 80 percent of infections are transmitted by hands.

The bacteria that cause diarrhea, pneumonia, skin and eye infections, and infectious disease are often passed along by hand. *Norovirus,* the most prevalent pathogen in foodborne illness, lives and thrives in the restroom. The path to norovirus contamination and illness is feces to hand to mouth and/or food. MRSA is often found on computer keyboards and under fingernails.[21] MRSA bacteria are so dangerous because they are resistant to most antibiotics.

Good hand hygiene is frequently called the "do-it-yourself vaccine," because this simple act can help protect you and your family from infection and disease. A thorough hand-washing reduces transient bacteria on the hands and prevents pathogenic bacteria from building biofilm under the fingernails. It also breaks the illness chain by preventing hand-to-hand transmission.

Hand-Washing How-To: Hand-washing is easy, right? Wet. Lather. Rinse. Dry. What else is there to know?

There is a little bit of strategy to the best hand-washing protocol. It is recommended to rub soapy hands together for at least twenty seconds. Remember to rub the tops of your hands and fingers! A nailbrush with natural bristles is a great tool for a deeper clean.

Skip the antibacterial soaps, sprays, and gels and stick with simple, pure soap. In a study comparing hand-washing products, volunteers washed their hands with regular soap, antibacterial liquid soap, alcohol-based hand gel, regular soap plus an alcohol gel, or regular soap plus a nailbrush. Regular soap plus a nailbrush eliminated the most germs. The alcohol antibacterial gel killed the fewest germs.[22]

Consider consecrating your hand-washing as a mindful moment, and come away with clean hands *and* a clear mind.

> *If by the quarter of the twentieth century godliness wasn't next to something more interesting than cleanliness, it might be time to reevaluate our notions of godliness.*
>
> Tom Robbins[23]

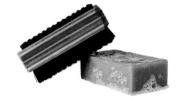

Nothing understands more what your skin needs and nothing understands the value of your skin more than your bacteria with its maternal microbiome imprint and its innate intelligence. No chemical cream will ever desire vitality for you more than a thriving microbiome. Replenish with bacteria-friendly botanicals so that you can meet the life of your skin and revel in the perfection you were born with.

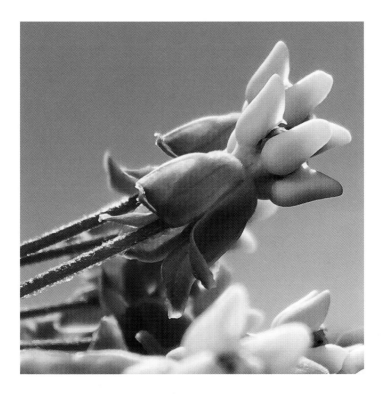

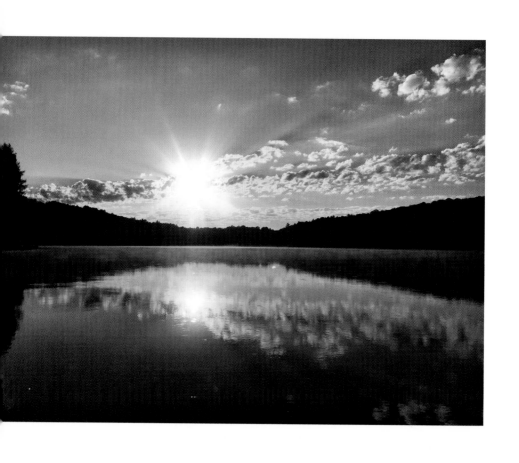

LET THE SUN SHINE IN

A candle has been lit inside me
for which the sun is a moth.[1]

The sun shines on everyone, graces all things green, and guides the growth of flora and fauna with its caress of warm wavelengths that coalesce from the solace of the celestial spheres. Life-giving solar rays penetrate the deep layers of earth to sustain the life of soil, and the same rays penetrate into the deep layers of our skin and bones.

Our bodies and bones need the sun. Our skin is designed for sunshine. Ample time in sunshine turns on a cosmic conversation, a banquet of information that percolates our pores, cells, and soul. When we merge our bodies with the sun's cathodic, cosmic rays, pores dilate deeply below the epidermis to receive the seminal influence of the sun's confluence, melting and melding with our body's ways to produce melanin and to lubricate the skin, organs, muscles, and marrow. These secretions turn sunlight into activating body electrons and substantive secretions for the immune, respiratory, digestive, and endocrine systems. Wise interaction with the sun presents revitalizing, illuminating nourishment for numerous body functions.

Currently, we live in a sunlight-deprived society; and according to the *Journal of Psychiatry and Neuroscience*, this deprivation is harming us,[2] as we deny our bodies and minds the recharging vitality of the sun. The fine filaments of our bodies are covered with thousands of vitamin D receptors designed as antennas for the sun's rays. Our cells have a DNA code and photons that require energy and information from the sun. Sunlight is a key that unlocks the nourishing energies that sustain our life.

While debates abound on if the sun is good or bad, we have forgotten our part: what do we offer these rays? It takes two to tango. The crux of our current crises is the sun as the culprit for skin carcinomas, mutating moles, wrinkles, and melanomas versus the sun as the giver of the sunshine vitamin D, a steroid hormone that illuminates our immune system and benefits every organ and cell.

HERE COMES THE SUN

The sun rises and sets with a stability and rhythm that is beyond the design of human time. This stellar star, our eternal sundial that charts the millennia of earth's existence, delivers its sustaining rays every single day. As I delved into the debates on sunbeams, I discovered a fascinating history of hope and healing. Early Egyptians worshipped the rising sun and created cosmetics to enhance their skin's interface with sunlight. "For the ancients there was little ambivalence about the role of the sun in their daily life; it was revered and the benefits conferred by it were considered unparalleled."[3] The citizens of Rome considered sun exposure so important that they had right-to-sunlight legislation,[4] and they built solariums on their homes and sunning terraces in their cities.

Sol est remediorum maximum.
The sun is the very best remedy.

Pliny the Elder[5]

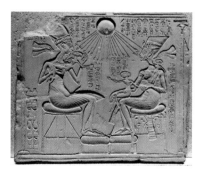

Ancient Greeks practiced *heliosis*, what they named therapeutic sun exposure via sunbathing and sungazing. More than 2,000 years ago, Greek historian Herodotus wrote that the "sun feeds muscles." Gladiators and Romans alike benefited from the sun's rays to strengthen their muscles. Herodotus also linked sunlight deprivation to brittle bones. He noted a marked difference between the bones of the Egyptian and Persian casualties he saw at the battle site of Pelusium: "I noticed the skulls of the Persians were so thin that the merest touch with a pebble would pierce them, but those of the Egyptians, on the other hand, are so tough that it is hardly possible to break them with a blow from a stone. I was told very credibly, that the reasoning was that Egyptians shave their heads from childhood, so that the bone of the skull is indurated by the action of the sun—this is why they hardly ever go bald, baldness being rarer in Egypt than anywhere else. This then explains the thickness of their skulls; and the thinness of the Persians' skulls rests on a similar principle: namely that they have always worn felt skullcaps to guard their heads from the sun."[6] Augustan ages of sun worshipping waned with the Dark Ages. The days of sunshine being the bearer of health and healing underwent a serious eclipse in the Industrial Revolution and in our current culture's consumption of sunscreen. Yet the sun dazzled for a few decades at the turn of the century.

DOCTOR SUNSHINE

My research on solar rays also led me to explore nineteenth-century heliotherapy. The work of two light-therapy pioneers, Drs. Finsen and Rollier, is highlighted in the article "The Rise and Fall of Sunlight Therapy."[7] Dr. Niels Finsen successfully employed light therapy in his treatment of patients with smallpox, lupus, and tuberculosis. He was awarded the 1903 Nobel Prize in Physiology or Medicine for his pioneering work in phototherapy. Soon after, Dr. Auguste Rollier brought heliotherapy into the mainstream.

Dr. Finsen, who suffered from Pick's disease, found heliotherapy as a result of his personal pursuit of a medical cure. As he explained, "My disease has played a very great role for my whole development . . . The disease was responsible for my starting investigations on light: I suffered from anemia and tiredness,

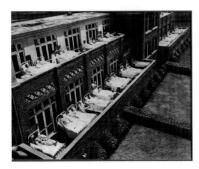

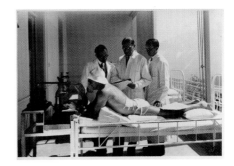

and since I lived in a house facing the north, I began to believe that I might be helped if I received more sun. I therefore spent as much time as possible in its rays . . . From this time (about 1888) I collected all possible observations about animals seeking the sun, and my conviction that the sun had a useful and important effect on the organism (especially the blood) became stronger and stronger."[8]

In the fresh air of the Swiss Alps, Dr. Rollier built solaria hospitals with walls of windows, southern balconies, and retractable roofs to maximize his patients' exposure to the sun, especially morning sun. His patients, mostly ill with tuberculosis and children plagued with rickets, were gradually introduced to sun exposure on their bare bodies in the cool Alpine air. In winter, the whole day could be spent in the sunshine. In summer, exposure was limited to the morning hours until solar noon. After a few weeks, patients were usually healthy enough to go home with the added benefit of a glowing tan.

Some children with rickets and tuberculosis would stay for a few months; the before and after photos of some of these children are astounding. The transformation from sickly, deformed bone structure, and deep, weeping wounds to healthy, glowing skin and straight spines is miraculous.[9]

Dr. Rollier said, "The sun is the best masseur."[10] He found, just as the ancient Greeks did, that when stimulating sunlight shines on bare skin in the cool air, it induces and maintains tone in the muscles without movement. It is a form of muscular activity essential for body heat, proper posture, and maintenance of bones (and such a fun way to work out!). He pointed out that every woman is careful to put her potted plants out into the sun—why not also her children? He knew that sunlight is especially important to the bone and ocular development of children.

Rollier's recipe for best results was sunbathing in the morning in combination with a nutritious diet. He insisted on wholesome meals, saying, "Well-nourished skin responds better to sunlight than mineral deficient skin." He did not calculate calories or micrograms of magnesium, simply wholesome foods and sunshine.

What surprised the medical community most about Rollier's therapy was that the sun's healing rays remained ineffective if the patients wore sunglasses.[11] Now we know that sunglasses block out important rays of the light spectrum that the body requires for essential biological functions. Interestingly, eyes do receive these rays even in the shade, just not when wearing shades.

In Rollier's days, the motto was "the deeper the tan, the better the cure." Today, diseases of darkness still exist. Deprived of sunlight, children still get rickets, and many people develop osteoporosis, dowager's humps, arthritis, hip fractures, brittle bones, tuberculosis, diabetes, and decaying teeth. When vitamin D is depleted, in the late winter of northern cultures, many folks experience increased diagnoses of influenza and cancer.[12]

As I looked at the photos of patients basking in the sun on balconies in the Alps, I recalled memories of my friends and me as we sat outside in the spring for lunch on the hillside of our school, rolling back every possible fiber of our navy-blue uniforms so that we could feel the warm embrace of the sun. We were not medical patients longing for a cure to a physical ailment. We were inmates of a school longing for any extra increment of freedom we could pursue for our spirits, minds, and bodies. Our mothers warned us about the sun's danger, and our schoolteachers attempted to ban us from basking in the sun. Yet, the feeling the sun gave, the cheeriness and warm rays, always made our days.

One person's pursuit of a cure led him to the sun. Another doctor, inspired by that discovery, made medical knowledge of the sun accessible to countless patients for a generation. Their experiences encouraged me to connect to my teenage self and confirm an intuition that reaches far beyond wanting a tan for my winter-white legs.

> The action of sunshine in the outdoors on the body is of such a nature that sun-baths have a triple significance—as a healing agent in the cure of disease, as a preventative to disease by building up body resistance, and as a sheer pleasure—giving tonic which increases the feeling of well-being.
>
> Edgar Mayer, MD[13]

Poetically, I have understood noetically that our skin's relationship to sunlight is our human form of photosynthesis. A recent remarkable study highlights that humans are indeed light-harvesters of chlorophyll pigments, and our bodies, through the mantle of melanin, can convert the sun's light into cellular, mitochondrial energy.[14] Plants can help us with this, too; eating plenty of

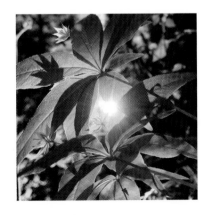

greens helps humans capture sunlight in our cells and translate it into energy via our mighty mitochondria.[15]

When we're outdoors, it's not just that we feel warm in the sun and get a suntan; a vibrational field actually merges with our own and enhances the quality or the flow of energy through our body. To put it in plain terms, the effect of sunlight on our energy system is similar to that of a battery being charged.[16]

Our evolution as mammals has always included being influenced by the lunisolar tides and being "bathed in photonic energy from the sun."[17] We can now add to this knowledge that the consumption of chlorophyll, the green "blood" of verdant plants, makes our mitochondria thrive. We optimize our biological potential nutritionally with leafy greens, green juices, and liquid chlorophyll, as they help us use sunlight as energy in lieu of relying solely on glu-cose for energy.[18] We can also correlate from this study that pigment-rich plants boost an internal SPF, a "sun-pigment factor" that enhances our engagement with the sun.

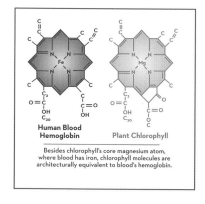

Human Blood Hemoglobin

Plant Chlorophyll

Besides chlorophyll's core magnesium atom, where blood has iron, chlorophyll molecules are architecturally equivalent to blood's hemoglobin.

SEASONS IN THE SUN

Although we now have a better under-standing of sunbeams' boon to our health, many may still be weary of wrin-kles linked to these light waves. Creat-ing concern about the sun's rays, most dermatologists and beauty magazines wax weary about ultraviolet hazards, and health campaigns advocate for avoid-ance of the sun. The sun has become the perpetrator of photoaging, wrin-kles, and hyperpigmentation, along with

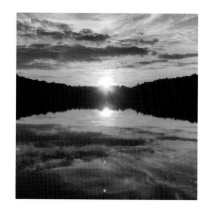

three types of skin cancer. There is the very serious and ever-increasing malignant melanoma, which is cancer of the pigment cells. It can infiltrate the lymph system, it spreads aggressively, and it can be fatal. Squamous cell carcinoma and basal cell carcinoma are non-melanomas. Basal cell carcinoma is the most common and the least dangerous, as it does not have the tendency to spread.

It is true that our skin can be vulnerable to sunburn, and repeated sunburns can cause visible damage, though despite the negative press linking sun exposure to skin cancer, there lacks consistent scientific evidence to support it.[19] For example, people with the greatest risk of melanoma are not those with the greatest cumulative solar exposure.

A sampling of a few research study conclusions sheds a different light on some common conceptions. One study found that malignant melanoma is less likely for adults and children who work and play outside. Another study showed that melanoma is far more common for people who work indoors.[20] A review of studies showed no correlation between sun exposure and melanoma.[21] In his extensively researched book *The Sun and the "Epidemic" of Melanoma: Myth on Myth!*, Dr. Bernard Ackerman, the founding father of the field of dermatopathology (the study of skin diseases), substantiated that "there is no proof whatsoever that sun exposure causes melanoma." He wrote, "The calculations now in vogue [about the incidence of melanoma] will be shown to have been inaccurate woefully . . . and that the sun, now incriminated as the major culprit responsible for an 'epidemic' of melanoma, will be rehabilitated from its status current of pariah, our worst enemy, to its place rightful, all things considered, namely, humankind's best friend."[22]

The results of a 1982 study conducted by researchers at the London School of Hygiene and Tropical Medicine and published by the medical journal *The Lancet* demonstrated that fluorescent light exposure from indoor work (and this was back in 1982 when most of the workforce was yet to stare at a computer screen all day) creates twice the incidence of melanoma than outdoor work in the sun. Office workers, exposed to high levels of artificial lighting during the day with minimal exposure to sunlight, had the highest risk of developing melanomas and mutations in their cells.[23]

Lack of sunlight and our culture's epidemic lack of vitamin D3 are linked to cancer, overwhelmingly, in more than 2,500 studies. Several studies confirmed that *appropriate* sun exposure actually helps prevent skin cancer. In fact, melanoma occurrence has been found to decrease with sun exposure, and increase with sunscreen use.

There is also a lack of scientific evidence that sunscreens prevent skin cancer. However, synthetic suncreams do prevent sunburns. Let's look at how this is achieved. When we apply sunscreen, sun-shielding chemicals that block UVB rays are absorbed into our skin; UVB rays do cause burns after extended time in the sun. SPF, sun protection factor, is a designation that can be used only for synthetic ingredients that have been laboratory tested to prevent sunburns. Yet SPF creates a false sense of security by disabling our skin's early-warning protection, the sunburn, against overexposure to the sun. Essentially, sunscreen anesthetizes skin. UVB rays—the rays blocked by sunscreens—are also the nourishing rays that spark production of vitamin D in the body.

UVA rays become harmful when they are separated from their UVB ultraviolet partner by sunscreens.[24] Current studies suggest that it is isolated UVA that damages DNA. So, slathering on sunscreen actually inhibits the much-desired vitamin D and allows the undesired penetration of isolated UVA while UVB is blocked. (Receiving hours of direct sunlight through a window will also separate the UVB and overexpose skin to UVA. Many drivers, for example, have one forearm that is more freckled than the other.)

> The scare tactics . . . adopted concerning melanoma include advocacy, in a manner verging on the hysterical, of the use of a sunscreen around the clock, even on cloudy days, and of garb protective similar to that donned by astronauts.
>
> Dr. Bernard Ackerman[25]

With ingredients of oxybenzone, polymers of petroleum, parabens, and PABA, these chemical-laden lotions also block our skin's ability to breathe; our skin's cellular-respiration process is inhibited from inhaling oxygen and exhaling toxins and carbon dioxide. Likewise, as we soak up the sun, these chemicals bake into our bodies. Oxybenzone, an active ingredient in many sunscreens, is a powerful free-radical generator that is noncarcinogenic—*until exposed to sunlight!*[26] These carcinogens are now being recognized as agents that actually increase disease by way of their free-radical-generating properties. Sunscreen ingredients are also known to accumulate in our lipid layers, increasing our intake of free radicals, xenoestrogens, oxidized amino acids, and damaged DNA. Promoted as necessary to preserve skin from aging, sunscreen ingredients actually alter the innate intelligence of our cells, increase carcinoma risk,[27] and prevent vitamin D production. Refuse to use sunscreens that restrain this vital cosmic connection, and let the sunshine in.

SUN-FLUID NUTRIENTS

Keep squeezing drops of the Sun.

Hafiz[28]

Our bodies are designed to be exposed to the rays of the sun, and our skin contains all the necessary mechanisms to extract and produce beneficial nutrients from it. The interaction of sun on skin is our human form of photosynthesis. Sunlight in the form of UVB rays touching the skin produces beneficial nutrients that our bodies require. Our skin converts sunbeams into regenerative substances of melanin, sulfur, and the steroid hormone, vitamin D. This distinct steroid hormone influences every cell in our body, and is easily one of nature's most potent champions. I think of vitamin D as golden drops of sun fluid that we all need internally to be optimally well-oiled.

The most natural and effective form of vitamin D is the type that we synthesize when our skin coalesces with the sun—without sunscreen. The best time of day to get out and play in the sun for making vitamin D is morning to solar noon. Time variances, existing melanin levels, geography, and weather are all factors in how much shine one would need to get a good day's supply of D—of course, there is an app for that.[29]

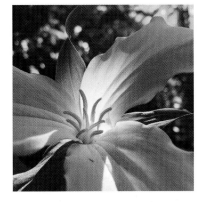

Our skin's exposure to sun produces two types of essential sulfur: cholesterol sulfate and vitamin D3 sulfate. Sulfur, cholesterol, and the vitamin D produced in our skin from sun exposure are necessary for optimal cellular health while protecting us from radiation damage. Sulfur and cholesterol protect our DNA from radiation damage that contributes to cancer. They "become oxidized upon exposure to the high frequency rays in sunlight, thus acting as antioxidants to take the heat, so to speak."[30] Vitamin D3 from oral supplements, which is unsulfured and fat-soluble, is helpful, but it is not bonded to sulfur to make D3 sulfate. Vitamin D3 sulfate is water-soluble and moves freely in the bloodstream, providing a healthy barrier against bacteria; it is "synthesized in the skin, where it forms a crucial part of the barrier that keeps out harmful bacteria and other microorganisms such as fungi."[31]

If we avoid the sun, we are missing out on this natural disease protection. When we circumvent this natural process, either by using sunblock or staying out of the sun entirely, we give free rein to a variety of disease activities. UV rays are potent disinfectants; they hinder the growth of bacteria, fungi, and viruses. Dr. Oskar Bernhard was a Swiss surgeon who would put his surgical patients out in the sun for a few minutes before suturing their surgical wounds to disinfect them.[32]

Our current sun-fear contributes to the soaring rate of vitamin D deficiency in North America. Nearly 75 percent of adults and teenagers are vitamin D deficient, and we have been on a two-decade-long slide.[33] Skin is like our solar panel, taking in the sun's energy, and a lack of sunlight disturbs normal cell growth. Research attributes health issues to low levels of D, including heart disease, osteoporosis, juvenile diabetes, multiple sclerosis, cancer, and more.

Vitamin D is designed to course through the body and facilitate various body functions. It repairs organs, boosts immune function, lowers insulin levels, reduces blood pressure, boosts neuromuscular functioning, and interacts with more than 2,000 genes. The sun, via vitamin D, lets the cells know when it is time to die; this healthy process is called apoptosis. Failure of apoptosis is one of the reasons for cancerous-tumor development. When cells stop dying when they are supposed to, endless cell division occurs and cells pile up in a disorganized body system.

Additionally, vitamin D (along with vitamin K2) is essential for proper absorption of calcium and other minerals into the bones and teeth. It promotes efficient neuromuscular functioning and plays a role in anti-inflammatory processes. Thousands of vitamin D receptors (VDRs) are found in our skin, in places where the sun doesn't shine, and in almost every single cell of our body, including the brain, breasts, bones, hypothalamus, prostate, pancreas, placenta, lymphocytes, heart, stomach, small intestines, colon, and more.

> The Sun is our most vital factor. Like sea water nourishes seaweed, so the Sun supplies the vitality that human beings live on. Bones and nails especially are concentrations of invisible sunfluid.
>
> Nobel lecturer Niels Ryberg Finsen[34]

With visions of vitamin D receptors and sunbeams swirling in my head, I wondered about the role of "empty" vitamin D receptors. What happens when these receptors are not filled with juicy sun secretions? I also wondered about the role of our gut bacteria and how they interplay with our skin and the sun's rays. I think we can trace many imbalances back to lack of intestinal integrity. So, I was excited to come across studies that tied some of these thoughts together.[35]

If our VDRs are brimming with the sunshine vitamin, this prevents the gene expression of a mind-boggling array of disease-causing genes. When our VDRs are not filled with active D3, bacterial ligands (which are sticky bacterial adhesions that affix to and stifle the receptors) enter, bind to, and inactivate VDRs. Subsequently, the ligands inactivate our innate immune response.[36] This hampers the VDRs' production of antimicrobial peptides, allowing microbes to proliferate and set up the environment for chronic inflammatory diseases. VDRs are at the heart of our immune system, and pathogenic bacteria thrive by going into the heart of our immune system and disabling the VDRs. A growing number of bacteria have been shown to downregulate the innate activity of the VDRs, including *Mycobacterium tuberculosis* and Epstein-Barr virus. This knowledge enhances why Dr. Auguste Rollier was able to cure tuberculosis with the sun and almost a century later we have the data to understand this on a scientific level.

In external environments, sunlight is a robust germicide and bactericide. Internally, the skin's secretions catalyzed by sunbeams are powerfully broad-spectrum antibacterial and immune regenerating. With VDRs present in every crevice of our body, we can trust this ancient relationship between the sun and our skin.

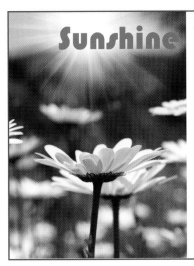

Sunshine Vitamin

- Organizes our biochemical processes
- Increases muscle tone
- Relaxes nerves
- Increases oxygen of blood & tissues
- Regulates and boosts hormones
- Supports eye health
- Lowers blood sugar
- Regulates basal metabolic rate
- Benefits thyroid
- Boosts immune and repairs DNA
- Antiseptic against pathogenic bacteria
- Necessary for normal cell division

Sunlight specific:
- Disinfectant and antiseptic
- Produces essential cholesterol sulfate
- Produces vitamin D3 sulfate
- Fills VDR with essential D3

Where I live in Canada, for about five months of the year the sun is not strong enough for skin to make vitamin D. Still, on sunny days I open my doors to the sunshine and I bask in the prana, the light, and the very fresh air. I make sure that my diet is rich in fats and greens, and I do find it essential to apply transdermal vitamin D cream and transdermal patches of vitamin D as well as supplement with an oral D3 and K2 combination.

Posidonius, a first-century BC Greek philosopher, astronomer, and mathematician, wisely wrote that the sun's rays were a "vital force" for all living creatures on earth. In my neck of the woods, the winters can be long and, for me, the warm solar rays of spring are a welcoming vital force. All spring, summer, and fall, when the sun shines I am sure to catch sun rays to store up vitamin D to carry me into the winter months.

Try as they might, scientists and pharmaceutical companies have yet to come up with a perfect sunshine vitamin. Supplemental fat-soluble vitamin D3 is a valuable and viable resource, yet the vitamin D that is produced by our bodies when the sun fuses with skin is a water-soluble form and it is stored in our cells as a rainy-day fund. Skin is innately designed to generate vitamin D in response to sunlight, not solely through digestive intake. Also, it is unclear if supplemental vitamin D ever reaches the upper layers of the skin, the keratinocyte layer, where it plays an important role in our immunity as a germ fighter and as a protector from sun overexposure.

My advice is to enjoy sun-kissed skin to create an ample supply of sun-made vitamin D reserves during the sunny seasons to resource you through the winter months.

ONE WITH THE SUN

Why deny our skin the sun's warm wavelengths of creation that blood and hormones need for cosmic pollination? Without sunbeams stimulating our skin, we drain our innate immunity and lose the lipids that lubricate our skin from within. Doctors of previous decades prescribed sunlight to heal injuries, strengthen weak skin, and prevent infections of acne, eczema, dermatitis, and tuberculosis. Yet in this century, we reject the sun's sustenance while injecting fillers into faces, applying chemicals to acne, and spraying on tans with dihydroxyacetone.

Although repeated sunburns are not ideal, sun-damaged skin actually comes from within: a depleted microbiome, a diet of rancid oils and processed food, washing repeatedly with surfactants, further exacerbated with chemical creams all baked in with synthetic sunscreen.

Including sunshine as part of our hygiene is one of the deepest ways to be clean. Sunshine purifies our blood and activates antimicrobial peptides that boost immunity by feeding and stabilizing the skin's flora. Sunlit skin becomes a lube for the microbiome. With our skin designed with receptors ready to receive these rays of restoration, we can be reassured that we are one with the sun.

Sunlight dominates the chemistry of the blood. People who do not get sunlight do not have the same richness and redness of blood as do those who secure plenty of sunlight. There is not a tissue or a function in the body that is not benefitted by regular and judicious sun-bathing.[37]

We do want to avoid sunburns, yet getting sunburned is actually easier on our DNA than processing the cell damage from being in the sun with synthetic sunscreen. Sunscreen blocks our biological mechanism called melanin[38] that was designed to guide our skin's interaction with the sun. When we get sunburned, our ancient photoprotective melanin ensures that only a tiny fraction of our DNA is damaged by the absorbed photons. Our DNA naturally transforms 99.9 percent of the photons into heat.[39] In this instance, heat is harmless! The remaining 0.1 percent of the photons is what causes sunburn. In DNA, this conversion of photons into harmless heat is extremely efficient. However,

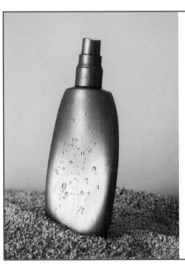

Sunscreens

- No proof of sunscreen preventing BCC
- Increase estrogenic activity
- Chemicals stored in fat tissue
- Generate free radicals
- Increase cellular damage
- Indirect DNA damage
- Absorb UVB rays, but let (most) UVA through
- 2007 study at U of C concluded significant correlation between sunscreen use and skin cancer
- No evidence sunscreen prevents melanoma
- Blocks production of vitamin D
- Carcinogenic ingredients
- Toxins inhibit skin's respiration cycle
- Disables skin's warning system

sunscreen damages DNA indirectly and without the warning signal of a burn. It is this indirect DNA damage that is responsible for mutations.

Sunscreen causes *indirect* DNA damage because the photons are not efficiently converted into harmless heat. This understanding of indirect DNA damage led to new research, like the 2007 study at the University of California, San Diego, that reviewed seventeen studies of sunscreen use and melanoma. The researchers concluded that there is a significant correlation between sunscreen use and skin cancer.[40] And in 1998, the *Journal of the National Cancer Institute* reported that children who were frequent users of sunscreens had a significantly higher chance of developing moles and freckles.[41]

Far more effective than sunscreen, protective melanin lingers on our skin and in our blood in the form of vitamin D long after the sun has set. To preserve the juiciness of sun exposure, lubricate with organic botanical oils before, during, and after sun exposure, and be sure not to soap the skin's surface, which disrupts the process of these regenerative substances.

SUN WISE: GRACEFULLY INTERFACE WITH SUNLIGHT

Imagine being at an appointment with your doctor, and you are advised to spend unblocked time in the sun to preserve the health and beauty of your skin. . . .

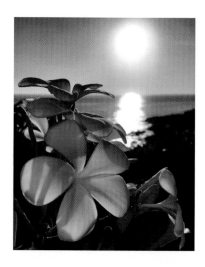

This renegade advice was written by an English physician, C. W. Saleeby, in 1923: "Properly aired and sunlit, skin becomes velvety, supple tissue, absolutely immune from anything of the nature of pimples, acne, and incapable of infection. Sunshine is the finest cosmetic. Skin, well-pigmented in response to sunbathing, becomes firm and strong, but at the same time delicate and soft. Followed by a filling out of the exposed skin and a smoothing away of wrinkles results from sunbathing. Increased beauty is the outcome."[42]

In contrast, today most dermatologists admonish us on ultraviolet hazards, and public-health advertising advocates for avoidance of the sun. While being campaigned into sacrificing sunlight, we have been told and sold on shunning the sun, and we fear exposure of the sun's rays reaching our skin. Although overexposure makes our skin vulnerable to sunburn, and recurrent sunburns can cause visible damage, there is more to the story than the sun being the sole perpetrator of hyperpigmentation and wrinkles. Our interaction with the sun need not be "all or none!" If we are wise, we can enjoy a healthy, happy relationship with our ancient friend, the sun.

Here are the best protocols for wisely imbibing solar wavelengths.

Eat Sun-Harmonizing Foods

Upon the altar of sunshine, what we ingest determines how our skin responds to sunlight. Skin cells must be strengthened and nourished internally with real food and water to receive the full blessing of interacting with the sun. Less food is needed when we are satiated with solar rays, and well-nourished skin responds better to sunlight. Sun-ripened food is also far more nutritious. We can create an internal SPF with an antioxidant-rich rainbow diet of sun-grown superpower foods, herbs, and luscious fats brimming with nutrients—all contributing to our internal sunscreen.

Summer is a great time to indulge in sun-ripened fruit, vegetables, and herbs that build an internal SPF. Take tomatoes, for example: researchers in

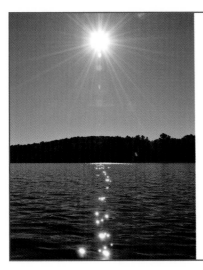

Sun Wise Interaction

- First recover integrity of skin's outer layer
- Topically use pure botanicals in sun and after sun
- Eliminate all processed PUFA vegetable oils
- Drink spring water
- Block: clothing, hats, zinc, & shade
- Enjoy sunrise & sunset
- Start tanning in spring
- Tan in morning hours until solar noon
- Gradually build melanin 5–20 minutes a day
- Expose as much of skin as possible
- Build reserves for winter
- Avoid soap and tap water after sunning
- SPF Diet: sunshine grown super-powered foods
- Antioxidants & iodine

the United Kingdom have demonstrated a 30 percent increase in sun protection after eating a tomato-rich diet. The key seems to be 16 mg of lycopene, the red antioxidant found in tomatoes.[43] Other SPF foods and beverages include pigment-rich, beta-carotene-bursting foods such as watermelon, green tea, turmeric, leafy greens, liquid chlorophyll, and berries. Also, save room for chocolate! Pure, unprocessed, and unadulterated chocolate has four times the amount of phenols and catechins as teas, and these compounds protect the skin against sunburn.

Many of the skin issues that are called "sun damage" are really the result of modern malnutrition. The recipe for wrinkles and dark spots is our current standard diet of processed food produced in the shadows of pesticides and factory farming. The trans fats, plasticizers, bromide, formaldehyde, coal-tar derivatives, color and flavor additives, and fluoride commonly found in these foods create reactions in our bodies that trigger collagen breakdown, inflammation, age spots, and hyperpigmentation. Adding to this are medications, chlorine, oral contraceptives, antibiotics, and the diuretic action of diet soda and coffee, all increasing our sensitivity to the sun. The rampant use of rancid polyunsaturated-fatty-acids, vegetable oils of soy, cottonseed, corn, canola, and Mazola found in every processed-food item impairs intercellular communication, suppresses immune functions, damages DNA, and this synthetic sundae is linked to wrinkles and hyperpigmentation. This is the difference between cooking with PAM or coconut oil and soaking ourselves in oxybenzone or sea-buckthorn berry oil.

The food industry falsely fortifies foods, and claims, "You may have been taught as a child that you need sunlight for your body to make vitamin D, because vitamin D is not found naturally in most foods. But today, many foods are fortified with vitamin D during the manufacturing process. So, sun exposure is not as important as it used to be."[44] Artificial fortification of most milk, baby formula, and cereal products is made with synthetic vitamin D2, which is not even the right kind of vitamin D! One issue with D2 is that it is way less biologically active than D3 and is inefficient at binding with our valuable vitamin D receptors, making room for those bacterial ligands to invade our VDRs.

Organic, healthy fats and fresh-pressed essential fatty acids, direly depleted in the North American diet, are really needed to amplify the benefits of the sun's rays.

Recover Your Skin's Integrity

The skin's outer layer, the epidermis, contains a thin coating of soothing sebaceous oils that provide natural antibacterial, antiwrinkle, and sunscreen protection. The integrity of this layer is damaged by surfactants, scrubs, chemical peels, and synthetic moisturizers. (These things also disrupt vitamin D production.) Washing and moisturizing the skin with botanical serums, as well as gently dry brushing, regenerates the skin's top layer, supports the collagen, and feeds the skin's immunity.

> A person has to be like a flower, open to the Sun in order to take in its energy, only this is capable of bringing the flower to fruition. The mind of a person has to turn to the Sun light . . . If a person takes in the Sun light, life unfolds correctly on its own.
>
> Beinsa Douno[45]

Sun Yourself Wisely

Start slowly but surely, and start in the spring so that you may create a protective tan with phased-in exposure. Melanin, the tanned-skin pigment, produced in the spring prevents sunburn in the summer. Melanin is our ancient biological mechanism of photoprotection designed exclusively to support our relationship with the sun. Melanin in the skin transforms 99.9 percent of absorbed UV radiation into heat that is easily dissipated, allowing us to sidestep radiation damage that contributes to cell damage. Far more effective than sunscreen is rebuilding your body's melanin base that further enhances the health of many body systems.

The D Minder app will calculate your geographic location, current cloud cover, and time of year to let you know how long to bask in the sun's rays and how much vitamin D will be generated that day. The best time of day for sunning is morning to solar noon. Bare as much skin as you dare. The dosage depends on the condition of your skin and your natural skin pigmentation. Tune in to your innate warning system; if skin starts to feel warm, seek shade. Start with a few minutes a day and build up. Remember to flip!

Recap on SPF

Sunscreens made from synthetic ingredients create a false sense of security by disabling our skin's early-warning system—the sunburn—which keeps us from indulging in too much sun too fast. Most sunscreens block only UVB rays, the rays that cause sunburn, but not UVA rays. Over the long run, people wearing synthetic sunscreens unknowingly overexpose their skin to UV radiation. Unfortunately, sunscreen prevents skin from receiving any of the benefits of engaging with the sun's rays.

Sunscreens are hazardous to our health and the vitality of the oceans. Scientific studies confirm that the synthetic sunscreen chemicals of oxybenzone, octinoxate, benzophenone, and butylparaben[46] wash off swimmers' and surfers' skin into the water, killing and bleaching coral reefs. An estimated *14,000 tons of sunscreen wash off annually into the world's oceans*, endangering the symbiosis of sea life. "Australia's Great Barrier Reef is undergoing the most severe bleaching event in its history, as corals along the reef expel the symbiotic algae that provide them both with their rich colors and food."[47] Beyond coral bleaching, studies also suggest oxybenzone is an endocrine disrupter among marine creatures such as shrimps and clams.[48]

To receive what the Sun is giving us, we should have a relation to it . . .

Beinsa Douno[49]

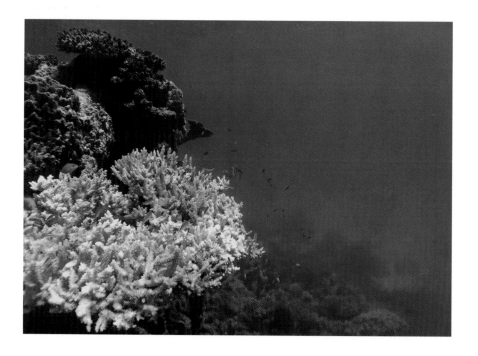

Bet on Botanical Oils

Botanical oils preserve the juiciness of your sun exposure. Plants, too, require wise interaction with the sun. Plants alchemize sunlight to create a verdant growth. This is the same star that stirs our skin cells and invites our bones to grow. What is on and in our bodies while engaging with sunshine is vital! Almost all plant oils offer some degree of ultraviolet protection to their own tissues— and ours.

> *Every kind of light ray has a different impact on the plant's life process. At the same time, the blossom leads a completely different life with regard to light than do the green leaves (the blossom consumes oxygen while the leaves produce it); it colors and unfolds itself differently within it.*[50]

Officially, the term "SPF" can only be used to reference synthetic sunscreen ingredients, yet plant oils do offer a range of protection that can gracefully extend our time in the sun. Plant oils of virgin coconut, jojoba, olive, and sea-buckthorn applied to the skin provide a measure of sun protection. Raspberry seed oil also has potential use as a broad-range sun protectant. Under a spectrometer, raspberry seed oil absorbed both UVB and UVC rays while scattering UVA; it may provide a botanical equivalent of SPF-25.

Essential oils, the distillates of plants, are especially adept at harmonizing the sun's rays with our skin and further enhance harmonizing our skin with solar rays when added to the lipid oils listed above. Rich in antioxidants and cell-regenerative activity, they nourish and heal the skin.

If you ever burn, aloe or jojoba mixed with a little peppermint, lavender, and/or seabuckthorn offers soothing relief, cooling and quickening healing.

The essential oils of sandalwood, geranium, frankincense, immortelle, and rose can fade hyperpigmentation and prevent abnormal cell growth. Scientific studies reveal that the alpha santalol and beta santalol in sandalwood essential oil are also chemopreventive, reversing the damage of skin lesions and tumors.[51] Other successful studies about skin cells responding positively to the botanical-biotics of essential oils have been conducted with lemongrass, frankincense, and others.[52]

We want to avoid sunburned skin, so for extended hours in the sun that exceed your natural melanin protection and plant oil oversight, wear a hat and cover your skin with clothing. Or use a natural, organic sunblock with zinc oxide as the active block ingredient. Uncoated, non-nanoparticle zinc oxide effectively blocks and reflects, rather than absorbs, the sun's rays. For waterproof sunburn prevention, mix pure vitamin C powder in a 10 percent solution with water; lightly mist onto exposed skin and allow it to soak in, and spray once again before sun exposure.

Learn from the Sun. When you see it in the morning, it greets you with a smile . . . To renovate yourselves, you have to get up early every morning to be able to receive the first rays of the Sun. They carry within them light and elevated thoughts. You may say that the rays of light are nothing more than vibrations, oscillations of ether. It is true that light is oscillations, vibrations, but these are life-bearing vibrations.

Beinsa Douno[53]

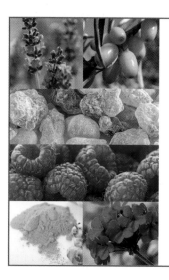

Sun Harmonizing Botanicals

Cell Regeneration—rose otto, lavender, sandalwood, myrrh, seabuckthorn berry, turmeric

Hyperpigmentation—frankincense, rose otto, cypress, immortelle, geranium

Sun Harmonizers—seabuckthorn berry, turmeric, carrot seed, immortelle, red raspberry seed, coconut oil, jojoba, olive oil, peppermint, geranium, sandalwood, frankincense

After Sun Care—lavender, aloe vera, frankincense, sandalwood, seabuckthorn berry

Sun Shade—zinc, vitamin C spray

Wear Sunglasses Only When Necessary

Our eyes need sunlight, too. Absorption of sunlight by the eyes is the most direct path of communication between the sun and our brains, and our good health and good mood hinge on it. When the full spectrum of light rays is intercepted in the retina, it is positively encoded in the brain and sets in motion the juicy hormones and neurochemicals that help us stay happy and healthy. This process works even if we are in the shade, yet not if we are *wearing* shades.

The blue part of the sunlight spectrum is absorbed by the lens at the back of the eye, which stimulates the suprachiasmatic nucleus (the body's master clock) in the hypothalamus and the pineal gland. In turn, they synchronize the production and release of neural and hormonal messengers, including melatonin (which is different from melanin). Melatonin is most widely known as the circadian-rhythm hormone that regulates sleep-wake cycles. It is also a powerful immune booster and antiaging antioxidant that protects nuclear and mitochondrial DNA and delays neurodegeneration. Wearing sunglasses and spending our days indoors blocks blue-light reception and reduces our nightly dose of melatonin.

As we rise in years, the photoreceptive lens may start to get cloudy, inhibiting the full absorption of the needed blue light. This leads to master-clock confusion and the underproduction of hormones, like melatonin, and neurochemicals. An average forty-five-year-old person's lenses absorb only half the amount of blue light as a child's lenses. The lenses of the elderly can be quite opaque, and this may explain why rates of sleep problems, immune issues, and some mood disorders, like depression, increase in the elderly. As your years increase, there is much benefit to being outside receiving the sun's fullest blessing and the night's best sleep.

Children also need to be outside in the sun, as natural light is crucial for healthy eye development. Ophthalmological research shows that spending three hours a day in natural light reduces the risk of nearsightedness in children. Sunlight triggers dopamine production in the eye, which stimulates normal growth.

We can safely satisfy our eyes' need for sunlight by practicing the ancient art of sungazing.

STARING AT THE SUN

Look to the sun for health. Another biological process of sun-energy absorption activates when we have the sun in our eyes. Sunlight enters our eyes and stimulates our pineal gland, which is connected to the hypothalamus, where sun-energy triggers vital magnetic, electrical, and chemical reactions in the human body. Science has revealed that sunlight stimulates the production of melatonin (a hormone that promotes calmness) and serotonin (a neurotransmitter that promotes well-being).

Practicing the ancient tradition of sungazing may meet all of your body's and spirit's sun needs. The practice is easy; simply look at the sun as it rises or sets. It is safe to look at the sun within the hour after sunrise or within the hour before sunset because ultraviolet levels are at zero.

You will want to begin sungazing slowly to acclimate your eyes to the sun. Start by looking at the sun, during one of the safe hours, for about twenty seconds and then add twenty seconds to your sungazing practice every day. At first, after years of indoor living and screen time, you may have to cover one eye with your palm and alternate eyes, so that you can take in the light without squinting. Allowing your eyes to increase their capacity for light absorption creates less squinting and hence less "crow's-feet," as the skin around the eyes is more relaxed. After three months, you will have built up to fifteen minutes a day, and you will likely feel the positive effects: less tension, fewer worries, a more balanced spirit, and increased vitamin D. The effects are truly positive and bring an ineffable brightness to the internal spheres.

Rejoice in the warm sunshine, and let the elements feed your skin and spirit. Engage it with grace. Greet it with self-knowledge, wisdom, and a well-nourished body, and all will be well.

Thank you, sun, that just miraculously happens to be precisely placed in the cosmos.

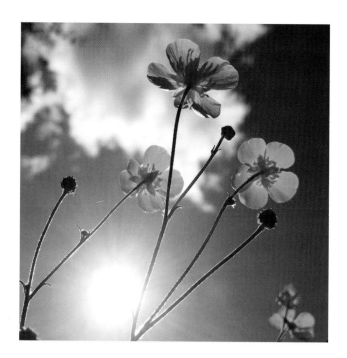

Why I Wake Early

Hello, sun in my face.
Hello, you who make the morning
and spread it over the fields
and into the faces of the tulips
best preacher that ever was,
dear star, that just happens
to be where you are in the universe
to keep us from ever-darkness,
to ease us with warm touching,
to hold us in the great hands of light—
good morning, good morning, good morning.

Mary Oliver[54]

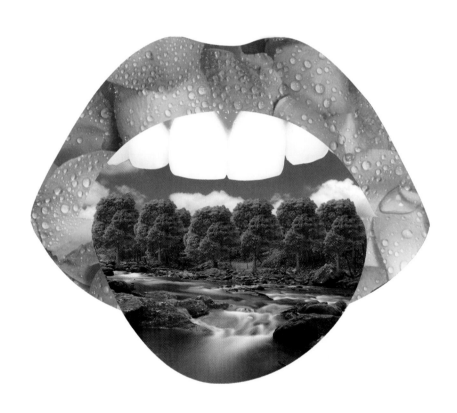

Chapter Eight

THE BONE–BEAUTY CONNECTION

Teeth and Oral Health

We have been taught to brush twice daily, floss, and visit the dentist to prevent tooth decay, yet the staggering number of cavities, crowns, root canals, and extracted teeth confirms that something is amiss. Although there are a plethora of periodontal promises ranging from fluoride floss to minty mouthwash, there is more dental decay now than in any previous century.

Wearily, we roam the drugstore dental aisles. Searching for solutions, we attain countless tubes of paste, we maintain the ingrained hygienist and dentist appointments, and we brush with daily diligence for decades. Even so, the possibility of periodontal disease percolates. Receding, bleeding gums are the norm. Unexpected cavities form, and millions of root canals are performed. The definition of insanity, doing the same thing and expecting different results, applies to our current state of dental care.

Our mouths are a microcosm mirroring the macrocosm of imbalances on our planet. Our dental dysbiosis reflects our lack of symbiosis in our relationships to our bodies, global food production, medicine, and the environment. On a microscopic level, everything that is going on in our mouth is going on in the world: enamel and topsoil erosion, systemic corrosion, crumbling bones, mold in our homes, triclosan in toothpaste, toxins dumped in haste, factory farms festering with fungi, pollutants in the sky, adverse effects of petroleum oil, glyphosates affecting our gums, guts, and soil; deforestation, fluoridation, pesticides, and antibiotics that mutate microbes, gum pockets that erode, chronic disease, mercury in our mouths and seas, environmental allergens, chaotic carcinogens, and invading pathogens. These things threaten the borders of our body and the boundaries of our planet.

The mouth is the principal portal into our bodies; it interfaces, absorbs, and assimilates our world. The endocrine, immune, and digestive systems are intimately bound to the microbiome of our mouths. By understanding the human microbiome, we understand that our health depends on a thriving microbiome; and as human hosts to this bacterial banquet, the key to vitality in our bodies and mouths is bacterial balance.

What we now know is that many of the periodontal procedures and medicants of modern dentistry disrupt the beneficial bacteria of our gums and mutate our mouth's microbes. Many of our oral-care practices suppress immunity. Instead, we need to reconcile with our bacterial community. We need to fluff our oral flora, and befriend our body's bacteria. We need to abandon the products, practices, and antibiotics that are making our microbes mutate, mottling our teeth, and deforesting the flora of our oral ecology.

On top of this microbe mutation, the profession put in charge of our oral cavity is shrouded in subjective science. Dental diagnosis can vary vastly from dentist to dentist. To demonstrate this, a researcher for the Canadian Broadcasting Corporation, armed with a hidden camera and a dental assessment from the University of Toronto, visited twenty dentists. Her mouth only needed a cleaning and a crown replacement, but if she had followed the combined recommendations of the twenty dentists, then nearly every tooth in her mouth would have been treated, including multiple unnecessary root canals, veneers, fillings, and crowns.[1]

Another journalist with a trusted dentist's confirmation that he only needed one crown on a molar traveled across the United States for fifty dental examinations. All fifty dentists examined the same mouth and the same X-rays. Their estimates ranged from $700 to $19,000, and the treatment plans ranged from crowning one tooth to having all twenty-eight crowned, from gum surgery to veneers! The actual molar that needed a crown was missed by fifteen of the fifty dentists. When asked about the journalists' findings, the American Dental Association was not surprised by the inconsistencies, as they claim, "Dentistry is an art based on scientific knowledge."[2]

This journalistic research illustrates that there is money to be minted from our mouths, which may be fiscally influencing some dentists. Although dentistry conjures images of the exactness of an X-ray, sterile environments, white lab coats, and advanced scientific equipment, it is not an exclusively objective vocation.

Clearly, there are fifty shades of gray affecting our pearly whites. Fifty interpretations from one X-ray! While we let that information sink in, it is easy to feel exasperated and to roll our eyes at such inconsistency; or we can see this as a crack for the light to shine in.

We can master the map of our mouths; with leading-edge information from compassionate, pioneering dentists, we can now understand how our bodies are designed with a dentinal fluid that acts like an invisible toothbrush, repelling cavities and synthesizing new dentin from odontoblasts. We can see that our mouths can be incubators of infection and that we need to create a microbe-topia for the multitudes of microbes in our mouths.

This is the triple threat to our mouths: the harmful procedures, the lack of understanding about the tooth-nurturing dentinal fluid, and the periodontal scorched-earth policy on bacteria. This trifecta is the perfect periodontal storm that fosters endodontic entropy, dental decay, and a system that settles for Band-Aid solutions of bleaching, gum grafts, veneers, and fillings.

Now let's look at some common dental procedures and weigh the pros and cons.

SILVER FILLINGS

Silver-colored dental amalgams have been used to fill cavities for more than 150 years. They are made from a combination of silver, copper, tin, and mercury. These fillings are more economical and durable than other filling materials. The American Dental Association recommends silver fillings for children who squirm in the dentist's chair because they are easier to place than composite fillings.

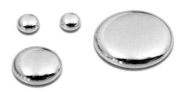

Silver Fillings: Cons

- Dentists must drill away healthy bone to prepare the tooth for silver fillings.

- These eighteenth-century dental solutions are 50 percent mercury, one of the most toxic substances on the planet; yet even though this toxicity is scientific fact, mercury is implanted in multitudes of mouths in the form of fillings. Mercury is also a cumulative toxin that passes through the blood–brain and placental barriers. It tenaciously binds to tissue, altering DNA, nerves, cell membranes, and mitochondrial function. Mercury toxicity is linked to dementia, multiple sclerosis, Parkinson's, and other degenerative disorders.[3] Mercury is also linked to periodontal disease, receding gums, and skin hyperpigmentation.[4] The U.S. Environmental Protection Agency (EPA) claims that the highest body-burden of chronic mercury toxicity comes from silver fillings. In addition, when mercury fillings are removed, even though there is not a metallurgic change to the mercury, the EPA considers it toxic waste, and fillings must be handled with a strict no-touch protocol to protect dentists and the environment from mercury poisoning.[5] The FDA states, "A person with four fillings has enough mercury to make a 20-acre lake unfit for fishing."[6] Yet, somehow, it is still okay for our mouths and tongues to touch it daily, and it is still not universally banned in dentistry.

- Both old and new mercury fillings release vapors twenty-four hours a day, with a 500 percent increase when chewing, teeth grinding, and drinking hot fluids. According to the *Journal of Dental Research,* gum chewing increases mercury-vapor release considerably![7]

OTHER FILLING OPTIONS

- Costly porcelain fillings are not 100 percent pure porcelain; they contain carcinogenic nickel and aluminum too. Most white composite fillings contain bisphenol A (BPA), formaldehyde, and aluminum. The best current filling choices are zirconium-oxide fillings, ceramic resins, and nondrilling techniques.

- Because all filling materials are foreign to the immune system, it is a best practice for dentists to do a biocompatibility blood-serum test. Ideally, preventing cavities is optimal! (We'll go into that soon.)

WISDOM TEETH

This third set of molars generally develops in the late teens and early twenties. These teeth are considered best to be removed as prophylactic prevention to avoid impacted teeth, and partially erupted wisdom teeth may be hard to clean or may affect neighboring teeth.

Wisdom-Teeth Removal: Cons

- A report published in the *American Journal of Public Health* deemed that 6.7 million out of 10 million preventive wisdom-tooth extractions are unnecessary.[8]

- The British National Health Service has stated that the practice of prophylactic removal of pathology-free impacted wisdom teeth should be discontinued. There is insufficient evidence that impacted wisdom teeth cause problems, and the expense and risks of the surgery are not justified.[9]

- We may need the wisdom of these teeth later in life for chewing surfaces; additionally, extraction alters the structure of the neck, jaw, and mouth.

- But that's not all. Multiple pathological bacteria are often found in the jaw on wisdom-tooth extraction sites. This is because it is standard protocol to leave the periodontal ligament in after extraction. Simply put, this causes a sluggish area in the bone marrow where virulent bacteria gather and eat away at the jawbone.[10]

- These jaw cavitations are a hidden consequence of wisdom-teeth extractions, as most of the time there are no visible symptoms. When a jaw cavitation shows up on an X-ray, the bone has already eroded by 50 percent.[11] These areas in the jaw are medically referred to as osteonecrotic lesions. Dr. Hal Huggins's research institute revealed that these jaw-cavitation sites are sanctuaries for serious pathogens that can lead to an array of autoimmune diseases.

Biological dentists can check for cavitations by making a small incision in the gum of the extraction site and examining for mushy pockets in the jawbone. If there is decay, a simple procedure can clear it up: the site is opened, the decay is scraped off the bone, bacteria are thoroughly removed, blood flow to the area is reestablished, and the site is treated with ozone. If you do need a tooth extracted, including a wisdom tooth, be sure to work with a dentist who will also be sure to remove the periodontal ligament as part of the protocol.

Through the dedicated research of dentists Weston Price and Ralph R. Steinman, we now know that proper nutrition is the key to keeping wisdom teeth. When enough nutrients are supplied to the jawbone during pregnancy and childhood, all thirty-two teeth have enough space in the mouth without crowding.

ROOT CANALS

A root canal is a procedure for infected teeth that kills the tooth by removing its internal structure, including the nerves, pulp tissue, and blood vessels. The hollowed-out tooth is rinsed, filled with latex and cement, and then topped with a crown. The purpose of a root canal is to hermetically seal the tooth and save the chewing surface.

Root Canal: Cons

Theoretically, a root canal seems like a good idea, but, clinically, it is a bacterial horror story. A dead tooth remains in the mouth as an incubator of infection, a bacterial breeding ground, and a necrotic nest for pathogens to grow and spread. This oxygen-starved stagnant tooth becomes a haven for harmful microbes. The whole goal of a root canal is to have a noninfected, sterile tooth; but the exact opposite is created. Each tooth contains three miles of microscopic dentin tubules that are impossible to sterilize! With the blood vessels removed, neither antibiotics nor white blood cells can reach the location to fight infection. Every time a root-canaled tooth is used to chew, bacterial toxins are squirted into the bloodstream. These toxins that flow from the anaerobic infection silently spread to the gums, ligaments, and jawbone. Because the nerve tissue is removed in the procedure, there will be no pain indicating infection. In an interesting correlation, physician Josef Issels in forty years of treating cancer found that 98 percent of his patients had root canals.[12] He insists that his patients remove root-canaled teeth before starting treatment.

Dr. Stuart Nunnally, a highly respected and pioneering biological dentist, conducted independent tests on root-canaled teeth.[13] To qualify, the teeth had to be symptom-free and show zero signs of pathology on an X-ray. One hundred percent of these root-canaled teeth, upon surface inspection and in X-rays, were textbook-perfect root canals yet lab tests revealed that the teeth harbored severe toxic pathogens. While this type of information has not permeated into every dental practice, and with the knowledge comes some ethical decisions for dentists about how to approach diseased teeth, thankfully there is vibrant discussion in endodontics journals about the impossibility of sterility in root-canal-treated teeth.

If you have a root canal and this information is unnerving, it is important to know that although root canals become focal infections that feed anaerobic bacteria 100 percent of the time, not all root canals are causing systemic health issues, because of an individual's epigenetics and because each person handles toxicity differently. If you are experiencing a decline in health (especially in the months preceding the procedure), or if you have an autoimmune issue, you may want to explore having root-canaled teeth extracted and the periodontal ligament removed. This is an easier decision if it is a back molar, as the space can be left as is, yet a difficult decision with a front tooth, as you may then need to explore a bridge or a zirconium post implant tooth.

It takes a special quality of mind to be schooled in certain methods yet hold the capacity to question these methods and to forge ahead to find new terrains of thought and scientific solutions. Fortunately, some dentists do, and there are new frontiers in dentistry that can help us all rectify the damage of previous decades of dental procedures. Some biological dentists are pioneering the way with the use of platelet-rich plasma (PRP) therapy that stimulates growth factors, and ozone injections and gels to clean infections and infuse surgical sites with a "breath of fresh air." These dentists are also leading the way with more biocompatible material choices.[14] Dentists that are leading the field with these innovations will be among the first to integrate successful stem-cell therapy for tooth regeneration, which will be a reality in the very near future.

FLUORIDE'S EFFECT ON BONES AND SKIN

If you suffer from cavities, then fluoride toothpaste and treatments *might* be right for you. Possible side effects may include bleeding gums, skeletal fluorosis,[15] sclerosis, dementia diagnosis,[16] pitted and crumbled teeth,[17] impaired myelin sheath, acne,[18] arthritis, gingivitis, bone-crippling disease, joint pain in your knees,[19] thyroid disease,[20] hip fractures, hyperactivity, damaged sperm motility,[21] increased infertility,[22] disrupted collagen synthesis,[23] gastritis, suppressed immune system, impaired glucose metabolism, skin rashes, damaged bone formation,[24] cell mutation, nausea, tooth discoloration, frequent urination, poisoning, DNA alteration, and reduced IQ.[25]

Go ahead and ask your dentist if fluoride is right for you.

Although we have been told and sold on fluoride in tap water and in dental products to strengthen bones, it actually makes bones brittle and stiffens skin by impeding collagen production. "Contrary to marketing madness, tooth decay is not caused by fluoride deficiency! The United States' EPA has fluoride on its 'substantial evidence of neurotoxicity' list. Fluoride appears to interfere with critical, bodily chemistry, damaging gums, disrupting collagen production, and reducing enzyme activity. Fluoride accumulates in the body, especially in the pineal gland, lowers IQ, forms deposits in the brain related to Alzheimer's, promotes early-onset puberty, and the list goes on and on."[26]

With all of these documented side effects, maybe fluoride isn't the answer. To truly grasp how cavities form, we need to understand how teeth are nourished and cleansed from the inside by a dentinal-lymph fluid.

Mottled, fragile, disintegrating, tainted teeth are the dental devastation from not understanding that our teeth are alive and intimately connected to the body, bloodstream, and lymph. It is through this systemic connection that some medications and chemicals, such as antibiotics and fluoride, contribute to brittle, discolored, and even crumbling teeth, by suppressing the dentinal-lymph system. This affects bone mineralization, nerve health, microbial diversity, saliva pH, and endocrine function.

THE INVISIBLE TOOTHBRUSH

Teeth are fed from their roots by the dentinal-lymph system, like tree roots drawing up nutrients via the sap. The dentinal-lymph flow is a toroidal system; lymph-liquid spins inward and upward into the tooth's core, the pulp chamber. It flows through the tooth and out onto the enamel. Like microscopic sweat, these tiny droplets coalesce on the surface of the enamel, forming a fluid layer that prevents biofilm formation and commingles with saliva to lubricate and communicate with the mouth's microbiome.

Operating much like the lymph system, there is a microscopic flow of fluid in the teeth that originates near the intestinal area and flows upward and outward through the teeth, flushing out toxins, providing nutrients for the teeth's mineral matrix, and repelling microbial biofilm on the tooth surfaces, preventing tooth decay and gum disease. When this dentinal-lymph secretion is properly metabolized and functional, it acts like an invisible toothbrush, preventing systemic decay, inhibiting the penetration of pathogens, and neutralizing acids on the

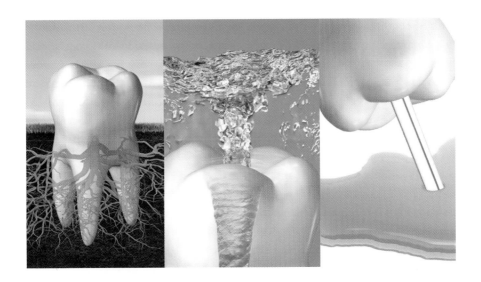

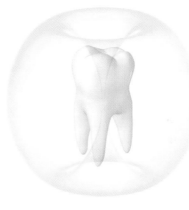

Dentinal Lymph System

tooth's surface. However, this dentinal-lymph flow can stagnate and even fully reverse. Diet and hormones are the principal activators of this self-cleansing system. Certain chemicals and medication, as well as a diet of processed food, sugar, and carbohydrates that spikes insulin levels and disharmonizes hormones, cause the dentinal-lymph system to reverse. When this happens, the capillaries in the tooth suck in bacteria, like a straw, and other microbes from the mouth into the tooth, causing infection and biofilm formation within the pulp chamber and dentin tubules. This self-contaminating system causes a "leaky tooth," and it is the genesis of cavity creation.

A cavity is an infection in the tooth. Like all wounds, it has the ability to heal. Teeth are alive! The current condition of your teeth and mouth can *evolve*. Dr. Ralph R. Steinman, the same dentist who scientifically proved the existence of the dentinal-lymph system,[27] showed that including dietary magnesium and phosphorus reduced the decay rate by 86 percent.[28] Dr. Melvin Page confirmed this by finding that when phosphorus blood levels drop below 3.5, cavities begin to form.[29] Additionally, the former president of the ADA, Dr. Weston Price, concluded that fat-soluble vitamins K2 and D3 reversed and inhibited decay. Fillings are Band-Aid solutions and are susceptible to recurrent decay. Yet, when the underlying causes of cavities are addressed and the dentinal-lymph flow is restored, teeth will remineralize and be more resilient to cavities in the future.

THE MOUTH'S MICROBIAL MENAGERIE

There are more bacteria in a kiss than there are people on the planet. Our mouths are a microbial menagerie. As holobiont human hosts to these microbes, we have forged an elaborate evolutionary and ancient alliance. A good host provides a stable, loving home and nourishing food for their flora friends. In

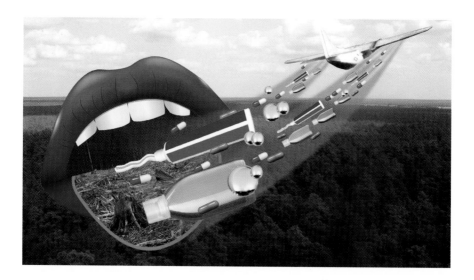

return, these microbes micromanage our bodies by digesting food and secreting beneficial biochemicals. They are also sentient sentinels that strengthen our immunity while preventing pathogenic periodontal party-crashers from proliferating and from excreting endotoxins and colonizing the community.

The key to oral health is maintaining an ecologically balanced and diverse microbiome. Contrary to this, we have been caught in the dross of carpet-bombing the biome—practicing a scorched-earth policy of periodontal care. Chemicals in teeth bleaching, fillings, rinses, and fluoride; the sudsy surfactants of toothpastes; the antibiotic atomic bombs on bacteria; masticating meals of glyphosates and pesticides; root canals festering focal infections; the metallic mass of mercury, titanium, and nickel—these have all scorched the hive intelligence of our oral habitat. This defoliation of our oral flora-nation has made extinct and mutated microbes, resulting in complex ecological shifts of resident microbiota, giving rise to gingivitis, halitosis, cavities, oral thrush, cankers, and bleeding and receding gums. Our mouth, once a moist microhabitat of homeostasis, becomes an oxygen-starved oasis of anaerobic activity eating away at our immunity and sending systemic disease throughout the body.

Just as toxic food and chemical irritants induce leaky guts by microscopically perforating the intestines, the scrubbing and rubbing of our gums with mutating medicants and caustic chemicals cause leaky gums. Bacteria from our mouth does not normally enter our bloodstream, but dental procedures and products can perforate the epithelium, the skin in our mouths, which is only one cell thick, providing a port of entry into the bloodstream. When the bacteria and plaque that cause tooth decay and gum disease enter our circulatory system, they cause a cascade of inflammation, releasing cytokines and C-reactive proteins.

A healthy mouth is a healthy gut and vice versa. We have gone from a seemingly Golden Age of Antibiotics to a very real Anarchy of Antibiotic Resistance. On average, a baby receives three courses of antibiotics in the first two years of life. By age ten, another eight courses. By age twenty, seventeen courses, and by age forty, thirty courses in total![30]

Antibiotic exposure is everywhere, in drinking water and in nonorganic supermarket food. All antibiotics have their allowable limits in the food and water supply. Antibiotics are indiscriminate assassins. Any surviving resistant bacteria mutate fast and bask in the empty niches the antibiotics made. Soon pathogenic biofilms bloom, and we no longer have protection from infection. It is important to save antibiotic use for life-threatening crises rather than ingesting them in daily doses that erode our immunity.

Our bodies will always contain a population of pathogens; the beautiful balance is to have the good bacteria far outnumber the bad. For example, even healthy mouths are homes to the cavity-causing *Streptococcus mutans*. Some research is positing that what might make *S. mutans* virulent is that it's missing its ancestral bacterial buddies. This particular pathogen only causes a problem when it forms a biofilm and adheres to the tooth's surface. Normally, pathogens exist in a free-floating planktonic state in our body's ecosystem. But when they grow in numbers, they are able to gain traction by communicating through quorum sensing, enabling them to colonize into a biofilm. Quorum sensing is the way in which pathogens communicate to coordinate group behavior and regulate gene expression. A biofilm is a densely packed colony of microbes that adhere to surfaces and surround themselves with sticky secretions. A mucopolysaccharide plaque layer is produced around the biofilm colony, which forms a barrier that is not permeable to antibiotics, yet antibiotics are often prescribed for oral disease.

Dental plaque is a biofilm that can either entrap existing oral pathogens from flourishing or provide a refuge for pathogens to hide from alkalinizing salivary flow. Under healthy conditions, an oral-ecological balance of bacteria keeps biofilms healthy and stable. But plaque is an ideal nest for germs. This blocks the teeth from respiration and prevents the saliva and dentinal-lymph fluid from doing its job of cleansing the teeth with a protective coating.

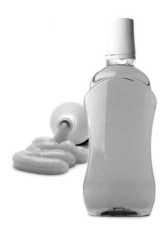

STOP

Dentinal Lymph Suppressors
Spiked Blood Sugar & Insulin Resistance
Mouth Breathing
Leaky Guts
Phytic Acid Consumption
Processed Food
Mercury Fillings
Microbe Mutators
Using Synthetic Dental Care Products

To restore balance to the mouth's microbiome, we need strategies to inhibit the quorum sensing that forms biofilms. We need to clear colonized citadels of their powerful cohesion on our mouth's surfaces and crevices. There is extensive research on strategies that inhibit quorum sensing. In various studies, essential oils such as cinnamon, peppermint, tea tree, frankincense, and clove showed promising results in reducing quorum-sensing activity. In one study, clove oil reduced quorum sensing by up to 70 percent![31] These essential oils indicate anti-infective activity that can coexist with our flora while cleaning up periodontal pathogens. Now we have scientific studies confirming the ancient wisdom of using botanical-biotics to maintain oral ecology.

ELEVATE ORAL ECOLOGY: STOP, SEAL, AND SEED

Stop

Start by ceasing many of the daily and dietary habits that are compromising to healthy oral ecology. Whatever improvements you make to your mouth will benefit your body's well-being as well.

Stop Dentinal-Lymph Suppressors of processed food, sugar, and chemicals that inhibit endocrine function.

Stop Spikes in Blood Sugar that create insulin resistance. Ideally, maintain blood sugar around 80.

Stop Mouth Breathing by assessing medications, food allergies and sensitivities, sinuses, and cranial balance. Chronic mouth breathing in children deeply affects the way in which the shape of their face grows. Myofunctional orofacial therapy is a revolutionary way to reeducate the habitual patterns of the oral and facial muscles and can help with teeth grinding, sleep apnea, headaches, and other health issues.[32] See "Breathing" in Chapter Seventeen.

Heal and Seal Leaky Guts by eliminating gluten, corn, and glyphosate irritants. See "Leaky Gut Syndrome" in Chapter Seventeen.

Stop Phytic Acid Consumption. Phytic acid is an antinutrient that plunders phosphorus stores in the body. Soak and ferment gluten-free grains, legumes, and nuts to reduce this antinutrient.

Remove Mercury Fillings. These silver fillings irritate gums and guts, cause gum recession, feed virulent pathogens, and more. Be sure to see a qualified biological dentist who follows the removal procedures of the Hal Huggins institute for your safety and the dentist's.

Stop the Microbe Mutators of excessive antibiotics, glyphosates, surfactants, and fluoride toothpastes.

Stop Using Synthetic Dental-Care Products from the "May Be Harmful if Swallowed" category.[33] Our gums and teeth are living tissue, and we want to approach cleaning them a little differently than we would scrub a countertop. If toothpaste is the magic cleaner for our teeth, then why are cavities at an all-time high, and why does toothpaste come with a big warning label: "May Be Harmful if Swallowed"?

Most toothpastes and rinses, including many of the brands sold in health food stores, use chemical and synthetic ingredients that are more appropriate for industrial purposes than for cleaning the delicate tissue of the body or cultivating oral health. Brushing with these chemicals may be harmful to our health. Absorbing through the mouth's mucous membrane into the bloodstream, these synthetic substances may lead to decomposing collagen, hinder hormones, damage the delicate epithelium, activate acne, disturb microflora in the digestive tract, and, in the end, encourage poor health.

Some toothpastes, rinses, and mouthwashes are better than others.[34] To help you make a wise decision about what you brush into your mouth (and apply to your body), there are oral-care formulas in Chapter Sixteen, "Renegade Beauty Recipes."

Commercial toothpaste gives an illusion of a fresh and clean mouth, yet it is the art of oral care, diet, and diligent brushing that actually removes the plaque. It is best to be a purist about oral health and diligently care with a toothbrush and a dab of salt or baking soda and a pure botanical serum. These simple, time-tested ingredients help prevent dental caries due to their buffering capacity, bacteriostatic nature, and alkalinity promoters that inhibit plaque formation and balance the mouth's microbiome. They also increase calcium uptake to the enamel, neutralize the pH in the mouth, and reduce the effect of harmful metabolic acids . . . and they are quite safe to swallow!

Hopefully, no one is gulping gobs of toothpaste! However, the rate of absorption is very high inside the mouth, where the moist tissue of the skin wall, the epithelium, is only one cell thick. This is very important if one has bleeding gums (and some of the surfactants in commercial toothpaste can cause gums to bleed, break down the phospholipids of our tongue and gums, and aggravate cankers) where anything in the mouth will have direct access to the bloodstream. We would not want to put anything in, on, or around the body that could not be swallowed. We can also maintain our molars with the molecular matter of phytonutrients; brushing with botanicals such as neem, cardamom, clove, peppermint, and mastic provides antibacterial and antifungal support while benefiting digestion and the rest of the body.

Seal and Heal

Bleeding, inflamed, and receding gums are signifiers of bacterial imbalance and that bacteria may be entering the bloodstream. Restore integrity to the oral epithelium by healing and sealing leaky gums and enabling the saliva's ability to protect enamel.

Gum Sealers are soothing serums with vulnerary botanical-biotics— seabuckthorn, rose otto, frankincense, and myrrh—diluted in a lipid such as coconut or MCT oil, as well as using ozonated oral gels. These botanical-biotics are rich in phytonutrients known for their ability to heal tissue, restore skin cells, foster phospholipids, and nurture the epithelium. When these soothing serums are applied, people often find a reduction in gum bleeding overnight.

Oral Alkalinizers of baking soda, sea salt, and magnesium are soothing in mouth rinses and effective as toothpastes due to their alkalinizing-exfoliating action that removes plaque. Their nutrients also switch on saliva's smoothing and soothing abilities. Saliva contains chemicals and enzymes that exist solely to take care of the teeth. Healthy teeth exist in a sea of saliva, a sea of saline

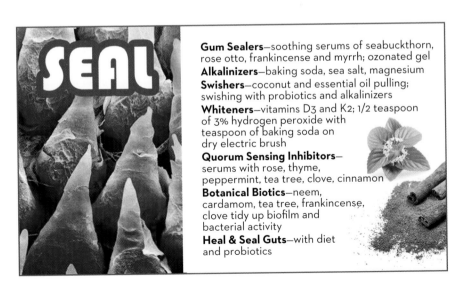

Gum Sealers—soothing serums of seabuckthorn, rose otto, frankincense and myrrh; ozonated gel
Alkalinizers—baking soda, sea salt, magnesium
Swishers—coconut and essential oil pulling; swishing with probiotics and alkalinizers
Whiteners—vitamins D3 and K2; 1/2 teaspoon of 3% hydrogen peroxide with teaspoon of baking soda on dry electric brush
Quorum Sensing Inhibitors— serums with rose, thyme, peppermint, tea tree, clove, cinnamon
Botanical Biotics—neem, cardamom, tea tree, frankincense, clove tidy up biofilm and bacterial activity
Heal & Seal Guts—with diet and probiotics

alkalinity. If saliva is too acidic, it dissolves the enamel on your teeth and creates an environment that supports bacteria. With decay, saliva jumps into action to coat the tooth with its beautiful healing fluid. The quality and quantity of saliva also hinge on hydration, so drink up!

Mouth Swishers of coconut or MCT oil imbued with essential oils work well for pulling and then spitting out. Or swish the oral environment with probiotics; simply pop a capsule in water with an **Oral Alkalinizer** and swish a freshly cleaned mouth and then swallow. See Chapter Seventeen for more on oral oil pulling.

Whiteness comes from within! Tooth enamel is actually transparent, and gray, glassy teeth denote a deficiency in the body of vitamins D3 and K2. These fat-soluble vitamins nourish the dentin, creating shiny, white teeth. Polish off plaque that can get stained by food pigments with one-half teaspoon of 3 percent food-grade hydrogen peroxide mixed with a teaspoon of baking soda on a dry electric toothbrush.

Quorum-Sensing Inhibitors are your beneficial bacteria's best friends. Erudite essential oils of rose otto, thyme, peppermint, cardamom, frankincense, tea tree, clove, and cinnamon can be used in diluted forms to brush teeth, as a rinse with oil or water, and in tooth serums to massage into the gums. Get really clean in between each tooth by sliding these serums across dental floss and upgrade your flossing routine.

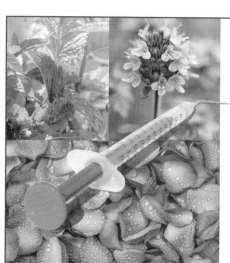

Ingredients for Optimal Oral Care

Brushing

Baking soda, sea salt. clay, charcoal. botanical-biotics
Neat trick: apply baking soda generously to teeth and then add a teaspoon of apple cider vinegar for a frothy, alkaline cleanser that lifts plaque off teeth and gumlines.

Flossing

Apply diluted botanical-biotics across floss to clean crevices

Rinsing

Water with salt water, baking soda, magnesium, essential oils

Swishing and Pulling

Add any of these alkalinizers to water: sea salt, magnesium salt, baking soda. Add any of these to MTC or coconut oil: probiotics, clay, charcoal, botanical-biotics

Massaging Gums

Botanical-biotic serums with coconut or MCT oils or ozonated gel

Implanting

Blunt syringe or water-pick with white iodine, probiotics, botanical-biotics, or 3% hydrogen peroxide

Botanical-Biotic Boosters

Tea tree, oregano, peppermint, frankincense, rose otto, cinnamon, clove, myrrh, cardamom, thyme, neem and/or mastic

Botanical-Biotics The aromatic compounds of essential oils act as bacteriostatic microbiome regenerators, and biofilm disrupters. Neem, cardamom, tea tree, frankincense, rose otto, myrrh, and clove are just a few of the intelligent essences that tidy up bacterial activity rather than indiscriminately bombing all bacteria. They effectively reduce biofilm formation, specifically biofilms formed by S. mutans. Cinnamon has shown the ability to penetrate pathogenic biofilms.[35]

Healing and Sealing the Guts with diet, herbs, and probiotics are also essential to optimal oral care. There is a relationship between the mouth and the metabolism of the rest of the body. Our teeth are connected to every organ and gland via the bloodstream. Any infection that the mouth harbors, any metals, and any toxins in our mouths affect our overall health.

Feed with Seeds

With so many agents in our society making our microbes extinct, from antibiotics to pesticide-laden processed foods, we need to build our oral bacterial bank account and fund it with investments of diverse flora.

PREBIOTICS AND PROBIOTICS

Maintain an oral microbiome of bustling bacteria with prebiotics and probiotics, as they are microbe multipliers. Prebiotics feed and enhance the growth of probiotics. Chicory root, available as an easy-to-use powder, is a prebiotic rich in oligosaccharides. Probiotics are food supplements with living microbes that are beneficial when used in adequate numbers. Lactobacilli (specifically L. fermentum, L. plantarum, L. casei, L. reuteri, and L. rhamnosus) and Bifidobacterium all showed the ability to adhere to saliva, inhibit the proliferation of periodontal pathogens, and reduce cavity-causing bacteria and plaque.[36]

A probiotic-dairy combination was found to reduce the cavity- and periodontal-disease-causing bacteria in the mouth. Providing Lactobacillus reuteri to children from the last trimester through the first birthday has been found to reduce cavities at nine years old. It can also help heal damaged gums and gingivitis.[37]

Researchers are looking for modes of delivery that increase retention and exposure times of probiotics to the mouth using lozenges. Yet we don't have to wait. Daily use in the diet along with swishing, seeding, and applying increase probiotic presence in saliva, dentinal lymph, and the entire GI tract. Successful experiments at some dental practices have applied a mixture of probiotics after scaling and root planing called Guided Pocket Recolonization.[38] This can be safely and simply carried out at home with a blunt-tipped syringe, filled with a mix of probiotics and a carrier oil, like MCT.

Seeding a Dental Diet: Switch on saliva and dentinal-lymph flow with wholesome sustenance, fermented foods, and balanced blood sugar. Healthy fats are where it's at, as a deficiency in the vital fat-soluble vitamins K2 and D3 can alter gut bacteria. K2 is a carboxylating osteocalcin, meaning it ushers key minerals like calcium and magnesium into the bones from the blood, preventing calcification of the soft tissues and inhibiting mouth plaque from turning into tartar. Certain enzymes, serratia proteolytic enzymes for example, can clean up plaque like Pac-Man and break down biofilm barriers.

Further boost the health of the oral environment with supportive vitamins and minerals of CoQ10, N-acetylcysteine (NAC), magnesium, phosphorus, amino acids, and vitamin C. Find superfoods, herbs, and supplements that have these nutrients, and flourish with food fares of smoothies, soups, and brews.

Our bodies are brilliantly designed. When we repopulate our mouth's microbiome and activate our invisible toothbrush by eliminating what hinders the innate functioning of our bodies, the external maintenance of brushing and flossing is so easy, because our teeth are alive and will respond to our efforts! The current condition of our mouth can *evolve*, as enamel can be restored, dentine can be reactivated, saliva can remineralize, and gums can be rejuvenated.

A mouthful of bustling bacteria just might keep the dentist away.

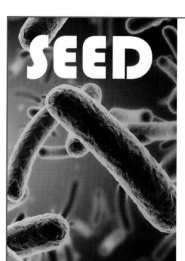

Prebiotics—chicory root
Probiotics—Lactobacilli of *L. Fermentum*, *L. Plantarum*, *L. Casei*, *L. Reuteri*, *L. Rhamnosus*, and Bifidobacterium showed the ability to adhere in saliva, inhibited the proliferation of periodontopathogens, reduced cavity-causing bacteria and plaque
Guided Pocket Recolonization—Use a blunt Vitapik syringe and pre/probiotic solution
Switch On Saliva & Dentinal Lymph—nourishing food and balanced blood sugar and hormones
Fermented Foods
Fat Soluble Vitamins K2 & D3—K2 is a carboxylating osteocalcin. It ushers key minerals into the bones from the blood, preventing plaque and calcification of the soft tissues
Enzymes—Serratia proteolytic enzymes can clean up plaque and breakdown biofilm barriers
Vitamins & Minerals—CoQ10, NAC, magnesium, phosphorus, amino acids, and vitamin C

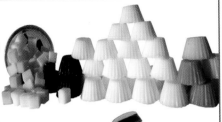

Probiotic Tooth-Butter Cups
for
Soothing and Swishing

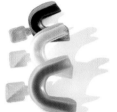

60 ml Coconut Oil
6 capsules of Probiotics
2 teaspoons Prebiotic Chicory Root
2 teaspoons Baking Soda
15 drops: Peppermint, Frankincense, Rose,
Cinnamon, Sea buckthorn and/or Clove
Optional:
2 teaspoons of Clay or Activated Charcoal

A BIT ON BONES AND OSTEOPOROSIS

Osteoporosis is a bone disorder that mostly affects elderly women. It involves a significant loss of bone density, most especially of the hips and spine, to the degree that they are vulnerable to breaks called "fragility fractures." A broken bone can be a serious challenge for an elderly person. The two-year mortality rate for women with a hip fracture is twice as high as for women of similar age without a broken bone.[39]

> *The longer I live the more beautiful life becomes.*
>
> Frank Lloyd Wright[40]

Osteopenia: *The Deficiency of Disease*

With proper nutrition and weight-bearing exercise, a woman continues to build bone density until she is twenty-five years old (a little older for men). After that, her job is to maintain bone density with the same good nutrition and weight-bearing exercise. Starting around menopause, as estrogen levels shift, bones lose some density, and this slight thinning is called osteopenia.

The label "osteopenia" was created by physicians and medical researchers at a meeting in 1992 hosted by the World Health Organization. These experts were charged with defining an international standard for osteoporosis. The experts had to decide at what point bone-density loss crossed from normal/

healthy to abnormal. After days of debate, they finally drew the line and set the standard for the defining factors for osteoporosis. For research purposes, they called the normal bone-density markers just on the other side of the osteoporosis line "osteopenia." The naming of osteopenia was not intended as a disease diagnosis or a determination of risk factors. These experts were simply giving a name to a set of reference points for lower bone density. Nortin Hadler, a doctor of rheumatology at the University of North Carolina, said, "Osteopenia is normal—it's like gray hair."[41]

However, now, after a pharmaceutical company started promoting peripheral-bone-density scans to boost their drug sales,[42] millions of women are being frightened with a diagnosis of osteopenia, and many are prescribed bone-mineralization drugs developed for osteoporosis. Several types of pharmaceuticals are used to stop the bone-destructive process of osteoporosis.

Bisphosphonates are currently one of the most commonly prescribed drugs, and they work by poisoning (promoting the death of) osteoclasts, which are bone cells that are responsible for clearing out cells that are no longer vital bone cells. Osteoclasts work together with osteoblasts, which are bone cells that make new bone cells. "Since the osteoclasts are killed off, old and sick bone cells are able to survive. This is what causes the bones to look denser on X-rays. In essence, the bisphosphonates create a skeleton of old, dying, decayed or sick cells. Although this type of bone looks denser on X-rays, it is weaker and potentially hazardous to your health."[43]

These risky drugs are promoted to prevent hip fractures, yet they are causing an unusual type of upper-thighbone fracture after normal actions like getting out of a chair. The more serious risks are ulcers in the esophagus, chest pain, problems swallowing, joint pain, dizziness, headaches, stomach pain, diarrhea, constipation, and nausea. A small study on this class of drugs in 2011 found that if taken for more than five years, the drug may cause fractures instead of preventing them. People who had taken the drug for longer than five years had a three times higher risk of a bone break.[44] They can also cause jawbone necrosis,[45] crumbling teeth, eye inflammation that can lead to blindness,[46] a bleeding esophagus, and an increased risk of atrial fibrillation.[47]

Dr. Zoltan Rona practices integrative medicine in Canada. He puts bisphosphonates in the same class of chemicals as scrubs used to clean soap scum from the bathtub. "The chemicals remove soap scum by basically dissolving dead skin cells that collect on the tub after taking a bath. If a substance is strong enough to dissolve skin cells, just imagine what it can do to your stomach when you swallow it. This is the reason the pharmacist will tell you not to lie down after taking any bisphosphonate. If you do, it's possible the drug will erode the lining of your esophagus, stomach or duodenum.[48]

There are a few other pharmaceuticals prescribed for osteoporosis. Here are a few along with their side effects:

- Selective estrogen receptor modulators (SERMs) are used in post-menopausal women. As estrogen levels drop, the capacity to build and keep strong bones also drops. These drugs bind with estrogen receptors in the bone and prevent bone loss. Side effects include hot flashes, dizziness, headache, joint pain, possible strokes, and gastrointestinal issues.

- Hormone replacement therapy works similarly to SERMs. It replaces deficient estrogen to stop bone loss and promote bone density. Side effects include bloating, breast sensitivity, moodiness, gastrointestinal issues, cramps, vaginal bleeding, and headaches. It may also increase the risk of blood clots and stroke.

- Biologics use human antibodies that prevent the development of osteoclasts, which are bone cells that break down bone. These drugs are riddled with risk: jawbone necrosis, swollen gums, loose teeth, infections, blood clotting, anemia, bladder infections, and pain.

- Synthetic parathyroid hormones mimic a hormone called parathyroid that exists naturally in the body. These natural hormones regulate the calcium level in all parts of our bodies, including the bones. The synthetic hormones stimulate bone-building cells called osteoblasts to rebuild and remineralize bone. Side effects include joint pain, muscle spasms, sore throat, head pain, gastrointestinal issues, fainting, confusion, and tiredness.

If you are concerned about osteoporosis and bone health, insist on a bone densitometer scan that examines the density of hip and spine bones in lieu of peripheral scans that look only at finger or arm bone density, which is not an accurate reflection of hip and spine health. Also, you can talk to your integrative medical practitioner about FRAX,[49] an online tool that measures your fracture risk based on a variety of clinical risk factors, including bone density.

There are also natural methods of bone-building that work with natural body processes that have no risks and no nasty side effects.

EAT YOUR WAY TO STRONG BONES
AND A WHITE SMILE

Nature has provided for us beautiful, colorful foods that enhance our health and bring about healthy bones. By following a few dietary tips, we provide our body with all the tools it needs for optimal health.

The first step is to significantly reduce, or better yet eliminate, consumption of nutrient-absent processed food. You want every bite to be brimming with beauty food.

A bone-healthy diet includes foods that are mineral rich and that are high in the fat-soluble vitamins E, D3, A, and K2. The type of vitamin A we get from eating vegetables, like carrots, is water-soluble beta carotene. Retinol-A, found in pasture-raised meat and dairy, has different biological activity than beta carotene. Both forms are important for health; beta carotene is a powerful antioxidant, and retinol-A is crucial for healthy eyes, skin, and bones. Fat-soluble vitamin E also promotes bone health by protecting the bone-making process from damage by free radicals.

Distinct from the vitamin K that we get from eating greens like kale and spinach, vitamin K2 is found only in grass-fed meat and pasture-raised animals that create eggs and dairy. Factory-farmed foods will be devoid of K2. You can see the vitamin richness in the dark orange and gold color of pastured butter, egg yolks, and cheeses. Vital for bone growth, K2 gets dietary calcium where it needs to go and removes the excess calcium from tissues. Vitamin K2 is also manufactured by intestinal flora; a couple of servings of fermented foods every week, like natto (fermented soy), sauerkraut, cultured grass-fed ghee, kimchi, and some cheese, like aged Gouda, are great sources.

Our bodies and bones also need vitamin D for efficient calcium usage, and vitamin A for both calcium and protein assimilation. Bone growth and maintenance are severely impaired by a vitamin D deficiency.

The standard Western diet is usually poor in bone-friendly minerals. Also, glyphosate, an herbicide, is used on genetically modified crops, and residue is found on the food products. This residue removes minerals in the gut, including bone-friendly calcium and magnesium.[50] Antacids, excess caffeine, refined carbohydrates, and sugars are also bone-mineral depleters.

There are also amazing vegetarian sources of calcium: leafy greens, spirulina, chia seeds, horsetail herb, algae, and nettles. One should avoid taking calcium carbonate supplements; predominately found in eggshells, seashells, limestone, chalk, marble, and other stones, calcium carbonate is not water-soluble or bioavailable, and when ingested it can cause calcifications, kidney stones, hypocalcemia, and joint problems. Calcium is futile in the body without silica, phosphorus, boron, strontium, and magnesium, and they are bone-healthy minerals that are deficient in a standard Western diet.

Hormones are also vital to bone health. Plummets in estrogen, testosterone, and progesterone around the time of menopause affect bone density. Herbs to boost healthy estrogen (estriol) and help with hot flashes include panax ginseng, black cohosh, and white kwao krua (*Pueraria mirifica*). Iodine, chamomile (acts as an aromatase inhibitor), and passionflower help to release excess estrogen and promote the best estrogen, estriol. Chasteberry stimulates progesterone, and maca helps as a general adaptogenic superfood to boost the body's DHEA. Pine pollen, tongkat ali, tribulus, nettle root, and weight-bearing movement encourage the body's natural testosterone, and supplementation with the bone mineral boron raises serum estrogen and testosterone levels.

Also, a healthy, diverse gut microbiome enhances the nutrition we get from the food that we eat, and probiotics along with prebiotic fiber may increase mineral absorption in the gut.[51]

These bone-boosting tips ensure a lifetime of beautiful teeth and bones.

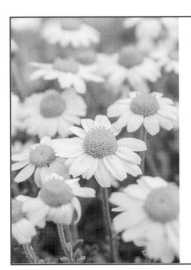

Herbs for Healthy Hormones

Estrogen (Estriol) Encouragers
Chamomile, *Anthemis nobilis*
Ginseng, *Panax ginseng*
Black Cohosh, *Actaea racemosa*
White Kwao Krua, *Pueraria mirifica*

Progesterone Protectors
Chaste Berry, *Vitex angus*
Maca Root, *Lepidium meyenii*

Testosterone Toppers
Nettle Root, *Urtica dioica*
Bindii, *Tribulus terrestris*
Tongkat Ali, *Eurycoma longifolia*
Pine Pollen, *Pinus pollen*

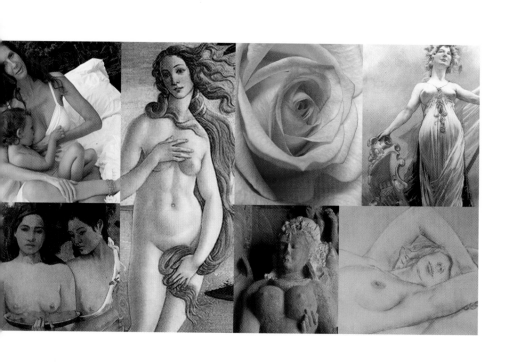

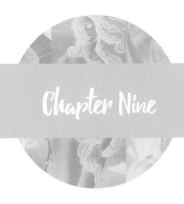

Chapter Nine

THE ALTAR OF OUR APOCRINE GLANDS

Breast Health

Mythologized, scandalized, and politicized; kept under wraps and veiled from view—our breasts. These cherished, tender tissues that embody both sensuality and sustenance have for many become a burden. Our A, B, C, and double D cups are lifted, separated, inflated, examined, and enshrined. Breasts ebb and flow with the moon and the tides of birth. They are strapped down and pushed up—all while being discouraged from their biological calling.

For many who live in fear of breast density, fibroids, and tumors, breasts have become a liability. There is an estrogenic epidemic in our erogenous zone, and our breasts are reacting; every twenty-three seconds a woman is diagnosed with breast cancer worldwide.[1]

As girls, we are taught that respectable young ladies make their bodies "polite" by applying antiperspirant, primping with perfume, and popping contraceptive pills. These preening paraben products create artificial estrogens that accumulate in the soft, lymphatic, fat-filled tissue of our glandular orbs. This altar of our apocrine glands pulls in pollutants like a pair of sponges, recording the history of our diet, drug use, dentistry, drinking water, deodorant, dry cleaning, home decor, and decades of DDT residue. They accrue bromide, benzene, chloride, radiation, and parts per million of pesticide and fluoride.

Estrogen is experiencing hormonal havoc; xenoestrogens (foreign estrogens), metalloestrogens (estrogenic compounds of toxic metals), and mycoestrogens (estrogen-producing fungi) accumulate in our body, affecting gene expression in ways that make breasts vulnerable.

There is good news, though. Cells in our breasts can regenerate. We will look into the etiology of breast imbalances, the promise of protective mitochondrial medicine, and breast regenerative strategies that release excess estrogen, encourage lymph drainage, and strengthen connective tissue.

In the last century, our mothers' bodies have experienced disastrous experimental medicine. In attempts to control the wily hormones of the feminine mystique, our mothers' bodies trialed new drugs, including thalidomide for nausea. To prevent miscarriages, doctors prescribed off-label use of diethylstilbestrol (DES) to five million pregnant women;[2] 46 percent of these women developed breast cancer,[3] and a decade later, their daughters developed vaginal cancer.[4] For years after, DES continued to be supplemented in livestock feed.[5] Our mothers were overprescribed and anesthetized; their generation swallowed the first birth control pills, Valium, and crude hormone replacement therapy. They received increased cesareans, episiotomies, lumpectomies, thyroidectomies, hysterectomies, and mastectomies.

Encouraged to feed their babies with formula, some mothers were injected with estrogen to dry up their breast milk. We now know that breastfeeding helps prevent breast cancer. It contributes to the full development of breasts and builds a child's immune system. In a perfect harmony of giving and receiving, breastfeeding gives beneficial strains of bacteria to our babies and to our breasts, because mothers receive the benefit of good bacteria passing through the breast ductal passages as well.

Our breasts receive misguided Las Vegas adulation while their biological purpose gets shrouded. Breasts, along with their undervalued role of sustaining life, are also canaries in a coal mine. They detect our environmental invasions and store the toxins of our trespasses for decades. Our breasts are barometers for the changing atmosphere of our planet.

Health professionals report increased infertility, miscarriages, record-breaking breast sizes, earlier menopause, and earlier puberty. (Gold, glittery maxi-pads are now marketed to eight-year-olds.[6]) The endocrine disrupters in many moisturizers, pasteurized milk, and sunscreens prompt earlier puberty. There is a delicate time in prepubescent girls during which chemical exposure from pesticides, processed food, and estrogen-mimics greatly influences breast health and gene expression later on.[7] All of this is linked to the residual results of marinating in the industrial flotsam of man-made chemicals.

We now know that most breast cancers are not inherited but are acquired from cell mutations. If a woman carries the *BRCA1* or *BRCA2* gene linked to cancer, she inherits only the risk *not the disease*. Prophylactic mastectomies may be overrated. Influential genetic links are now reported to be as low as 5 percent.[8] Women who carry this genetic risk must also develop a second mutation before tumors will form, and epigenetics reveal that these secondary mutations are from environmental exposures.

Confounded by causes, doctors tout that the best prevention is early screening with mammography—a fifty-year-old technology. Think of all of the technological advances we have seen in the last fifty years! Yet mammography remains the same: archaic and deeply flawed. It scans for cancer by blasting radiation ions 1,000 times greater than a chest X-ray[9] into breasts at 42 pounds of pressure.[10] A decade of annual mammograms in premenopausal, asymptomatic women results in radiation exposure similar to the radiation received by women just outside Hiroshima's atomic epicenter.[11]

Mammography compresses breasts tightly (and often painfully), which can lead to a lethal spread of cancerous cells should they exist. Even the United States Preventive Services Task Force has recommended since 2009 that women avoid getting mammograms until age fifty.[12]

There are quite a few studies that support avoiding mammograms, including these samplings:

- The *Cochrane Database of Systematic Reviews* concluded in a 2009 meta-analysis that breast-cancer screening led to a 30 percent rate of incorrect diagnosis and overtreatment.[13]

- A Norwegian study published in 2010 concluded that the reduction in mortality as a result of mammographic screening was so small as to be nonexistent—2.4 deaths per 100,000 persons.[14]

- A study published in 2014 by the *British Medical Journal*[15] and reported by the *New York Times* further confirms, "One of the largest and most meticulous studies of mammography ever done, involving 90,000 women and lasting a quarter-century, has added powerful new doubts about the value of the screening test for women of any age. It found that the death rates from breast cancer and from all causes were the same in women who got mammograms and those who did not. And the screening had harms: one in five cancers found with mammography and treated was not a threat to the woman's health and did not need treatment such as chemotherapy, surgery or radiation."[16]

Extensive mammography has also led to an 800 percent increased diagnosis of ductal carcinoma in situ (DCIS),[17] a benign zero-stage cancer that currently constitutes 25 percent of all breast-cancer diagnosis.[18] It is called cancer, yet doctors still debate what constitutes this noninvasive ductal-cell abnormality. As random as a coin toss, 15–25 percent of all DCIS is misdiagnosed as a false positive,[19] prompting women to go through the treadmill of needless invasive biopsies and lumpectomies. For some women, this also means radiation, tamoxifen, and mastectomies.

Adding to this, mammography has a 50 percent false-positive rate,[20] with 1 in 12 leading to a biopsy.[21] Biopsies can lead to infection and cancer recurrence along the biopsy needle track at an alarming 50 percent rate.[22] Most biopsy procedures of the past decade also include the insertion of a breast marker clip to mark the biopsy spot for future review. However, these clips are known to migrate[23] and are made of stainless steel, titanium, or plastic. Breast marker clips are promoted as nonreactive, yet blood levels of leached implant chemicals and related infections are documented.[24]

Medical solutions fumble around in the dark. The cell line culture used for breast-cancer research over the past twenty-five years, with results published in more than 650 studies, was recently discovered to not be breast-cancer cells but melanoma cells.[25] The debates continue: Why does breast cancer go systemic? Are mastectomies, lumpectomies, or super-radical mastectomies the solution?

The leading remedy in tackling tumors continues to be the knife. Some doctors are now questioning that course of action. In 1994, a link was discovered between the removal of the primary breast tumor *and an increased growth of metastases*[26] (the spreading of microscopic malignant tumors characteristic of late-stage cancers). A protein called angiostatin was discovered to be secreted by the primary tumor. This protein moves freely throughout the circulatory system suppressing the spread of microscopic tumors. When the primary tumor is surgically removed, and this source of angiostatin dries up, the tiny tumors go into high gear, creating uncontrolled metastases.[27]

Some doctors think that the problem with breast cancer is not in the breast, but in the soil in which it grows. It is claimed that the etiology of breast disease is unknown, and of course every disease is multifaceted. We endlessly debate risk factors, running around for the cure, blinded by pink. Pink ribbon campaigns sponsored with plastics and parabens and *laced* with pesticides are the belle of the charity ball. Yet the answer to cancer is not found in a pink bucket of fried chicken, pink water bottles, or pink lipstick.

As I pondered breast health, especially as my mother was in the final stages of breast cancer, I saw a clear pattern in the recipe that makes breasts a liability. This trifecta of excess estrogen, heavy metals, and mycotoxins creates the perfect storm for breast imbalances. Diseased breast tissue seems to be a repository. When examined:

- 99 percent had parabens.[28]

- 100 percent had fungal spores of *Staphylococcus* and *Ascomycetes* fungi.[29]

- Tumorous breast tissue had higher aflatoxin levels than did normal tissue of the same person.[30]

Our breasts are organs that are designed to be incredibly, biologically responsive to signals inside our body, to our babies, and to our outside world. Breasts have a dense supply of estrogen receptors that sit on cell walls like flowers ready to catch the "bees" of passing molecules of estrogen. However, these sensors also corral heavy metals and synthetic estrogens. Our breast receptors latch on to these synthetic carbon ring structures—an action that may prove harmful to them.

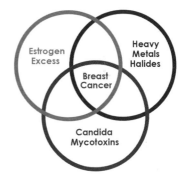

In earlier times, the only estrogen-mimics we experienced were plant based. For eons, our breasts could trust what they received because we coevolved with plant estrogens; but modern mimics come to us in a deadly daily drip.

Excess estrogen tips the delicate balance of hormones by outweighing levels of progesterone, thereby throwing all other hormones off kilter. Contributing to excess estrogen are the synthetic hormones in agriculture, birth control pills, IUDs, and hormone replacement therapy, along with xenoestrogens (the foreign synthetic-estrogen mimics in PCBs), BPA, parabens, and phthalates. We are soaking in the false estrogens of deodorants, perfumes, and creams. The average cosmetics consumer is exposed to 126 unique chemicals per day and five pounds of dry chemical weight per year.[31] All of this accumulates in breast tissue and may lead to abnormal cells and detectable changes in DNA!

There are hundreds of chemicals used to make plastic that have estrogenic activity—including in BPA-free bottles. Numerous studies confirm that BPA activates estrogen receptors, causing normal breast cells to act like invasively growing cells. BPA, a by-product of petroleum processing, was actually identified in the 1930s as a powerful synthetic estrogen.[32] It is now in everything from money to dental fillings. Slowly, BPA alters our cells by turning off suppressor genes and turning on tumor promoters called oncogenes.

Adding to the daily drip of endocrine disruption is high sugar consumption, which spikes blood sugar levels, contributing to insulin resistance and, in turn, estrogen spikes. If the liver is carrying a full load of modern-day detoxification, it can struggle to process all these estrogens, leaving us in excess.

Next, we have heavy metals and halides.

Heavy metals are toxins that accumulate in our tissues and bones. Once they penetrate, toxic metals compete with and displace much-needed minerals. Mercury, the same mercury that is in eco-lightbulbs and silver fillings, was found in all cancer and precancerous cells by Dr. Yoshiaki Omura in 1996.[33] Mercury is also a metalloestrogen, a type of metal-estrogen-mimic. Aluminum, cadmium, and lead are also metalloestrogens. If you have heard of the gender-bending effects of pesticides, these are the metalloestrogens in action. One such product is atrazine, which chemically castrated 75 percent of adult male frogs.[34] It is an endocrine disrupter in humans, too, and can alter genes that regulate hormone signaling and may influence infertility.[35]

Halides are from the halogen family of metals, consisting of fluorine, chlorine, and bromine. Bromine is pervasive in the form of BVO (brominated vegetable oil), used in breads, sodas, and sports drinks. It also appears in the form of the PBDEs (polybrominated diphenyl ethers) in flame retardants found in kids' pajamas and almost everything we touch, from laptops to Legos to lint. This chemical is not molecularly bound, so it migrates and attaches to dust in our homes. PBDEs are also goitrogenic, lipophilic, fat-loving toxins that have an affinity for breast tissue. A small study showed that bromide levels are two times higher in women with breast cancer.[36]

Last, we have *Candida* fungi, invasive pathogenic yeast that excretes a mycotoxin waste product. In advanced stages of overgrowth, *Candida* fungi grow root-like filaments that dig tiny holes in the intestines. This can cause leaky gut syndrome, when food, bacteria, and toxins escape the gut through tiny perforations and flow into the bloodstream. The mycotoxins *Candida* releases mimic estrogen and may deactivate our *p53* gene, which is our anticancer superhero gene.[37] These mycotoxins also contaminate our food chain; it is in moldy corn and grains and in tainted meats from pharmaceutical mycoestrogens added to animal feed. A 2001 study of New Jersey schoolgirls found that 78 percent had synthetic mycoestrogens in their urine.[38]

For the sake of our health, and our breasts, we must eliminate these things, because even with attentiveness, synthetics and carcinogens seep in. Studies show that it is well worth the effort.[39] With this inevitable seeping of synthetics, I wondered: What could we do to sharpen our breasts' sensory receptors? What could activate their discernment? Could we possibly refine our breast receptors to not latch on to every carbon ring structure that passes by?

There is a simple solution, a powerful pillar, an antidote that addresses all three contributing patterns of excess estrogen, mutant metals, and chronic *Candida*. This substance fine-tunes estrogen-receptor sensitivity. It returns tender breasts to normal tissue. It chelates halides and heavy metals gracefully from the body. It protects the guts. It refines insulin sensitivity, and it is found in every cell of our body.

This ancient antidote is iodine.

Iodine sensitizes our receptors, harmonizes hormones, metabolizes estrogens, and positively alters the gene expression of breast cells. It effortlessly cleanses bromide, mercury, fluoride, and more from the body.

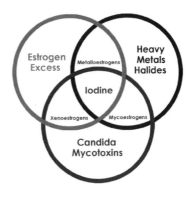

Although iodine may conjure images of the red medicine painted on soldiers' wounds, it is actually an electron-rich essential mineral used by every hormone, every organ, every tissue, and every cell of the body. Iodine is a potent ancestral antioxidant—more potent than vitamins C and E.

Iodine comes from our planet's original rock formations. Ice-age erosion of these rocks dispersed this water-soluble ion into the briny oceanic depths. Iodine began to concentrate in algae and then seaweeds. Seaweed has a membrane-capturing system that extracts iodine 20,000 times the ocean's concentration. Iodine came first, and through the complex evolution of cells, the very first hormone to form was thyroid hormone. The main function of iodine is the secretion and synthesis of thyroid hormone. The thyroid's main purpose is to survey each cell, keep the genome stable, and allow each hormone to perform perfectly.

The thyroid, breasts, ovaries, and prostate are all iodine dependent. Iodine kindles the flame of vitality by igniting our thyroid. Every seventeen minutes, every drop of blood passes through the thyroid. If our thyroid has an adequate supply of iodine, iodine is carried to nourish every cell. Only after the thyroid gland gets saturated can iodine then be absorbed and used by the breasts, ovaries, intestines, nasal cavities, stomach, bones, extracellular fluids, connective tissue, hormone receptors, cerebrospinal fluid, gastric mucosa, and salivary glands. Iodine is the Where's Waldo? of minerals; it shows up everywhere in a healthy body.

- Approximately 1.5 billion people live in countries that are iodine deficient.[40]
- Over the past forty years, iodine deficiency has increased 400 percent in the developed world.[41]
- 74 percent of healthy adults may not get enough dietary iodine.[42]
- World Health Organization and United States Recommended Dietary Allowance (RDA) recommendations for iodine are based on the minimum needed to prevent goiter and cretinism and are not for sufficiency for optimal health.[43]

Thirty years ago, when only 1 of every 20 women had breast cancer, iodine consumption was twice as high as it is today. Thirty years ago, iodine was used widely in dairy farming, and bread makers switched from iodine to potassium bromate as an anticaking agent. This absence of iodine causes dysfunction that can be seen with practically every hormone inside the body. The entire endocrine system, brain, and immune system need far more iodine than is being consumed.

Iodine is the gatekeeper of our breasts' glandular integrity. Iodine deficiency increases estrogen production. Iodine sufficiency maintains the correct balance of the three estrogens (estrone, estradiol, and estriol), helping us metabolize the estrogens in favor of the safer, protective form of estrogen, estriol. Iodine sufficiency is necessary for the normal growth and development of breast tissue.[44]

The breasts, like the thyroid, have a system for absorbing, storing, and secreting iodine. The ductal cells in the breast, the ones most likely to become cancerous, are equipped with a sodium-iodide symporter; this is the same type of iodine pump that soaks up iodine in the thyroid.[45]

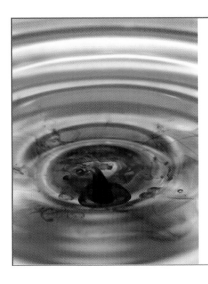

Iodine

- Used by **every** hormone, organ, cell
- Regulates metabolism
- Cell differentiation
- Boosts enzyme systems and immune
- Ancestral antioxidant
- Antiseptic to fungi, bacteria, viruses
- Detoxifies heavy metals, halides
- Triggers apoptosis
- Improves insulin sensitivity
- For fibrocystic breasts
- Shrinks ovarian cysts
- Improves estrogen receptor sensitivity
- Breast ductal cells equipped with an iodine pump
- Iodine can cause tumors to shrink
- Iodine concentrates in and is secreted by mammary glands

As iodine consumption drops, there is a significant increase in diseases of the endocrine system. A malfunctioning thyroid is a precursor to many female disorders. Iodine, together with thyroid hormone, acts as a surveillance team against abnormal cells by inducing apoptosis (natural cell death). Also, in an iodine-deficient state, the breasts and thyroid will compete for what little iodine is available. Iodine deficiency can lead to both thyroid and breast imbalances. When there is a deficiency, the breasts, the thyroid, the ovaries (and perhaps the prostate too) enlarge to compensate. Swollen ovaries are very similar to a swollen thyroid—a reaction to iodine deficiency. The thyroid is sometimes referred to as the third ovary. The connection between hypothyroidism and breast cancer was first reported in 1896!

Fibrocystic breasts occur in about one-third of women of childbearing age,[46] and when women are supplemented with iodine, fibrocystic disease often reverses.[47] Fibrocystic breasts, a condition whereby swollen breasts have cysts and are usually tender to touch, are thought of as a benign condition, although many physicians consider it a precursor. Several studies discovered that the greater the iodine deficiency, the greater the amount of estrogen and increased cysts in breasts.[48] The amount of iodine needed to control breast cancer and fibrocystic breasts is twenty to forty times the amount of iodine needed to prevent goiter; doses above the RDA are needed to reach saturation. Low-sodium diets and low levels of iodine in iodized salt contribute to our deficiency.

Our bodies' stores of iodine are further crowded out by daily exposures to bromide, fluoride, and chlorine. These halides are antagonists of iodine. If a body is iodine deficient, these halides happily attach to the vacant iodine receptors. In a fascinating molecular harmony, iodine is also from the halide group of elements, and it is the antidote for chelating the toxic halides from the body.

Supplementing replenishes our iodine stores while flushing out heavy metals and halides from our glands and connective tissue. After only one iodine dose, bromide and fluoride begin to excrete via the urine. Dr. Guy Abraham found that some patients began to excrete lead, cadmium, and mercury after one day, and aluminum began to excrete after one month of daily iodine.[49] Most people do not experience any negative detox effects unless they are unloading extremely high levels of bromine. Many people experience better sleep, energy, and mental clarity.

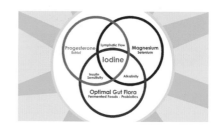

The best types of iodine are atomic, nascent forms of iodine with better uptake and a high electromagnetic charge and alcohol-free/aqueous iodine. When our glands are satiated with iodine, our constitution and connective tissues are strengthened.

Iodine deficiency aggregated with xenoestrogens, metalloestrogens, and mycoestrogens creates a pattern of prolific breast imbalances. We can understand where our bodies are at with laboratory analysis of our blood, saliva, urine, and hair.

This is our effective early-screening program.

MITOCHONDRIAL MEDICINE

As we consider best-breast practices, we also want to think in terms of mitochondrial medicine.

Mitochondria are our cell's energy-makers, and until recently, that is all that was known about them. Now, researchers across all disciples of medicine have discovered that mitochondria have their own sets of DNA beyond the DNA in the cell nucleus; they communicate with each other, regulate gene expression, control synapse firing in the brain, trigger systemic inflammation, and contribute chemicals that play a role in tumor formation. We know that DNA defects and mitochondrial dysfunction contribute to common diseases studied in genetics, neurology, immunology, and oncology.

In many ways, mitochondria are more like bacteria than mammal cells. Dr. David Perlmutter wrote that "mitochondria can in fact be considered a third dimension to our microbiome; they have a unique relationship to the microbiome of our guts."[50] Healthy gut bacteria support mitochondria, but when bacteria are out of balance they can damage our mitochondria either with toxic waste products or by triggering systemic inflammation.

Furthermore, our mitochondria, the protector of our genes, our guts, and our brains, are more vulnerable than we realize. Research published in 2016 found that commonly prescribed antibiotics induce reactive oxygen species, a.k.a. free radicals, in bacteria thus causing harm in our tissues, and antibiotics deteriorate mitochondria.[51]

Increasing mitochondrial strength is vital to shielding our cells from the mutations of toxins. Iodine is mitochondrial medicine. There are several ways to protect mitochondria.

- Maintain fasting blood sugar levels at 80.
- Magnesium is like the light in each cell, and is essential to mitochondrial function. Once iodine starts excreting heavy metals and halides, you will want to refill cells with magnesium, along with selenium and trace minerals.
- Natural terpenes protect against mitochondrial dysfunction.[52]

TERPENES: BREAST BOOSTERS

Nature provides us with a gentle yet potent answer in plant terpenes. These powerful pillars for health are found abundantly in essential oils. They improve the liver's ability to break down carcinogens, stimulate cell death (apoptosis) in abnormal cells, facilitate healing, reduce inflammation, and selectively block the division and multiplication of abnormal cells.

Terpene is the fancy word for a medicinal compound found in essential oils. Terpenes are produced by a variety of plants, especially conifers, and they are the oldest group of small molecular substances made by plants. They are chemically composed of only hydrogen and carbon atoms structured as an isoprene unit, the building block of plants.

As these isoprene building blocks link up, they are classified by the total number of units in the chain. Monoterpenes consist of two isoprene units, and they are especially breast-boosting.

Isoprene

When a monoterpene enters the body, it is processed and broken down, mostly by the liver, into various, more water-soluble components. For example, perillyl alcohol, a well-documented potent anticancer metabolite of limonene, is transformed by our liver enzymes into perillic acid. These components vary in their affinity with types of tissues. For example, limonene is especially lipophilic and accumulates in fatty tissue where it lingers longer than most other essential oil constituents. Research continues to look for ways to use limonene as a means of enhancing pharmaceutical absorption through the skin because it interacts well with the lipids that coat the top layer of our skin to facilitate drug diffusibility.

Interest in monoterpene research was aroused by the discovery that limonene prevents mammary cancer in mice. Until the mid-1990s, research journals brimmed with studies on monoterpenes and their influence on cancer development and progression. The research stalled out after a few clinical trials reported less-than-stellar results. One of the problems in these clinical cases was that the monoterpenes were metabolized into components considered to be less bioactive.

Now, with innovative technology to guide the way, a new era of research has begun. Recent developments suggest that monoterpenes prevent both the initiation and progression of cancer, offering at least chemopreventive benefits today and perhaps cancer treatments tomorrow. And—surprise!—researchers have discovered that many of the digested monoterpene metabolites, such as perillic acid, are just as potent against particular cancers—including cancers of the breast—as their precursors.[53]

Monoterpenes influence cancer and cancer cells in multiple ways by inhibiting particular cell-signaling pathways and by counteracting metabolic changes that occur in breast disease.

Breast cancer is hormone dependent, and among all of the chemical carcinogens we are exposed to, excess estrogen is a doozy.[54] Limonene, as well as other monoterpenes, stimulates estrogen detoxification via enzymes in the liver, thus restoring hormonal balance in the body.[55] In other words, monoterpenes detoxify our tissues of cancer-causing chemicals, including our own excess estrogen. The monoterpene alcohols carveol, uroterpenol, and sobrerol are also carcinogen detoxifiers.[56]

Tumors occur when cells multiply faster than they die off. Apoptosis, or programmed cell death, is the body's method of maintaining tissue homeostasis. When apoptosis is curbed, there is fertile soil for tumors to grow. Monoterpenes trigger apoptosis and suppress tumor formation via the inhibition of cell growth-regulating proteins.[57] Linalool, a monoterpene alcohol, is also cytotoxic to cancer cells and activates antitumor immunity in the body.[58]

For those who like to dig deeper into the details, here's a list of studied anticancer monoterpenes and alcohols:[59]

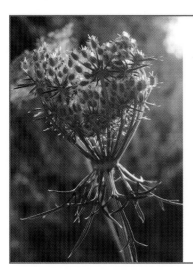

A list of studied anticancer monoterpenes and alcohols:

- Alloocimene
- Ascaridole
- Borneol
- Camphor
- Carvacrol
- Carvone
- Cineole/eucalyptol
- Citral
- Cymene
- Dolabrin
- Geraniol
- Limonene
- Linalool
- Linalyl acetate
- Menthol
- Mycene
- Perilla aldehyde
- Perillic Acid
- Perillyl Alcohol
- Pinene
- Sobrerol
- Terpenene
- Terpineol
- Terpinolene
- Thujaplicin
- Thymol
- Thymolhydroquinone
- Thymoquinone
- Uroterpenol

A research team at the University of Arizona led by Dr. Jessica Martinez found that orange peel oil, which is about 90 percent d-limonene monoterpene, administered either orally or topically to female mice, showed *preferential absorption of limonene into breast tissue.* They discovered that this occurred independently of the method of administration.[60]

Dr. Martinez and her team then recruited a group of healthy women to determine the safety and feasibility of topical application of orange oil. The women applied to their breasts orange oil diluted to 10 percent or 20 percent in coconut oil. No safety or practical issues were reported by the women.[61]

In yet another clinical study, women newly diagnosed with breast cancer ingested 2 grams of limonene every day for two to six weeks. The study reported that the limonene concentrated in their breast tissue, and there was a

22 percent reduction in cyclin D protein expression. Cyclin D plays a role in the rate of cell growth and proliferation and is overexpressed in hyperplasia (the initial stage of cancer) and in intraductal carcinoma of the breast.[62]

SOOTHE YOUR CELLS

Strong, healthy tissue is vital to our health. Weak tissue—weak breast cells—is vulnerable to disease, and inflammation is commonly considered a culprit for frail and diseased cells. Inflammation is not always unhealthy, though. It is the body's natural response to an injury. Acute inflammation is part of our innate immunity; it helps to protect the body against toxic substances, remove injured and dead cells, and begin the healing process.

On the other hand, medical journals have documented well the pathological consequences of *chronic and systemic* inflammation. Enduring inflammation is a marker of autoimmune and degenerative diseases, and research suggests that it may cause everything from Alzheimer's to irritable bowel syndrome, rheumatoid arthritis to depression, and cell senescence to cancer. Chronic inflammation also seems to promote cancer's progression.

Many of the pharmaceuticals recommended after an injury or prescribed for chronic inflammation and pain are called nonsteroidal anti-inflammatory drugs, including Tylenol and Celebrex. These drugs are helpful at reducing

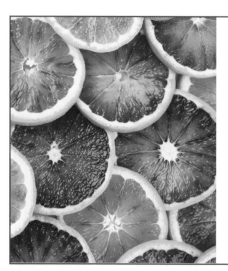

**Beautiful Breasts
Therapeutic Massage Oil**

55 ml Jojoba
5 ml Orange essential oil
10 drops Laurel essential oil
10 drops Frankincense essential oil

Massage inward and upward stimulating lymphatic drainage.

The higher concentrations of essential oils in this massage mix are therapeutic. Best used just on breasts. Orange oil is photosensitive at higher dilutions; do not apply this oil and expose skin to direct sunlight afterwards. Orange essential oil contains high levels of the constituent d-limonene monoterpene (approximately 90%) . Limonene, as well as other monoterpenes like those found in frankincense, stimulates estrogen detoxification by way of enzymes in the liver. Laurel essential oil contains a diverse mix of monoterpene esters that stimulate the lymphatic system.

inflammation, but they also inhibit healing and they are not without serious side effects. Research now supports the use of other means of analgesia if a healing process is needed. (Monoterpenes are also being explored as medical therapies for pain. The monoterpene alcohol menthol in peppermint comes to mind as a good option.)

Monoterpenes are uniquely gifted at soothing the cells while also encouraging tissue to heal. Their potent anti-inflammatory plant power probably results from the regulative and restorative effects of inhibiting cell-signaling proteins involved in inflammation: tumor necrosis factor alpha (TNF-α), Interleukin 6 (IL-6), and Interleukin 1 (IL-1). One or more of these cell signalers is often elevated in weakened, frail tissues.[63] Clinical reports have reported application doses for anti-inflammatory active healing to be 10–50 milligrams per kilogram (mg/kg) of body weight per day.

Our immune system starts with healthy skin, which keeps invaders at bay. Yet we trespass daily by applying pounds per year of toxic cosmetics to our skin that sink deep into the underlying mesoderm. An issue with our breast tissue is the cellular penetration of xenoestrogenic and metalloestrogenic cosmetics, embalming us with formaldehyde and propylene glycol. How many more blogs and studies do we have to read about the chemical menace of moisturizers and the poison of perfumes before we understand that transdermal absorption is our kryptonite if we dose daily with parabens and soak in the halides of municipal tap water? Yet with the right stuff—monoterpene-rich oils

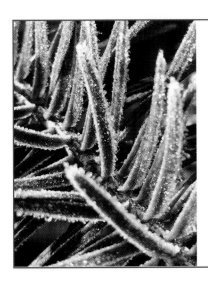

Monoterpenes, found abundantly in essential oils, ally with our bodies boosting breath health by

1. Removing toxins
2. Turning on protective genes
3. Improving the liver's ability to break down carcinogens
4. Stimulating apoptosis
5. Inhibiting cell division in abnormal cells
6. Reducing abnormal cell signaling pathways
7. Soothing pain and inflammation while encouraging tissues to heal

and mitochondrial-protecting iodine—our skin contributes to the strength of our immunity.

BOOSTING BREAST HEALTH

At the heart of basic breast care is real food, sunshine, iodine, and being sure your skin drinks in bodycare that is brimming with botanical medicine.

Breast-health solutions include stimulating the lymph, strengthening breast tissue, and feeding breast receptors the right genetic information. This means we need to step away from the cosmetics, chemicals, and toxic metals that unlock secondary cell mutations, and bring in the confluence of the cosmos.

Our breasts need life-affirming bodycare that protects the mitochondria, encourages the lymph, and boosts immune and liver function. Nature provides this simple solution with monoterpenes.

An issue with our breast tissue is the cellular penetration of commercial cosmetics. Transdermal absorption can be our kryptonite or it can be our caregiver—if the right substance is applied to strengthen our cells. In the realm of scientific study, monoterpene research is still nascent. Scientists are developing ways to deliver monoterpene medicine to us, yet we don't have to wait! The safety, efficacy, and availability of monoterpene-rich essential oils invite us to be plant pioneers and to nourish our tender tissues with frankincense, grapefruit, cypress, orange, lemon, laurel, and rose otto essential oils.

Breasts contain an abundance of lymph vessels that support the circulatory system in maintaining proper fluid balance and carrying away intracellular waste. The health of our lymphatic system is intimately connected to our breast health. Lymph flow can be obstructed by poor posture, lack of exercise, shallow breathing, and tight neck, shoulder, chest, and back muscles.

Bras can also constrict our lymph system, causing a toxic backlog in our breasts. This is an easy fix. Look for red marks on your skin after removing your bra to determine if it is too tight and needlessly burdening your breasts. Consider wearing softer yoga tops and bras.

Massaging our way to healthy breast tissue is a simple strategy. Breast massage lubricated with essential oils regenerates our cells and supplies monoterpene medicine to where it is needed most. Be sure to massage *inward and upward* to stimulate lymphatic drainage, release excess estrogen, firm connective tissue, and enhance elasticity.

Cypress, yarrow, and laurel oils stimulate the movement of the lymph fluid to remove toxins and supply fresh nutrition to the cells. In *Advanced Aromatherapy*, Dr. Kurt Schnaubelt wrote that simply "rubbing a few drops of bay laurel on swollen lymph nodes may have an immediate, noticeable effect."[64] These oils would be a beautiful addition to breast massage oils.

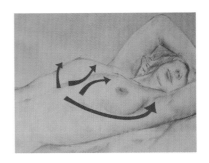

Tumors in the lateral aspect of the breast, a.k.a. the armpit, have been linked to paraben and aluminum in antiperspirants.[65] Consider sandalwood essence for a deodorant instead. Unlike chemical-based, cancer-correlated deodorants, sandalwood oil contains rather rare sesquiterpene alcohols (alpha santalol and beta santalol) that are, like their monoterpene cousins, chemopreventive agents. Also, sandalwood oil has an affinity for the armpit because it contains phytoandrogen. When it mingles with the androgen exuded by our armpits, our pits become a pheromone perfumery that creates captivating aromas.

Beyond mitochondrial medicine and monoterpenes, my other breast-health strategies are sunshine and iodine. Keeping vitamin D levels optimal reduces breast-cancer risk![66] My basic daily breast care is consuming only pure food and water, employing mitochondrial medicine, soaking in the sunshine and iodine, and surrounding my skin in my beautiful oils. I soak in frankincense and rose baths, and my skin drinks in only botanical medicine in the form of real body-care serums that are cell enhancing and breast-health boosting.

Our breast health is a barometer. Breasts are pranic channels; they give and receive life force. Take these things into consideration for your breasts, and your whole being will benefit.

It's in the arch of my back,
The sun of my smile,
The ride of my breasts,
The grace of my style.
I'm a woman
Phenomenally.
Phenomenal woman,
That's me.

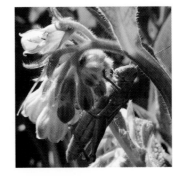

Maya Angelou[67]

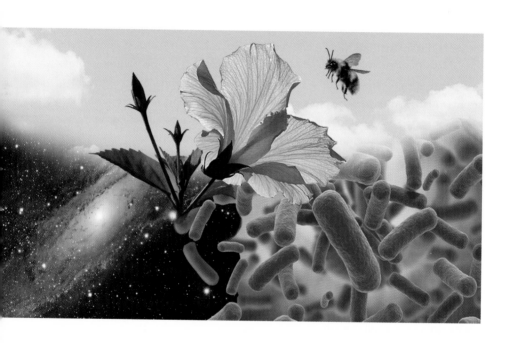

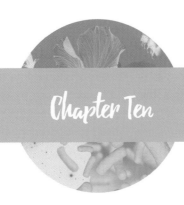

Chapter Ten

BACK TO THE GARDEN

Tending to the Virtues of the Vagina

The vagina, the savory peach, the fertile crescent of our femininity, is not merely the reproductive plumbing that reductionist science would have us believe. Neither are the jewels of the nether region a receptacle. The vagina is, in fact, a gateway and a passage to the brain, the body, and the spirit. It is also a sublime portal where the form and formlessness of a soul can coalesce.

The geography of a woman's vagina is much more expansive, diversified, multifaceted, and nuanced than has been imagined by medical study, the far-reaching foibles of Freudian philosophy, and the mass marketers of feminine hygiene.

We are taught to skip past our lunar rhythms, the waxing and waning of our womb. When we trade in our uterus's compass for synthetic birth control, our estrous becomes rhythmless. We trade the wisdom of knowing when our eggs are in full bloom for dangerous products to consume.[1]

Periods are plugged with the unsterile fibers of rayon, plasticizers, and cotton made of GMOs as our vaginal canals drink in their dioxins, bleaches, pesticides, and molds,[2] subjecting us to the risks of toxic shock syndrome, disease, pelvic inflammation, and bioaccumulation. Could we be so bold as to celebrate our monthly cycle as gold?

We grew up as a nation out of touch with ovulation. We have accepted artificial assistance that has proved time and time again to be more treacherous than trustworthy:[3] from the contraceptive contraptions that cause uterine perforations,[4] to the plethora of birth control pills that have made us hormonally ill, provoked pulmonary embolisms,[5] disrupted the thyroid's metabolism, and caused blood clots. These false pharmacy plots have proven to increase breast and cervical cancers. Eliminating periods and preventing ovulation are just not the answer.

Arrays of industrial tricks promise to perfume and make polite the effluvia of feminine fluids. We submit our secretions to be technologically tamed. Shamed, we attempt to scrub clean in a dangerous daily routine of douches, deodorants, wipes, powders, and shower gels—drenching us all to glorify some advertiser's dream of holy hygiene.

These devices—sprays, foams, spermicides, and gels—invented to sanitize smells and prevent pregnancy cause our vaginal cells to atrophy, devitalize, recoil, shrivel, and shrink. We used to think of our yonis as a perfumed garden with *kulamrita*[6] nectars, nectars so divine they were thought to originate in heaven. Once revered, now sheared, promises of self-esteem are smeared on with vaginal-bleaching cream.

Our lovely labia, we have become afraid of ya'. With the surge of internet pornography and vaginas now airbrushed as a commodity, we have newfound fears about our genitalia's geography. We have come to doubt the design of our lady lotus, leading to an epic increase in the plastic surgeries of labiaplasty, vaginoplasty, "revirgination," and G-spot augmentation. This mutilation includes female circumcision; although often thought of as something that happens in distant lands, it was covered by Blue Cross and other health insurance until 1977 in America.[7] A 1973 issue of *Playgirl* magazine promoted the article "Circumcision for Women: The Kindest Cut of All."[8] Now female circumcision falls under the category of FGCS, female genital cosmetic surgery, where the surgeon plays god.

The clitoris has the unique history of being both the encourager of masturbation and the physiological cause for a woman's orgasmic failure. In the past, circumcision was performed to prevent masturbation, and now "clitoral unhooding" is fashionable as a sexual-enhancement therapy. The American Congress of Obstetricians and Gynecologists cautions that women seeking "designer vaginas" should be "informed about the lack of data supporting the efficacy of these procedures and their potential complications, including infection, altered sensation, adhesions, and scarring."[9]

The sacred Venus mound has become a modern dumping ground of negative thoughts, surgical alterations, and a receptacle for industrial violations. The thing is, it likes fresh air and rebels at polyester underwear.

I like to use the term *yoni*, the sacred Sanskrit word for vagina, because it is a fun word that prevents me from schoolgirl giggles and also because the meaning expands to include the creative force that moves through the universe: the vagina as the "origin of life," the "divine passage," and "sacred temple." I will use yoni and vagina interchangeably as umbrella words for the whole region including the vulva, clitoris, labia, vaginal canal, and womb. We all came into being through a womb and, whether we bear children or not, this divine passage resides within us.

In ancient Taoist and Tantric texts, the vagina was held in reverence as a source of wisdom connected to the female mind as precious, unique, fragrant, a treasure, a seat of divinity, a gateway to the Atman, the True Self. These texts describe it as: sweet, juicy, succulent, a precious pearl, a jade gate, the mysterious valley, and the lotus of her wisdom. In poetic detail, the yoni was described as a "flower [that] loves to absorb the sun's rays . . . [And] her juices have the fragrance of a freshly blossoming lotus flower."[10]

In the sacred Taoist texts, the Great Medicine of the Three Peaks highlights the regenerating, vital fluids that women secrete from their vagina. It is written that the lover's goal, for the sake of his own health, is to unlock the "mysterious gateway" in order to stir the release of these precious fluids. The secretions are seen as mystical medicine and called Moon Flower. As the woman's fluid-gate opens and her secretions overflow, qi is released and her fluids strengthen the man's primal yang and nourish his spirit.[11]

Let's now look at Western history for a vast contrast. It begins with the vagina dentata and Freud's declaration that women's bodies are the genitally deficient "dark continent."[12] This historical sediment swept women's pleasure and precious fluids under the rug of time, leading to a cascade of cultural impulses that maimed and defamed the juice jewel of our body. This history leaves us vulnerable to the modern marketing maze that socializes our fertile fluids into shame, scrutinizes insecurities, and holds our bodies to blame. It is a dangerous game that has led to depression, disease, and death.

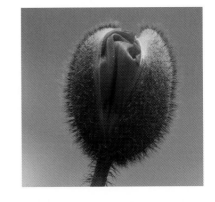

Denuded of mystery, the power of our petaled pool is tamed with names like "kitty" and the faux-empowerment of commercial labels such as "froo-froo," "hoo-haa," and the infantile "la-la."

The yoni is celebrated only when its vitality is sealed in Saran and the menstruum, ovum, and orgasmic broth are captured by toxic tampons, obliterated by the Pill, or impeded by tubes of petroleum lube. The loquacious liquids of our womanhood get curtailed by chemicals that deodorize and by cute maxipads that accessorize as the life force gets civilized. In this, women are empowered solely as consumers of manufactured choice.

HIGHLIGHTS FROM THE HYSTERIA OVER FEMININE HYGIENE

Here is a brief history of some of the insane recommendations made for our delicate mucous membranes. One of the earlier commercial douching products for birth control was Lysol, which focused its fearful ads on the reality that women would wreck their marriages if they neglected their intimate feminine hygiene. "Gentle, non-caustic Lysol will not harm delicate tissue . . . Many doctors advise patients to douche regularly with Lysol just to ensure daintiness alone . . ."[13] Historical hindsight shows that Lysol douching caused 193 poisonings and five deaths.[14]

Once Lysol douches were deemed caustic, Listerine filled the void with this campaign: "Intimate use of harsh antiseptics leads to untold damage. Women now hail a gentle, safe means . . . Its effect on tissue is soothing and healing. It deodorizes instantly. Listerine for Feminine Hygiene."[15] We now know that alcohol-based mouthwashes, such as Listerine, contribute to an increased risk of oral cancer.[16] My guess is that Listerine, containing alcohols linked to oral cancer,[17] is not so soothing in the vaginal canal.

As women's liberation lit up the 1960s, the marketers at Massengill made "the freedom spray." The ad states, "We make it with hexachlorophene . . . You like freedom, don't you?" Harsh hexachlorophene is a disinfectant that can be lethal when absorbed through the skin. In France in 1972, due to a manufacturing error, hexachlorophene was added to baby powder and killed thirty-six children.[18]

Raising female "consciousness" through heightening insecurity, feminine-hygiene product ads pointed to odor as a serious issue. A 1969 Bidette ad (imprinted with a Good Housekeeping Seal of Approval) called it "the odor problem men don't have."[19] A Pristeen ad reads "the trickiest deodorant problem a girl has *isn't* under her pretty little arms."[20] A 1968 Pristeen Feminine Hygiene Deodorant Spray ad also promised to keep "girls" "fresh and free of any worry-making odors" and stated that it had been "tested in leading hospitals under the supervision of gynecologists."[21] In reality, we soon learned that these products are beyond silly; they are dangerous. In 1970, Dr. Bernard Davis, a gynecologist, reported in the *Journal of Obstetrics and Gynecology* that he had treated about twenty-five women who used a feminine-hygiene spray daily and who reported "itching, burning sensations in the vulvar area." A fourteen-year-old girl arrived at her appointment with an "incredibly" swollen labia, and even after treatment her clitoris and labia were "peculiarly" abnormal.[22]

"Honey," said Bill Blass when asked to explain why his line of cosmetics included a so-called *private* deodorant, "if there's a part of the human body to exploit you might as well get onto it."[23] Many manufacturers do. Norforms Feminine Deodorant Suppositories promise "easier, *surer* protection for those most intimate marriage problems."[24] This "germicidal protection" promise is made with these ingredients: PEG-20, PEG-32, Benzethonium Chloride, Methylparaben, Lactic Acid, and Fragrance.

Summer's Eve Douche, as well as other brands of douches, has this warning on the label: "An association has been reported between douching and Pelvic Inflammatory Disease (PID), ectopic pregnancy, and infertility."

Recently, FemFresh extolled its deodorizing product as "one of the kindest ways to care for your kitty, nooni, lala, froo froo!"[25] These are some of the ingredients: Sodium Laureth Sulfate, Triethyl Citrate, Parfum, Polyquaternium-39, Glycerin, Dichlorobenzyl Alcohol, Sodium Carbonate, 2-Bromo-2-Nitropropane-1, 3-Diol, Maltodextrin, Methylparaben, and Propylparaben. Um, no thanks.

Vaginas are supposed to look and smell like vaginas. Keep your strange scented washes away from me, women's magazines.

Amy Schumer[26]

Do you think that pay equity is a serious issue? Well, the solution is simple: douche more! In 2010, Summer's Eve placed a big ad in women's magazines suggesting that women could boost "their confidence at work" and "ask for a raise" by douching.[27] If the cleanliness of our private parts plays such a pivotal role in getting paid more, it begs the question: where does one have to sit to get a raise?

The U.S. Department of Health now warns against feminine-hygiene products as interfering with the vagina's self-cleansing system and as harmful to the natural bacterial strains that prevent infections.[28]

THE FLORA OF OUR FLOWER

Let's get back to the garden where our lotus blossom is understood to be the seat of our wisdom, strength of self, and connection to life, love, and divinity. Whether you are a maiden, mother, or maven, let's delve into understanding and harmonizing our yoni's elegant ecology so that we may thrive and be energized by this mysterious gateway.

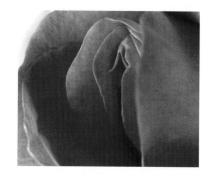

I like to keep things simple. So when it comes to my body wisdom, I look for the self-organizing principles that activate the innate intelligence of the body. When it comes to the self-regulating system of your yoni-land, nothing is more important than understanding its unique microbiome.

What do yeast infections, vaginitis, cervical dysplasia, vulvodynia, pelvic inflammation, premature births, miscarriages, dryness, and bacterial conditions, including vaginosis, postpartum bacteremia, *Trichomonas vaginalis*, and other invasive vaginal infections, have in common? They all share vaginal microbiome imbalances.

Microbiologist Gregor Reid insists that not placing "a huge focus on the vaginal microbiome is like putting human survival at risk."[29] Indeed, vaginal microbes are paramount to our survival, because they affect our vitality and immunity and also our fertility, the health of our babies, and the genetic wealth we bestow to future generations.

The vaginal microbiome has a signaling capacity that connects to the guts, immune system, and brain. It regulates pH, hormones, and lubrication. This gateway of our genitalia acts like air traffic control for many microbes. The flora of our flower colonizes and protects the vagina; they shield the vagina by producing lactic acid, which lowers the pH, making it slightly acidic and less hospitable to pathogens. These friendly bacteria create the yoni's self-organizing system that naturally seeks optimal balance by monthly flushing out dead skin cells and bad bacteria.

Everything that has been invented for pristine feminine hygiene disrupts the very mechanism that actually keeps us clean—the vagina's own microbiome. These modern, invented practices contribute to our missing microbes, and they are becoming endangered species due to the overuse of antibiotic medication, hormonal contraception, overzealous sanitization, hazardous lubrication, and chemical-laden products for menstruation care.

No two women have the same flora fingerprint, and the diversity is easily influenced for good . . . or not so good. A plethora of factors sway our bacterial balance: ancestry, diet, hormone levels, stress, antibiotics, sexual partners, hygiene practices, epigenetics, and adverse exposures. Your bacterial fingerprint is also contingent on if you were breastfed and if you were birthed via cesarean section, as well as your blood sugar levels and immunity status.

Our dynamic vaginal microbiome can transform in a mere twenty-four hours, and the lunar rhythms of a woman's cycle guide bacterial population shifts throughout the month. In response to the rising and falling tides of estrogen, the yoni's microbial population goes through distinct changes at conception, birth, puberty, and menopause.

Yoni microbial health is important before, during, and after pregnancy. It influences fertility, full-term deliveries, healthy postpartum recovery, and even the baby's health. All babies receive their first anointing of beneficial bacteria for their skin and gut as they slide their way through the birth canal. A baby girl's vaginal colonization also occurs at this miraculous time. In childhood, a girl's microbes will be diverse and her vaginal pH relatively neutral. When puberty arrives, estrogen will rise, creating a new vaginal ecosystem along with a lower pH from lactic-acid-producing bacteria. Therefore, it is crucial that a baby's body is seeded with healthy, beneficial bacteria, inside and out. Yet, according to the Centers for Disease Control and Prevention, in 2006 as many as 16 percent of pregnant women in America had bacterial vaginosis.[30]

The good news is that if microbial health and diversity are a problem, one can course-correct. The microbial superhighway moves microbes from mouth to gut to vagina. Oral doses of *Lactobacillus bifidus*, fermented foods, and soil-based probiotics increase the friendly microflora in the vagina. See Chapter Eleven for more information.

Menopause creates a microbe-pause; and it is thought that as estrogen levels fall, the vaginal microbe population shifts away from lactic-acid producers to other species of microbiota. As a result, the vaginal lining changes and the pH rises, making the menopausal yoni vulnerable to vaginosis and dryness.

Many women douche because their yoni ecology is off kilter; and they are caught in an endless loop of douching and deodorants that, in the end, exacerbate the microbial imbalances that contribute to infections. These women may be repeatedly prescribed antibiotics and vaginal creams. If a woman uses lubes or spermicides and has a partner with *Candida*, she will continue the cycle until the root cause is addressed.

A 2004 study reported that 30 percent of American women had bacterial vaginosis.[31] Might this be the result of an unending microbial assault from feminine-hygiene products? What about the perplexing ingredients mixed up in the material of nonorganic tampons and pads? Bleached, genetically modified cotton was found to contain traces of eight microbe-killing pesticides, rayon, plasticizers, and petrochemical additives.[32] In addition, there are traces of damaging dioxides in the cotton, and the FDA knows it and allows it even though the EPA declares any exposure unacceptable.[33] Inserted into the apex of our body temple, all of these substances enter the bloodstream through our highly permeable petal.

You really need to understand what you put on, in, and around your yoni! Just as garden soil needs good bacteria and appropriate pH to thrive, so does our goddess garden!

The pubic hair that covers our lady lair is not just a biological mishap that propels women to wax. It serves the paramount purpose of protection. The hair down there is a pheromone blanket ensorcelling the scents that lead potential partners to the promised land. Cameron Diaz advises, "Pubic hair also serves as a pretty draping that makes it a little mysterious to the one who might be courting your sexiness . . . Consider leaving your vagina fully dressed, ladies."[34] Waxing and shaving irritate and inflame hair follicles, leaving microscopic open wounds. Combined with a moist environment, perhaps exacerbated by unbreathable polyester underwear, this creates a breeding ground for bacteria and STDs.

Birth control pills have a microbe-disrupting effect on our body similar to the effect of antibiotics. Besides disrupting the endocrine system, the Pill puts the body into a chemically induced menopause by signaling the ovaries to not release eggs. These precarious pills also reduce colonies of good microflora via surges of synthetic hormones, and this cultivates yeast and bacterial infections.

With further study of the vagina's microbiome, we will discover that, similar to our GI microbes, our flower's flora provides essential input to the rest of our body.

JOUISSANCE JUICE

A balanced, healthy vagina contributes to healthy secretions. I like to think of lubrication as an internal and external juiciness that is reflected in our relationship to life. The French word *jouissance* describes this perfectly. Jouissance is sensuality beyond pleasure, and engaging with the rapture of being alive. It is the fusion of all the senses—emotional, physical, and mystical. Jouissance juice is how I define the exquisite, essential lubrication that consecrates the yoni, connecting juiciness to life, creativity, and health.

The vagina is a naturally moist environment. It is delicate yet exceedingly elastic, expanding up to 200 percent when aroused. The vagina's tissue lining is similar to skin, though much more pliable and highly innervated. There are 8,000 nerve endings in the clitoris alone! The vagina is also highly vascularized, containing miles of blood and lymph vessels.

The vaginal lining is thin like the epithelial lining of our mouths, measuring only one cell thick. It is highly absorbent and allows naturally occurring moisture to pass through it. It is much more permeable than our skin; the mucous membranes in the vagina absorb chemicals quickly. It is so efficient that researchers are exploring the opportunity of dosing drugs vaginally. The *American Journal of Obstetrics and Gynecology* published a study that found that blood levels of estradiol are ten times higher when applied vaginally in lieu of taken orally.[35]

Ribbons of nerve cells weave through the vagina in an intricate communication pathway further connecting it to the body and brain. "The vulva, clitoris, and vagina are actually best understood as the surface of an ocean that is shot through with vibrant networks of underwater lightning—intricate and fragile, individually varied neural pathways . . . Among the many incredible things about your incredible pelvic nerve and its lovely multiple branches is that, as we saw, it is completely unique for every individual woman on earth—no two women are alike."[36] These nerves transmit sensation and regulate the vagina's engorgement with blood. With arousal, blood flow to the area increases, and microscopic pores secrete a soothing lubrication. The amount of lubrication produced in arousal is responsive to a very important peptide, called vasoactive intestinal peptide (VIP). This VIP is a genetically encoded neuromodulator and neurotransmitter produced in the brain, gut, and pancreas. It regulates biophysical responses and secretions from skin cells. Research reveals that when healthy women have VIP in their bloodstream and are aroused, their natural lubrication doubles! This field is still very new, and there is still much to be learned.[37] Jouissance juice is affected by emotional and relational issues. Stress affects the endocrine system and contributes to low levels of VIP. Depletion in the juiciness of daily life, depression, and anxiety can lead to the feeling of a loss of soul succulence.

Silly marketing schemes, ranging from the absurd to the seriously perilous, have sold us on caustic cleanses and perfumed petroleum products as expert care for "down there." In reality, a healthy yoni is self-cleaning (the original self-cleaning oven), and feminine douches and deodorants disrupt this innate process. Besides brutal bioaccumulation, these detrimental douches contribute to dryness. The same ingredients that you avoid in skincare are best avoided in yoni-care.

Those tubes of genital lubes all contain chemicals that irritate, inflame, dry, and disrupt this delicate area. There are three main types of lubricants: petroleum, glycerin, and silicone. We have all witnessed what an oil spill does to the ecosystem of an ocean. Petroleum, dimethicone, nonoxynol-9, and glycerol monolaurate have no place in the vagina. There is not a single cell in our body that thrives on petrochemicals and synthetic silicone.

Although water-based lubes sound safe, the main ingredient, glycerin, and the preservatives used are toxic. Glycerin is heavily processed and contains residual chemicals. Additionally, glycerin is a sugar, which contributes to the development of infections, as sugar feeds yeasts and bacteria.

Synthetic lubes are momentary petal-plumpers, offering only a very temporary lubrication with the consequence of long-term drought. Researchers have demonstrated that the ingredients of drugstore lubes dehydrate and disorganize cells.

Remember the high school chemistry class on osmosis: our cells seek a state of equilibrium. Synthetic ingredients throw our cells off kilter due to osmolarity; to maintain balance on both sides of the cell wall, the cell releases water to dilute the sugar, glycerin, and other synthetic substances outside of the cells. This dehydrates the cell and causes cellular and epithelial damage to the vagina. Charlene S. Dezzutti, a professor of obstetrics, gynecology, and reproductive sciences, reported that these substances make the "cells shrivel up to the point that they look like little raisins under a microscope."[38] Cellular raisins! It does not seem sensual to use a love lube that actually produces parched cellular raisins in the yoni.

When these cells dry up, they die and exfoliate from the epithelium, weakening the yoni's defenses and making it increasingly vulnerable to disease and infection. K-Y Jelly killed all three species of *Lactobacilli* on contact. Another experiment with K-Y Warming Jelly increased herpes transmission.[39] Richard Cone, a biophysicist at Johns Hopkins University, has stated that "virtually all sex lubricants need to be reformulated."[40]

Furthermore, these cell-shriveling lubricants are known for their fertility failure. Researchers found that all commercial lubricants impaired the sperm's overall motility.[41] As an interesting side note, mustard seed oil, used for centuries in Ayurvedic medicine, inspired the sperm to go into high gear.[42]

Spermicides are no friend of the yoni (or penis) either. The active ingredient in over-the-counter spermicides is nonoxynol-9, a detergent. Similar to synthetic lubes, nonoxynol-9 irritates and disrupts the membranes of the cells that line the vagina, gradually eroding its integrity. This in itself is unhealthy, and it also makes the vaginal cells vulnerable to viruses and bacteria that cause sexually transmitted diseases.

Optimize your jouissance juice by attending to these guidelines:

Soak up plenty of sunshine, baring as much skin to the sun as possible. Shailene Woodley knows what to do: "Another thing I like to do is give my vagina a little vitamin D. [Laughs] I was reading an article written by an herbalist I studied about yeast infections and other genital issues. She said there's nothing better than vitamin D."[43]

It is time to refine our concept of feminine hygiene and elevate our daily devotion to something more serene. With this divinity in mind, the best dew for our petals is edible. Succulent plant secretions are safe and sensual. Flowers

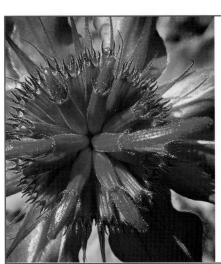

Jouissance
Life Lubrication

Yes

Live in Jouissance
Plenty of Probiotics
Abundant Healthy Dietary Fats
Balancing Herbs: vitex, black cohosh, wild yam, evening primrose, pueraria mirifica
Baths: sea salt, magnesium salts, essential oils
Soap: wash with a natural bar soap and follow with a botanical oil
Lube for play or day-to-day yoni protection: aloe vera; oils of coconut oil, cacao butter, or jojoba with tissue rejuvenating essentials of rose otto, frankincense, ylang, myrrh, sea buckthorn, and/or schizandra berries

Avoid

Endocrine Disrupters
Synthetic Lubes & Spermicides
Tampons (use organic when needed)
Douching
Synthetic Soaps
Chemical Bath Additives
Shaving Pubic Hair

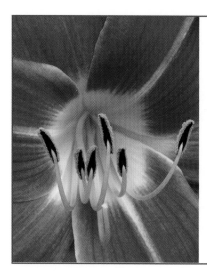

Soothing Suppository
30 ml Cacao Butter
30 ml Coconut Oil
20 drops Seabuckthron Berry
20 drops Frankincense
20 drops Tea Tree
10 drops Peppermint
Gently melt together, pop into freezer to solidify

Yoni Serum
60 ml Jojoba or Coconut Oil
10 drops Ylang
5 drops Rose Otto
20 drops Frankincense
20 drops Schizandra Berry
Combine in a glass bottle

See Chapter Fifteen, "Renegade Beauty Secrets," for more yoni care creations

are the reproductive organs of plants, and their oils are the *love liniments of nature*. Petals, sepals, stamens, and pheromones are attuned to one objective— attracting pollinators into the flower to revel in the percolating pollen. *Can that be said for petroleum?*

Distilled from the sex glands of flowers, many botanicals are aromatic aphrodisiacs, such as jasmine; just one honeyed whiff will deepen breathing and unwind the mind. Euphoric ylang and rose oils are delightfully heart-healing and tissue-toning. Frankincense is fortifying. Luscious, red schizandra berry is used in Traditional Chinese Medicine to build up body fluids. Seabuckthorn is lush in lipids and miraculous for mucous membranes.

Mix these euphoric essences into the luxurious oils of aromatic cacao, creamy coconut, and juicy jojoba to saturate tissues with deep moisture for long-lasting lubrication and to provide beneficial barriers. These oils inspire fragrant ways to consecrate the fertile crescent of your femininity. Sensually soothing, these botanicals are beautiful to use as daily yoni serums and to consecrate your love life.

Release your jouissance juice and imbibe life's sensuality, all while protecting the flora of your flower.

Take a moment to connect to the wisdom of your womb:
Close your eyes.
Feel your breath, feel life breathing you.

With each breath, drop deeper into the flower of your womb, and drop
deeper into the seat of your root chakra.
Visualize yourself bowing to the wisdom, to the supreme strength, to the
alchemy of your womb.
Bowing in reverence to the life force of this cauldron that can gestate and
bring forth life and creative fertility
Bowing to the womb from whence you came.
Acknowledging the interconnectedness of your womb as contained within
a cosmic womb, your womb as part of the creative force that moves
through the universe.
Feel life's innate wisdom, its infinite intelligence, its beauty and
benevolence,
Feel the sparkling effervescence of life in your yoni and womb.

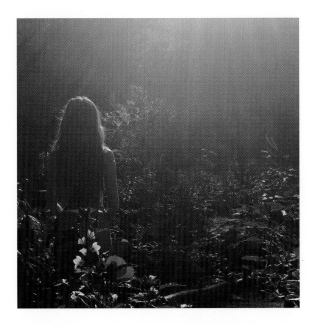

We are stardust
We are golden
And we've got to get ourselves
Back to the garden

Joni Mitchell[44]

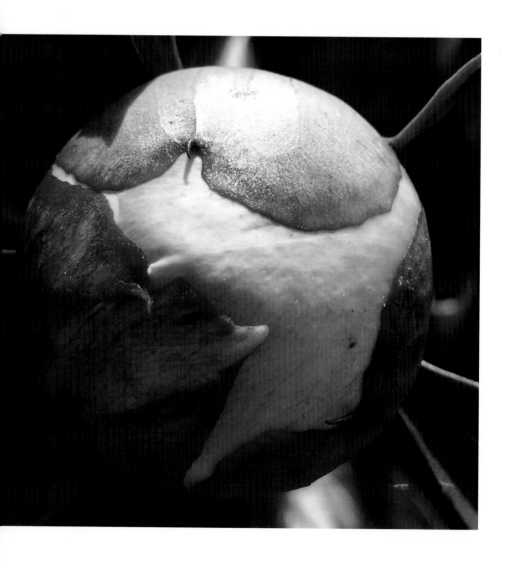

Chapter Eleven

GREAT EXPECTATIONS

Embracing the Expansion of Pregnancy

Do you remember being born?
Are you thankful for the hips that cracked?
The deep velvet of your mother, of her mother and of her mother?
Your mother is a woman, and women like her cannot be contained.

Beyoncé[1]

THE BLESSINGS OF BOTANICALS FOR PREGNANCY

When does it start, that soul that circles your heart?

Naturally, as your baby grows your belly expands, and this new soul captures your heart. Your desire to nurture and protect your little one grows, too. Increasingly thoughtful about your health and what you put on and in your body, you may now wonder how botanical oils will affect your pregnancy. Delightful and intuitive, essential oils are an unparalleled gift for our beauty, and they are life-nurturing elixirs for expectant mothers.

Many women ask me if essential oils, or if any specific oils, should be avoided during pregnancy. Aromatherapy books and bottles make sweeping disclaimers, cautioning us of the potential risks of using essential oils and extracts during pregnancy. It is true that the pure plant potency of essential oils uniquely interacts with and influences our bodies, our brains, and our cells, and this does raise interesting questions for expectant mothers:

Could essential oils disrupt the normal outcome of pregnancy?

Could they harm the baby?

It is really important to know the source of the essential oils that you use; you want to know exactly what is in that little bottle of oil. The essential oils that are readily available in the market, even those sold in health food stores, are often less than pure and true. Mass distilled for the food and perfume industry, these oils are cheaply produced and may even be imitations. It is inadvisable for safety and effectiveness for anyone to use low-quality oils. Only authentic oils that are distilled carefully from organically grown plant matter can provide the benefits of plant wisdom. Know your source.

There are hundreds of essential oils available in aromatherapy. Most of the oils are elegant and user-friendly, and only a handful of them are best avoided. With so many choices, it is easy to avoid these oils, and most of the essential oils in the avoid category are not commonly available.[2]

What about the other essential oils?

In a healthy pregnancy, a woman naturally has more of the hormone progesterone in her body than estrogen. There are a few essential oils, including clary

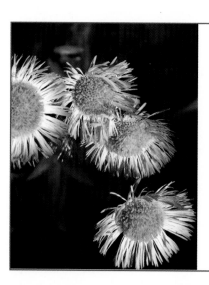

Essential Oils Best to Avoid When Pregnant

- **Mugwort**
- **Thuja**
- **Tarragon**
- **Pennyroyal**
- **Parsley leaf**
- **Parsley seed**
- **Oakmoss**
- **Savin**
- **Hyssop officinalis**—not *Hyssop decumbens*
- **Lavandula stoechas** and **Lavender cotton**
  These hybrids are quite different than classic Lavenders: *Lavendula officinalis* and *L. angustifolia* and generally not available.
- **Dalmatian Sage** and **Spanish Sage**
  These sages are unrelated to safe clary sage, salvia sclarea, and common sage, *Salvia officinalis*.

sage, anise, and fennel, that contain phytoestrogens that closely resemble the natural estrogen produced by the body. The concern raised in aromatherapy books is that there may be a chance that the oil will tip the scales toward estrogen, thereby destabilizing the delicate and perfectly calibrated balance of hormones and putting an expectant woman's body into an unwanted estrogenic phase.

Many plants have estrogenic actions, and many of these plants are common, such as potatoes and soy. It is unlikely that a doctor or midwife will request that you refrain from eating or touching potatoes while pregnant to prevent an estrogen imbalance (although I highly recommend never eating nonfermented soy). Like potatoes, the estrogenic property of essential oils is mild when used in moderation as a drop or two. Even the estrogenic oils that are on the do-not-use list in aromatherapy books are safe to use metered as a few drops. When these oils are used in moderation, you receive all of the blessings of the plant oil without creating an estrogen issue that would disrupt your pregnancy. Historically, most of the attempts to use essential oils for abortions have flopped.[3]

Another concern is that essential oils may cross from the mother's blood through the placenta and affect the baby. For a substance to cross through the placenta, its molecular weight must be under 1,000, and the molecular weight of all essential oils is well below 500.[4] So, it is best to assume that every essential oil can cross the placenta. Exposing a fetus to essential oils is only risky if specific components of some oils reach a toxic level. There is minimal data on the effects and concentrations of essential oils, or drugs for that matter, on a human embryo, because of the ethics and complications of experimenting on babies in utero.

Pregnant women who use essential oils responsibly and properly diluted—enjoying one drop, not guzzling or rubbing on half a bottle of undiluted essential oil—can continue to enjoy essential oils throughout pregnancy. Instead of worrying about specific oils (in fact, worry can be harmful to a pregnancy!), simply use oils that you are comfortable with and keep the concentration at or under 2–5 percent for a generous application, such as a full-body massage. A 2 percent dilution contains 15–20 drops of oil for every ounce of carrier base, such as organic jojoba, virgin coconut oil, and olive oil.

You can continue to enjoy all of the elixirs and creations that you employ in your daily ablutions and meditations. If you loved particular oils, such as ginger and rosemary, before you were pregnant, you can still inhale or apply the oils, or even add a single drop to culinary creations, without issue.

If you are a newcomer to the wisdom of essential oils, a reasonable approach to explore the world of botanicals is to introduce into your daily life a few drops of the well-known health-tonic oils.[5] These oils are broad spectrum and life sup-porting, and they will keep your body strong and centered throughout your pregnancy. Over time, as you try out different oils, you will develop a feel and an intuition for the oils that are best for you.

You can always start with your favorite scent; if you love rose, use rose. All essential oils are antibacterial, antifungal, and antiviral, and more impres-sively, they fortify and stimulate the immune system so that you are resistant to pathogenic bacteria and bugs. A playful and preventive use of your favorite oil throughout your pregnancy will balance your mind and spirit while reducing the odds that you will contract an illness.

Many of the plants and oils that are used in aromatherapy and aroma-medicine have cared for people and blessed their beauty for thousands of years. Below are a few simple and elegant ways you can include essential oils during pregnancy to bless your health and baby.

I see the beautiful curve of a pregnant belly
Shaped by the soul within.[6]

GRACE BELLY AND SKIN WITH BENEVOLENT BOTANICALS

Your belly is expanding with you, so it is important to keep it happy and your skin well lubricated. Lavender, neroli, frankincense, seabuckthorn, or rose oils diluted in jojoba oil are great for the skin, prevent stretch marks, and are safe to use frequently. I have made many blends of these oils for hundreds of beautiful bellies; and when they are applied early and daily, every women has been free of stretch marks.

Dry brushing is also a great practice during pregnancy; it stimulates the endocrine, circulation, immune, and detoxifying systems. For more information on dry brushing, see Chapter Seventeen.

BE A BATHING BEAUTY

Baths are a remedy of relaxation and indeed a wonderful way to drink in needed nutrients by activating the action of transdermal absorption via the skin. Quenching the skin with magnesium benefits both you and your baby in

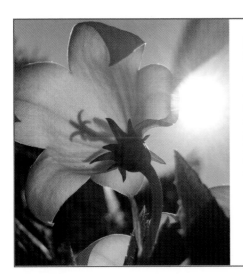

Health Tonic Essential Oils for Pregnancy and Beyond

Chamomile	Lavender
Cape Chamomile	Neroli
German Chamomile	Myrrh
Cypress	Palmarosa
Eucalyptus	Patchouli
Frankincense	Rose Otto
Geranium	Sandalwood
Ginger	Seabuckthorn
Laurel	Sweet Thyme

the belly. Much magnesium is needed during pregnancy, and this vital nutrient is often quite depleted in our modern diets. Medical opinion finds that magnesium is critical to all stages, from fertility to birth: "The evidence is clear that inadequate magnesium intake is common during pregnancy and that the plasma levels of magnesium tend to fall, especially during the first and third trimesters of pregnancy."[7] Magnesium is essential to hundreds of body interactions, including preventing early childbirth, building and healing skin tissues, effectively eliminating, normalizing blood glucose levels, and maximizing mitochondrial function. Enjoy warm baths during this blossoming time by adding a cup of magnesium salts, a cup of baking soda, and a few drops of iodine and frankincense to your bathing ablutions.

A MOTHER'S MICROBES

Microbial health is crucial before pregnancy, and a healthy proliferation of microbes is now scientifically understood to make pregnancy possible, whereas a lack of microbes makes fertility a challenge. Australian fertility specialists observed bacteria in healthy ovaries that likely travel up through the vagina. They discovered that the women with *Lactobacilli* in their ovaries had more successful rates of pregnancy. Furthermore, the women with high counts of *Lactobacilli* throughout the reproductive tract early in pregnancy were more likely to have a healthy, full-term pregnancy than women with lower counts.[8]

An expectant mother's bacterial balance has generational consequences for her offspring, potentially affecting fetus brain development via nutrient absorption and later through signaling pathways in the child's gut. A recent study correlated inflammation of the placenta to asthma.[9] This may occur if bad bacteria slip through the cervix into the uterus, causing placental inflammation and vaginosis, which increases the risk of asthma.[10]

One out of every eight American infants is born premature, which is the leading cause of infant mortality and developmental disorders.[11] Uterine infection, which usually stems from an imbalanced microbiome, is ripe grounds for premature birth. In full-term labor, an immune response in the uterus helps to expel the baby. However, if this response is triggered by invading germs earlier in the pregnancy, it may stimulate premature labor and birth. Any inflammation in the body during pregnancy can trigger labor—even gum disease.[12] In addition, the antibiotics prescribed in pregnancy to treat infections also negatively influence the diversity of the infant's (and mother's) oral and gut bacteria.

All babies receive their first anointing of beneficial bacteria for their skin and gut as they slide their way through the birth canal. As the mother's cervix dilates in preparation for delivery and as labor begins, bacteria from the birth canal coat the baby's body, enter its mouth, and are swallowed into the digestive system. This primes the baby with bacteria, which is perfect and ideal as long as there is friendly flora, not pathogens, in the birth canal. If the mother's body is not brimming with beautiful bacteria, then she cannot pass them on to her baby.

The good news is that you can reseed the vagina with friendly flora if microbial health and diversity are an issue. There is a microbial superhighway with stops along the gut, vagus nerve, and vagina, so one can course-correct with oral doses of *Lactobacillus bifidus*, fermented foods, and soil-based probiotics that increase the friendly flora in the vagina. The technology is still in development, yet soon probiotic vaginal suppositories will be available over the counter.

For cesarean deliveries, researchers have found that simply swabbing babies with the mother's vaginal microbiome fluids helps to colonize babies' bodies with the microbes they would normally receive in a vaginal birth.[13] The small study found that the swabbed babies harbored skin, gut, anal, and oral bacterial communities that were similar to those of infants that had been delivered vaginally, compared to the C-section-delivered babies who did not go through the procedure.

"It's something that, on first principles, just makes evolutionary sense," says Rob Knight, a microbiologist at the University of California, San Diego. "Until very recently, every surviving mammal that was delivered into the world was essentially coated in its mother's vaginal community."[14] This is such a simple step that parents or health practitioners can do immediately after the birth to boost and build a lifetime of better immunity.

After you have given birth, be sure to boost your bacterial bank account with extra probiotics and prebiotics. This special time requires extra flora to nourish your vaginal, breast, and body's biomes. Also, pregnancy and delivery are physically laborious, and new babies promise that moms will get less than the optimal eight hours of nightly sleep, which puts your strength and immunity at risk. Daily doses of pre- and probiotics and fermented food will supply your extra postpartum needs and keep you healthy.

GARDENING YOUR GUTS

Nausea, heartburn, and upset tummies are common occurrences during pregnancy; and probiotics, prebiotics, enzymes, and fermented foods will help with this too. The beneficial bacteria found in fermented foods, such as kimchi, and probiotics will keep your digestive system working efficiently.

Also, the carminative oils—cardamom, chamomile, coriander, peppermint, and ginger—soothe and smooth the gut and digestive tract. A single drop of any one of these oils in a glass of water, on a piece of fruit, or added to a spoonful of honey will settle your tummy.

HARNESS FLOWER POWER DURING DELIVERY

Essential oils are aromatic attendants during labor and delivery. Use a diffuser to fill the air of your birthing space with any oil that has an aroma that you like and that creates a relaxing atmosphere. Frankincense, neroli, rose otto, lavender, and chamomile are good oils for the birthing process. As a portal oil, frankincense is used to welcome us to new places and open us to transitions.

Marjoram essential oil is a potent analgesic and muscle relaxant. When I was delivering my baby, Ron, my partner, massaged a special, much-stronger 20 percent dilution of marjoram and lavender in jojoba oil onto my back, right in the pelvic region, for about an hour. It was essential to my birthing process!

Preparing the perineum is of practical importance too. Much of modern birthing has been stripped of the wisdom of women's and midwives' knowledge. Wherever and however we choose to give birth, it is important to revive much of this sage birthing body of intelligence.

Prime your petals and tone the tissues of your lady garden with the **Perineum Petal Preparer.** This loving lipid can be used daily to tone and strengthen yoni tissue and help prepare it for the passage of birth. This birthing blend keeps the delicate tissues resilient and most likely without the need for a mend. Begin to use it three months leading up to birth. Tend to the labia by applying this soothing serum topically after bathing. Also apply it with a deeper perineum massage to encourage elasticity and deep-tissue lubrication.

PRE-BIRTH YONI MASSAGE

Perineal massage can be performed individually or with a partner. If you will be serving as your own masseuse, be sure to have a mirror handy so you can become better acquainted with your perineal area.

1. Begin with clean hands. You will be massaging inside and outside your yoni, so you may want to trim your nails before the massage begins. Choose a comfortable place to recline with your legs bent and knees apart. Place the mirror between your legs, and position it so you can see the entire perineal area.

2. Place a generous amount of **Perineum Petal Preparer** on your fingers and then lubricate the entire perineal area (the entire area surrounding the vagina and anus).

3. Place both of your thumbs about one inch inside your vagina. Use the strength of your thumbs to press downward, stretching toward your rectum. Continue to gently stretch the tissue until you feel a slight discomfort. Hold the stretch for two minutes.

4. Gently move your thumbs to the sides of your vagina, keeping them inserted at least one inch. Pull the tissue, following the motion of childbirth, gently stretching the sides in a forward then downward motion. Your goal during this stretch is to imitate the movement of the baby through the birth canal, so pull the tissue in the direction of the baby's

head. Continue this stretch for three to four minutes. Gently massage the area between the vagina and anus for another one to two minutes, pressing in a downward and forward motion.

Remember to be *extremely gentle* to prevent swelling or bruising. Avoid the urinary opening during massage so that oil and any bacteria are not pushed into the urethra.

After your babe has been birthed into being, apply the **Peppermint Petal Cooler** for calm, cool relief in this area that has just expanded beyond belief. This simple blend delivers the medicine yonis need to rapidly recover and eases the body back into its daily rhythms.

A relaxed and responsible use of essential oils lets you enjoy your pregnancy with balanced health. Always trust the intelligence of your intuition and common sense as you care for your body. Your baby is the "book" and as your baby grows, your awareness of and attunement to your needs and your baby's needs will also strengthen. Let your body speak to you and guide you.

The day came when the risk to remain tight in a bud
was more painful than the risk it took to blossom.

Anaïs Nin[15]

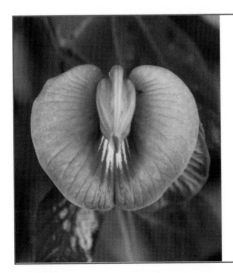

Perineum Petal Preparer
55 ml Jojoba
20 drops Seabuckthorn Berry
20 drops Frankincense
20 drops Ylang
10 drops Rose Otto

Peppermint Petal Cooler
55 ml Jojoba
5 ml Peppermint essential oil

Breast Balm
30 ml Cacao Butter
25 ml Coconut Oil
5 ml Seabuckthorn Berry

THE BIRTH AND BEING OF BABES AND THE BEGUILED CHILD

You are the bows from which your children as living arrows are sent forth.

Kahlil Gibran[16]

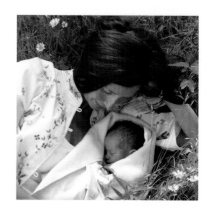

Plants and flowers brim with vigorous, ever-renewing life, and they symbiotically lend their life energy to sustain us. The life force of plant oils in aromatherapy and aroma-medicine makes them natural and wise attendants to births and babies. Following a few simple guidelines and your own intuition, essential oils will bless your birthing rite and befriend your new little one.

Before you put anything on yourself or your baby, you want to know that it is pure and really real. Issues with safety and effectiveness make it inadvisable to use low-quality essential oils. Only authentic, artisanal oils distilled carefully from organically grown plant matter can fulfill the promises of plant wisdom.

Prepping the Nest

Essential oils are natural and reliable helpers as you prepare yourself and your home for your new arrival. Diffusing the air with a natural forest of fragrance creates a welcome reception, and a few drops of tea tree oil in warm water are all you need to clean and disinfect your baby's world (starting with a drop on the baby's fresh belly button to clean it and to assist the skin to heal). You can make a spray of water and tea tree oil to wipe down any baby accoutrements.

Let Bath Time Wait

The first few precious moments after birth are a time of celebration and bonding with your baby. Try to let this moment last for hours! It is common for medical staff to whisk away the newborn for a quick bath. Washing a baby's skin immediately after birth is unnecessary and perhaps even counterproductive. Bathing lowers the baby's already falling body temperature, and infants have a very limited ability to create their own body heat in the first few hours of life. Neonatal experts urge us to let bath time wait: "Washing a baby soon after birth clearly contributes to a fall in body temperature, and for this reason it is difficult to justify this practice."[17] Instead, let your baby rest on your belly under a warm, dry blanket and let the skin contact keep the little one's body temperature up.

The *American Journal of Obstetrics and Gynecology* gives an even-stronger reason for delaying that first bath. Researchers reported that the white waxy substance, called vernix, that coats a newborn's skin is a valuable part of the infant immune system. Vernix is a wide-spectrum antimicrobial agent that protects against bacterial and fungal infections, such as B streptococcus and *E. coli*. The researchers also advised, "Delaying the bath and keeping the newborn together with his or her mother until breastfeeding is established may prevent some cases of devastating infections caused by these bacteria."[18]

Another key thing you will want to wait on is cutting the umbilical cord.[19] Most midwives know, and obstetrics is catching up to the fact, that delayed umbilical cord clamping is the way to go. When babies are carried away to clamp the cord, this delays fundamental skin-on-skin contact time for parents and their newborn bundle. Umbilical cords are also a vital source of oxygen for the baby. This is why babies can be birthed in water, as a baby's breathing reflex is activated only when it is first exposed to air. Unless there is a medical issue, it is best to wait until the cord stops pulsing; allowing for even just a few more minutes of cord connection permits more blood to flow from placenta to baby. One study demonstrated that babies born with delayed clamping also have higher iron levels and higher birth weights too.[20] There is also the more traditional lotus birth method, which follows the birthing flow of the body's design, of leaving the umbilical cord uncut until the cord naturally separates at the perfect place from the navel three to nine days after birth.

Mother Love

The days following birth are a tender time of elevated emotions, new family rhythms, and new beingness in your body. If you are a first-time mother, it is quite a trip to feel the expansion and contraction of hip bones and skin and as breasts become ripe with manna fluids produced by the body. Here are a few botanical tips to help to harmonize your new life:

- A few drops of neroli, bergamot, and frankincense oils in a diffuser or as a pillow spray will help the family ease into new rhythms and will delight the senses as you cuddle with your bundle.

- One drop of fennel oil taken internally in a glass of water or with a spoonful of honey will increase breast milk production.
- Reduce the pain, inflammation, and itching of hemorrhoids by applying the **Peppermint Petal Cooler** to the area.
- For caring for C-section scars, see the **Beloved and Benevolent Beauty Spot Treatments** in Chapter Sixteen.

Look in a clear mountain mirror—
See the Beautiful Ancient Warrior
And the divine elements
You always carry inside
That infused this universe with sacred Life
So long ago

Hafiz[21]

Breastfeeding for Baby's Immunity

When possible, breastfeeding is the best thing that you can do for your baby's health. Each drop of breast milk contains more than a million white blood cells, and it actually builds antibodies through all the years of breastfeeding. The substances in the milk shift and change along with the child's changing needs.

Breastfeeding is also of prime importance in taking care of your baby's teeth. Generally, newborns are born without teeth, yet they are already form-ing. Nutrition is key for tooth development, so make sure that Mom is getting enough of the fat-soluble vitamins A, D3, and K2 in her daily diet to pass on to baby. Tooth decay in babies and toddlers is *never* caused by breastfeeding.[22] Nighttime nursing, which has been done since the beginning of time, has never caused a cavity. However, juices are very acidic and can promote cavities, so limit nighttime drinks to breast milk and water.

Bouncy Baby Biome

Maintaining and developing the baby's microbiome are key to a lifetime of health and longevity. The first few days after birth, mucus begins to form on the lining of the baby's gut, and bacteria nestle in and grow in this warm, secure surrounding. All of these new bacteria must be fed as well.[23] Breast colostrum and milk supply unique sugars that feed the beneficial flora that aid the baby with good diges-tion and a resilient immune system. Babies who begin life without a full array of beneficial bacteria may experience reflux, gas, colic, diarrhea, pathogenic bacteria, and poor digestion, and later in life this may demonstrate as food allergies and possibly even behavioral issues.

Understandably, there are various reasons why women sometimes cannot breastfeed or continue to breastfeed. If this is the case, please do due diligence on what to feed your baby. Most infant formulas offer meager (if any) amounts of the specific sugars, polysaccharides, that feed new microflora but contain chemicals of perchlorate[24] (rocket fuel), BPA, melamine,[25] calcium chloride (classified as an irritant), cupric sulfate (a common pesticide), and ferrous sulfate (a by-product of steel, classified as a harmful irritant),[26] to name a few. Furthermore, rather than prebiotic polysaccharides to spark the baby's biome, most infant formulas are made with approximately 40–50 percent high-fructose sugars. The phytoestrogens in soy formulas are also an issue for girls and boys. A study published in *The Lancet* found that infants fed soy formulas have a blood concentration of estrogen 13,000 to 22,000 times higher than babies that are breastfed. This high amount is sufficient to exert negative biological effects on the development of girls and boys.[27] Another study linked soy-formula consumption as a baby to uterine fibroids in adult women.[28] You can give your baby's bacteria a boost by giving them teaspoons of cultured vegetable juice and diluted milk kefir, which are rich sources of prebiotics and bacteria. Also, the Weston A. Price Foundation has information on how to make baby formula at home that is more similar to breast milk than commercial formulas.[29]

When the baby is old enough to be introduced to food, you can feed softly cooked egg yolks from pasture-raised hens, which are great sources of protein and fat for good brain development as well as essential vitamins D and K2. Small amounts of ghee, raw butter, cod fish oils, and extra-virgin olive oil are also wonderful fats for babies, along with avocados, coconut pulp, and coconut oils. You can also make your own baby food by steaming organic vegetables, pureeing them, and then letting them ferment for extra microflora TLC.

Botanical Baby Care

Essential oils provide simple solutions to common childhood susceptibilities. There is a bounty of effective and easy-to-use essential oils. My favorite oils to use with babies are Roman and German chamomile, lavender, frankincense, eucalyptus, and rose otto. The general guideline for using oils on infants and young children is to keep the mixture of oils and carrier oil to a 1–2 percent dilution: 7–12 drops essential oil per ounce (2 tablespoons or 30 ml) of organic carrier oil.

There are only a handful of oils best avoided by little ones younger than two years old. These oils are: anise, citronella (which is not an authentic essential oil), clove (undiluted), laurel, lemongrass, melissa (lemon balm), oregano, savory, and pines and spruces. Avoid applying peppermint directly to an infant's skin, as it is very cooling, like an ice cube, and can unsafely lower body temperature. Use spearmint instead. As the child grows and is able to more efficiently regulate body temperature, you can start using peppermint—it is an effective first-aid essence and a pain reliever for boo-boos.

It is very important to store your temptingly pretty bottles of essential oils out of the reach of children. Essential oils are very potent! Most oils taste like a pine tree, so they are unappealing to a child's palate. Even so, for safety and ease of use, be sure to store all essential oils away from curious children, and keep them in bottles with integrated drop-dispensing lids.

Teething

Teething can often challenge a baby's immune system and may be accompanied by swollen gums, ear infections, colds, diarrhea, and irritability. Raising your little one's dietary intake of phosphorus and vitamin C can be helpful during teething (and if you are breastfeeding, raise your intake too). To relieve discomfort, massage into the cheeks and jaw one drop of chamomile or lavender essential oil diluted with one drop of jojoba oil. To calm inflammation, half a drop of organic clove and/or rose otto essential oil diluted in virgin coconut oil can be applied to the gums. These oils will also boost the child's immune system.

Congestion

Eucalyptus oil has a long history as a treatment for congestion from colds, infections, and allergies. There are two great ways to use this oil. Sprinkle a few drops of eucalyptus essential oil all over the bedsheets rather than directly on the baby. Or add a few drops to an aroma diffuser throughout the day and night. As the baby inhales, the nasal passages will open and clear so that your baby can breathe freely.

Earaches

Earaches can also be treated with eucalyptus oil. Place 1-2 drops on a cotton ball and gently insert it into the ear for a few hours. You can also massage diluted lavender around the jaw and the area behind the ear. Learn more about ear health in Chapter Seventeen.

SKINCARE

Babies' soft, delicate skin is sensitive and can be easily irritated. It is great to engage these fresh souls in the elements of water, sunshine, and fresh air and to let these liniments of nature help with your care. Except for the area of their derriere, which needs some extra tender loving care, babies do not need soap and sudsy baths. Add a little sea salt to bathwater but leave the bubbles aside. When you clean and moisturize your little one, it is vital to avoid petroleum-based products frequently marketed for babies, such as baby oil. Infants need to be cleaned, though, and essential oils can help you with that. A warm, damp cloth with a squirt of oil is the perfectly gentle, skin-microbiome-nourishing way to completely clean and care for baby's fresh skin.

Instead of soaping baby's bum, a squirt of oil on a cloth is far more effective and simply protective against diaper rashes. We cut up an old flannel sheet into squares[30] to use as wipes and used a little warm water and a squirt of jojoba oil for our derriere care. If a diaper rash occurs, let the baby have a few diaper-free hours, allowing fresh air and sunshine to be the rapid cure.

After I gave birth, the midwife advised me to keep Leif's belly button clean. I put one tiny drop of tea tree oil (widely heralded as a gentle cleaner) on his belly button, and then I put him in the warm sun for just two minutes. When the midwives returned the next day, they were amazed to find that his little belly was clean and his belly button was totally healed and formed. Normally it can take about two weeks to heal.

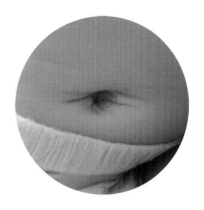

We all love a good massage, and babies do, too. Massage stimulates circulation, gets the lymph system moving, improves the immune system, and relaxes and calms baby, preparing her for deep sleep. I like jojoba oil as a massage oil, adding a little bit of lavender oil as I massage the baby's feet.

Colic

Colicky tummies are unpleasant for babies and tough on parents. A change in Mom's diet is the first step to easing colic. Try eliminating from your diet the common childhood allergens to determine which foods upset your baby's tummy. These foods are: dairy, nuts, soy, eggs, wheat, and fish. Also, you can add ginger and fennel to your diet to pass along the tummy-calming elements to baby through your breast milk. If colic continues, give the baby a teaspoon of diluted water kefir or fermented vegetable juice to give the gut microbes a boost.

In the meantime, as your diet takes effect, you can help your baby's digestion by dabbing a few drops of **Colic Calmer** on your little one's lower back and feet—places where her little wandering hands can't reach.

There are many ways to prepare for birth and just as many ways to give birth. They are not all like the birth scenes from movies like *What to Expect When You're Expecting*. I highly recommend exploring the childbirth wisdom of other cultures to glean wisdom on subjects such as: baby-carrying slings that keep babies near the heartbeat of the father and mother and offer ease of access to breast milk; multitudes of massages for mothers before, during, and after birth; and creating space for the mother and family to be reprieved from household chores for the first moon cycle as a new family. As much as childbirth is exhilarating, there is much that is exhausting; and holding the space for the

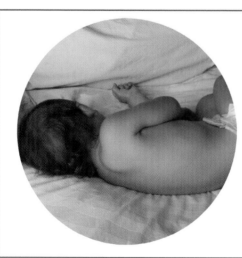

You Are My Everything Oil

For cleaning skin and massages
60 ml Jojoba
20 drops Seabuckthorn Berry
10 drops Frankincense
10 drops Lemon
10 drops Chamomile

Colic Calmer

30 ml Jojoba
2 drops Chamomile
3 drops Lavender
3 drops Cardamom
3 drops Fennel
3 drops Ginger

reception of rest in the first months creates beautiful bonding and long-term fortification for the family.

The Beguiled Child

With the birth of a new baby, you have a fresh opportunity to endow your child with a legacy of understanding of the body and the mouth. They can learn that their bodies are dynamic and regenerative.

Botanical Blessings for Bath and Bed Time

Commercial soaps, bubbles, powders, and shampoos can disrupt the delicate pH of a child's skin. Add salt and baking soda to bathing waters to cleanse and refresh body and spirit. Splashing around in a salt bath may be all young skin needs to be clean. Hair washing need not be done daily either. It may sound strange, yet we wash our son's hair only a couple of times a year, and his first hair washing was when he was three years old. By not beginning the cycle of shampooing, hair and scalp regulate their own oils, and all that is needed to refresh hair and "dust it off" is water. His hair and scalp never look unwashed, and his scalp is super healthy.

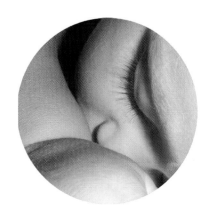

Lavender's Lullaby

Sleep is one of the sweetest elixirs for any parent, and ensuring your child is soundly slumbering helps you get yours. Sprinkle sheets, infuse bedtime baths, and diffuse with drops of lavender, tangerine, and marjoram. This quiet, comforting combination will be an aromatic lullaby for sweet sedation.

Teeth Tips

As teeth start to come in, wipe the teeth with a cloth dipped in saltwater and a tiny dash of baking soda. This will help clear plaque and neutralize acids. Teach children to swish with saltwater and spit it out, which will do most of the work. Later, brushing can begin, using salt and baking soda. At this time it is also awesome if you can teach your child how to do oil pulling, as a thorough brushing and flossing is, for any young child, practically impossible.

Around two to three years old, the permanent teeth are forming and calcifying into the jawbone. If there is a nutritional deficiency of minerals and vitamins C, D3, K2, and A at this time, the teeth that are being formed will be less resistant to decay. Include plenty of food rich in fat-soluble vitamins and minerals in the child's diet.

Childhood cavities are not inevitable. If a carie (a dark spot on the tooth) forms, this does not necessarily mean a permanent cavity is unavoidable. Brown enamel lesions can be halted and reversed from becoming a full-fledged cavity.

Healthy Teeth Tips for Children

1. Avoid bonding molars. This traps bacteria in the tooth.
2. Offer zero processed food.
3. In the beginning, stick to breast milk and water.
4. Floss when the teeth start getting close together.
5. Avoid fluoride-treated water and treatments.
6. Help ease teething with phosphorus and vitamin C.
7. Soak all grains and beans overnight before cooking to get rid of phytic acid.
8. Avoid all commercial toothpastes—stick to the basics: salt and baking soda.

Dive Deeper: For more on teeth and creating an optimal oral environment, see Chapter Eight, and refer to my book *Holistic Dental Care: The Complete Guide to Healthy Teeth and Gums.*

Responsible use of essential oils will bless you and your baby with good health. You will discover how these plant gems are handy household friends that provide restorative remedies that help keep a family's health buoyant and balanced. Always trust your intelligence and common sense as you care for your child. As your knowledge of plant botanicals grows, your intuition and attunement to your child's needs will also blossom. Let your parental intuition guide you.

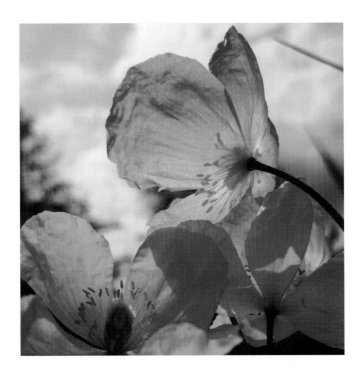

Your deepest presence is in every small contracting and expanding, the two as beautifully balanced and coordinated as birds' wings.

Rumi[31]

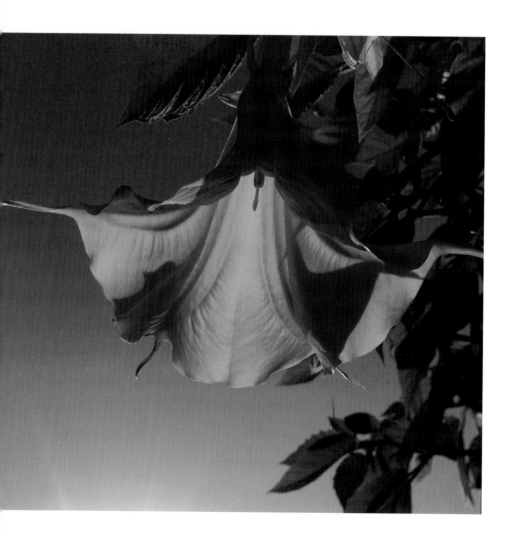

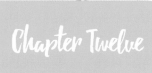

Chapter Twelve

FLORAL CONSCIOUSNESS

Perfumes are the feelings of flowers.[1]

Humankind is about to enter the floral stage of its evolutionary development.[2]

Perfume was birthed in infinite purity and from a sacred desire to connect with the botanical realms and ethereal nature of the heavens. Its origin is so pure, the very essence of life and beauty, it was devoted and purposed to purifying the body, mind, and spirit. Humans turned to aromatic unguents and oils to help us heal, mourn, worship, love, birth, meditate, celebrate, purify, comfort, and revivify. Esteemed as precious, they were offered as royal gifts and sacred libations.

Perfume. The word originates from Latin: *per* means "through" and *fumus* means "smoke." Long preceding the Latin language, perfume was one of humanity's first discoveries as ancient plants and flowers were incensed, primitively pressed, exuded in enfleurages, and extracted in alembics to collect and consecrate their sacred scented oils. Aromatic preparations perfumed the paths and baths of the many nations that weave through our recorded history. Let's take a quick redolent romp through our perfumed past:

A frankincense footpath traversed the trade routes with ancient wise men.

Myrrh from the mysterious Land of Punt was coveted by Egyptian Queen Hatshepsut.

Rose oil scented the sails that carried Cleopatra to greet Anthony.

The woman with the alabaster jar, Mary Magdalene, became the patron saint of perfumers after using her mane to shroud the feet of Jesus with soothing spikenard oil.

Poseidon's waves presented Phoenician glass bottles of perfume to Greece.

Hellenic distillers deferred to Theophrastus's "Concerning Odors," the first written perfume-mixing protocol.

Avicenna, Persian poet and physician, distilled potent perfume-pharmakons to restore his patients.

Egyptians embalmed with extracts of myrrh, galbanum, cinnamon, and cedarwood to prepare and preserve bodies for the rites of passage to the afterlife.

While invading India, Alexander the Great found himself pervaded with the fragrance of spikenard crushed out of the plants by the feet of his elephants.[3]

Caravans carrying silks and spices carved paths from China to countries desiring exotic Eastern aromatics.

Merchants of Sheba bore bottles of alabaster and boxes of chalcedony filled with aromatic extracts.

Lavish Greek banquets were replete with fluttering fragrant doves whose wings were soaked in perfume, and myrrline perfumed wines poured forth from goblets.

Roman perfumers, with the title of unguentarii, set up unctuariums[4] where alabaster vessels containing solid (hedysmata), powdered (diapasmata), and liquid (stymmata) unguents were offered.[5]

Tantalized by thyme, the Greeks perfected perfume as medicine and titled it thymiatechny.

Jasmine journeyed the seas with the Moors, riding the winds from Arabia to Europe.

Primitive perfume bottles and the oldest, large-scale essential oil distillery dating back to the Bronze Age were unearthed on Aphrodite and Queen Artemisia's island of Cyprus.

The biblical Balm of Gilead was a market commodity of Ishmaelite merchants who used the balm to baptize and eulogize.

Pauchaput (patchouli), grown by the Ganges in India, was distilled to perfume and protect exquisite shawls from moths.

Pomanders packed with aromatic offerings to inhale were popularized and prescribed in times of plagues to ensure good health.

Antibacterial plant perfumes protected medieval perfumers, distillers, and aristocrats (who balked at bathing) from the bubonic plague's Black Death.

When King Tutankhamun's tomb was excavated, hundreds of aromatic alabaster jars still containing potent fragrances were unearthed.

Fragrance-frenzy swept through fourteenth-century France, and the glorious gardens of Grasse were planted to provide plant oils.[6]

Napoleon declared, "Water, air, and cleanness are the chief articles in my pharmacy." Also, a connoisseur of cologne, he used upward of sixty bottles each month for dousing his skin and pouring into hot baths. The composition of his cologne was a refreshing accord of lemon, bergamot, rosemary, and citron essences.

Empress Josephine Bonaparte's passion for perfume required vanilla and clove extracts sent from Martinique. She grew more than 200 varieties of roses at her Malmaison estate for their essences, and her boudoir "was so saturated with musk that sixty years after her death it was still redolent of it."[7]

Fanatical for flower essences, King Louis XIV demanded a new scent daily, earning his court the label "la cour parfumée."[8]

French aristocrats had their own distilling rooms with stillroom women attendants who distilled fresh floral waters for bathing and perfumes.

Foreshadowing today's polluted perfumes, scent was scandalized in the "Affair of the Poisons" when fragrance turned fatal as a front for lethal poisons.

For scent was a brother of breath. Together with breath it entered human beings, who couldn't defend themselves against it, not if they wanted to live. And scent entered into their very core, went directly to their hearts . . . He who ruled scent ruled the hearts of men.[9]

PERFUMED PORTALS TO THE IMMORTALS

Ovid declared of frankincense, "If it is pleasing to the gods, it is no less useful to the mortals."[10]

Aromatic ethers are a bridge between material and nonmaterial realms: invisible yet influential, intangible yet molecularly tangible, unseen yet inhaled in an ephemeral form of olfactory intercourse. Our ancient ancestors knew perfumes opened pathways of communion with the 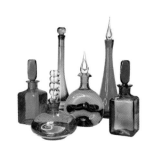 etheric realms. They altered minds, purified the times, and pleasured the senses of gods and mortals.

Aromas open a door to the soul. The presence of the gods of antiquity was sensed as emitting fragrances, and worshippers were enraptured in receiving them. Perfume preparations, indivisible from medical ointments, were consecrations of divinity made by priest-perfumer-physicians. South American shamans, called *perfumeros*, used fragrant fumigants and the perfumed juices of jungle plants as remedies. The Greeks envisioned Elysian fields to be made of hundreds of perfumes flowing with aromatic rivers and misty fragrant dew.[11]

In the Divine Commandments, Moses was directed to make altars of incenses and holy anointing oils: "Take the following fine spices: 500 shekels of liquid myrrh, half as much of fragrant cinnamon, 250 shekels of fragrant cane, 500 shekels of cassia, and a hin of olive oil. Make these into a sacred anointing oil, a fragrant blend, the work of a perfumer."[12] Egyptians perceived perfume to be the fragrance of the gods, and if wafts of aromas were sensed, the gods were present. Cleopatra had a stillroom for making fresh cosmetics, and Egyptian priests compounded perfumed preparations in temple laboratory chambers as part of their adept ecclesiastical medicinal mysteries.

Sufi mystics, in their spinning desire to become the divine not merely meet it, often described mysticism as catching a fragrance from the effable that arrives through presence and through the senses.[13] Rumi's father, Bahauddin, affirmed, "I am composed of this beauty, the attar of pressed plants, rose oil, resinous balsam: live essence, I am the intelligent juice of flowers."[14]

Our early ancestors knew aeriform aromatics were medicine for the mind and could regulate the body, alleviate pain, inspire emotions, and elevate moods. Perfumes were birthed on this planet to purify. Yet presently, fragrances are figments of their fertile floral history and filled with formaldehydes as cologne cocktails that toxify.

PERFUME'S PROVENANCE: FROM THE FLORAL PHENOMENON OF PHARMAKONS TO FRAGRANT FALLACY

Our flower-petaled scent trail hits a historical dead end in the late nineteenth century. Scientist Albert Bauer, while attempting to improve the effectiveness of TNT, noticed that the by-products of the petro-based nitrobenzene used in the explosive smelled like musk. He began chemically formulating nitro-musk or Bauer's Musk, which was quickly adopted by fragrance companies for perfumes and colognes. Laboratory accidents like this one spurred the development of a few synthetic scents: Jicky (1889), L'Heure Bleue (1912), and Shalimar (1925). And with that, perfumers abandoned plant oil to the past.

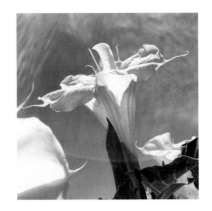

Today, the aromatic molecules used in fine perfumes, processed foods, cleaning products, air fresheners, cosmetics, and medicines are composed of laboratory-made scent molecules. Single chemicals, called isolates, are engineered to resemble the primary aromatic component found in the original source. For example, the primary aromatic component of lavender oil is linalool. Chemical and biotech engineers have discovered methods of making linalool-isolate apart from a lavender plant and divided from all of the other components of really real lavender oil.

There must be a thousand online articles about perfumes and their caustic-chemical dangers. As public awareness grows, department-store retailers and some of the big perfume manufacturers are introducing "natural" lines of perfumes to meet the public's demand for safe scents. What they consider "natural" may surprise you. Currently, fake-fragrance manufacturing falls into three categories: chemical synthesis, microbial platforms, and plant tissue cultures.

ORGANIC PERFUME? CHEMISTRY, *E. COLI,* AND CULTURE

Most department-store and drugstore perfumes are complicated formulas composed of hundreds of synthetic chemicals like phthalates, acetones, and petroleum by-products. To transform individual chemicals into one compound, they are exposed to a variety of proprietary catalysts and chemical reactions, including various enzymes, metals, extreme heat, and pressure.

The clean, fresh scent of citrus is widely used in perfumes, skincare, foods, and household cleaners. A chemical engineering company formulated a method to make barrels of citrus scent without using any citrus fruits or plant material. They make this citrus-like odorant, called citral, by joining isobutene and formaldehyde under high pressure, using metal as a catalyst. Isobutene is "cracked" from naphtha, which is a liquid mixture of petroleum. Citral can be chemically modified to produce other aromatic substances like linalool and geranial, which are single constituents of lavender and rose odor molecules.[15] The most obvious issue with citral is the use of formaldehyde, a known carcinogen, allergen, and irritant.

Hundreds of odor compounds are made synthetically like this, full of undesirable chemicals and residuals from processing. The odor compounds may lawfully be listed as "fragrance" or "perfume" on the ingredients label without mentioning any of their chemical components.

Perfume Thyself with E. Coli?

Growing public awareness of the issues with synthetic perfumes has motivated scientists and biotech firms to find a way to produce aromatics without the chemicals. Over the last few years, they have discovered a way to genetically engineer microbes (bacteria and yeast) on a large scale to produce key aromatic isolates.

Bacteria such as *Escherichia coli* and yeast like *Saccharomyces cerevisiae* (baker's yeast) are used in the process. These host microbes are used because they are easy to cultivate and grow on cheap media, and they are easy to genetically modify. The exact process used by biotech companies to develop their "microbial platform" is proprietary. In general, the process works like this: *E. coli* and *S. cerevisiae* are grown in a rich medium to encourage rapid multiplication to build the "platform."[16] *E. coli* is grown in amino acids, yeast extract, sodium chloride, distilled water, and an antibiotic. *S. cerevisiae* is grown in a similar medium with the addition of hydrochloric acid. Yes, highly corrosive hydrochloric acid.

These microbes are turned into odor-molecule factories; they are implanted with the genetic pathways that have been removed from the plants that naturally make the targeted scent. The genetic code for making the enzymes that joins all the odor molecules together is also removed from the plant and inserted into the microbe. These genetically modified (transgenic) fungi and bacteria are then fed inexpensive sugar-based agricultural and food by-products to stimulate fermentation. The result from the fermentation process is terpene, a constituent of most essential oils. The terpene is then put through another process (hydroxylation, isomerization, oxidation, reduction, or acylation) to make it into a usable substance.[17]

One example of this is Valencene Pure™ made by Isobionics. Valencene is one part of the scent compound naturally found in oranges and grapefruit and is a common base note in perfume. They claim that this trademarked product has "odor and taste similar to valencene from oranges."[18]

The odor compounds produced via microbe fermentation can be labeled in the United States as "natural" even though the compounds are produced by genetically modified organisms that are grown in antibiotics and chemicals like hydrochloric acid.[19]

Compare the contrived process of microbial fermentation with the natural scent-producing relationship between plant and bacteria. Scientists have discovered naturally occurring bacteria on vetiver roots, which are the part of the plant that is distilled for the oil. The root cells work symbiotically with the bacteria to create a complex and fragrant oil.[20] (All microbes also emit their own type of aromatic molecules that are part of the organism's communication pathway with its environment.) Naturally occurring microbes on the floral phyllosphere (phyllosphere is the microbiome of all aboveground plant parts) also influence the volatile, aromatic emissions from flowers. A group of scientists from Spain tested this by spraying a black elderberry flower with three broad-spectrum antibiotics: streptomycin, oxytetracycline (trade name Terramycin), and chloramphenicol (trade names Chloromycetin, Econochlor, and Ocu-Chlor). Afterward, they measured the floral emissions and discovered that four aromatic compounds had been suppressed by the antibiotics, and the total scent emission was reduced by two-thirds. The floral tissues were intact, so the reduction was not caused by damage to the flower. The scientists propose that the microbes living on and in the flower are responsible for producing and emitting those four missing major compounds that contribute to the overall aromatic bouquet of the elderberry flower. Without a flower's native phyllosphere, its aroma is just not the same.[21]

Petri-Dish Perfume

In the mid-1900s, university botanists began cloning plants in petri dishes using cells taken from roots and growing tips. Soon, botanists were delivering brand-new species of plants by mixing plant DNA using *in vitro* fertilization. In the 1980s, what began as an academic experiment to learn about how plants grow became a boon for horticulturists and agriculturists who adopted the plant-tissue-culture process to promote plant-species improvement as well as rare and difficult-to-propagate plant reproduction.

Biotech companies are now trying to use this technology to selectively grow the plant tissues and organs that make the desired oils. The end goal is to grow and sustain these organs in a sort of organ farm to produce industrial quantities of specific plant oils—totally separate from the rest of the plant, the dirt, fresh air, and sunshine.

Nature-Identical?

Never does nature say one thing and wisdom another.

Juvenal[22]

If your jaw is agape and you are asking, why?? Why go to all this trouble to make a scent-mimic in lieu of using the real-deal plant oils? Why invest so much time, energy, and money into a biotech-produced scent that nature effortlessly produces and graciously offers us? It seems backward, upside down!

The bottom line is the bottom line: the food and fragrance industry is looking for larger quantities of odor compounds that are cheaper than synthetic chemical fragrances and essential oils distilled from plants. Also, the industry needs a solution to the increasing economy for natural products. The marketing madness is legal, allowing laboratory-made scents to be labeled as "natural," yet I suspect that this is not quite what savvy consumers have in mind.

Microbial-platform- and plant-tissue-culture-produced scents are referred to in the industry as "nature-identical" or "bio-identical" because the chemical structures are "identical" to those produced by plants grown naturally. In fact, these products can be legally labeled as "natural" in everything from perfumes to drugs to cleaning products. Some may even be bottled up and sold as a plant's essential oils. The fragrance industry touts that these products will be pure because they will have no pesticide, herbicide, or petro-by-product residues.

If the substance is actually identical to the natural one, then why does it need the label "nature-identical"? If it were really real, wouldn't it just be called the name of the real thing instead of having a copyrighted name, such as Isonaline 70®?[23] The reality is that bio-identical isolates and fragrances are like cheap, brand-name knock-off purses sold on city sidewalks; the surface-level sameness collapses upon closer inspection. There are major differences between plant oils from nature and those made in the laboratory. For starts, laboratory fragrances will have by-products not found in nature, and they will require fuel and resources for production beyond sun, rain, and soil.

Mimicking Mother Nature's Molecules

There are numerous hitches in trying to re-create plant oils in a lab. The fragrant oils distilled from plants, called secondary metabolites, are part of a plant's defense system against pests, predators, microbes, sunburn, and drought. They are also part of the plant's reproductive system used to lure in friendly pollinators. These plant mechanisms are complex and are interconnected with metabolic challenges as well as free-radical and oxidative stress in the plant.[24] The potency and qualities of the secondary metabolites made by the plant are unique, reflecting the subtle differences in the plant's environment, influenced by the soil it grows in and even by what is growing next to it. All of these factors contribute to the exceptional qualities of pure plant oil, and they cannot be re-created in a lab.

Perfumes made with only really real essential oils are magnificently multifaceted and unequaled by anything produced in a laboratory. A true, pure essential oil is greater than the sum of its parts. Lavender essential oil is more than just linalool, which is the component that most laboratories are producing under the guise of lavender scent. True lavender oil also has traces of other compounds like α-pinene, limonene, and 1,8-cineole. All true essential oils are complex mixtures of phytochemicals and phytonutrients that work synergistically. "The property of the whole essential oil results from the limitless rearrangement and permutations of the basic components."[25] All of the trace components contribute significantly to the fragrance of the oil *and* how the fragrance affects us physiologically.

PURIFYING PERFUMES

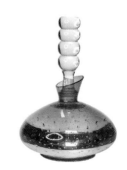

The aroma of flowers, from which we have borrowed our perfumes, while extremely powerful, has been from the beginning entirely seductive in its intentions. A rose is a rose is a rogue. Perfume, fundamentally, is the sexual attractant of flowers.[26]

While artificial and contrived perfumes affect us physiologically with sneezes, light-headedness, headaches, hormonal imbalances, and in countless other ways, pure plant perfumes silence sneezes and sniffles, ease sensitivities, cool aching heads, and fortify minds and emotions. They are immune enhancing and are the *remedy* to many synthetic-stimulated issues caused by modern-day synthetics.

Whole worlds twirl on the tip of a leaf, in the cosmos of a seed. Tendrils of petal firmament-fumes blushing with pollination-invocations emit ambrosial aromas that invite us to breathe in blooms and become one with the perfume. Pure plant distillations have been captured for eons, and these emanations are a gift to engage with as a perfume. With an ode to Kahlil Gibran, I ask, "For what is perfume but the expansion of oneself into the living ether?"

LIVING ETHER: LET PERFUME BE YOUR MEDICINE

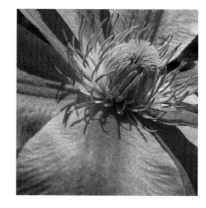

The wisdom of ancient Egyptian cosmetics, early Ayurvedic medicine, and physicians like Avicenna, Pliny the Elder, and Hippocrates knew that perfume and medicine are a blended bond of beauty and remedy. To feed the spirit is to feed the body.

It is written in the Flower Adornment Sutra (an ancient scripture that is estimated to have been written in the fourth century), "I know about all fragrances—and how they are compounded and used. I also know the sources of all fragrances. I know celestial fragrances, I know the fragrances that cure illness, I know the fragrances that remove depression, I know the fragrances that produce mundane joy, I know fragrances that incite passions, I know fragrances that produce pleasure in enjoyment of various created things . . . I also know the external appearance of these fragrances, as well as their source, production, manifestation, perfection, purification, removal, application, use, sphere of action, efficacy, nature, and root."[27]

"The fragrance always stays in the hand that gives the rose."[28] This lovely proverb eloquently expresses why as a perfume formulator, I am loyal to plant purity; the aroma from every bottle "stays on my hand." Truly, what is more grand than working with fresh exudates pressed from the pheromones of flowers, the amber ambrosias of resins, and the sweet sweat of sap gleaned from many lands? Knitting a natural mix, playing with the delicate essences born from soil, sunshine, and rain, is one of earth's most elegant endowments. To anoint a drop of floral oil or to fuse a perfume is to weave a smelling harmony between the known and the unknown. The craft of perfumery involves precision and a translation of plant breath.

To anoint yourself in natural perfume, you can easily apply a drop of a full-bodied aroma such as vetiver, rose, sandalwood, jasmine, rose, or neroli. To prepare a blended perfume, fine-tune your sense of smell with a dose of curiosity. The creation of perfumes, while an art and a science, is also a playful experience. Use these suggestions as a guide, and then abandon them as you splash and dash your way through bottles of botanicals.

When fragrance vaporizes and intermingles with life, different nuances of the scent become apparent. Throughout time, these nuances have been placed on a scent scale and called notes. This scale is divided into three categories that describe the depth of smell: top, heart, and base notes. Berries, citrus, and some flowers, smells with brightness, clarity, and sparkle, are top notes. They are the first aroma invitation to tingle your nose and the first to evaporate. The heart notes awaken the more receptive elements of the heavier base aromas and push forth the delicate strands of the top scents. Leaves, seeds, grasses, flowers, and herbs can be found in the heart note ensemble. The tenacious aromas come from full-bodied base notes that ground the bouquet. These long-lasting chords can be found in oils from resins, woods, roots, vanilla beans, and some flowers. Each essential oil, perfection in its own creation, has elements of all the notes, which take turns playing hide-and-seek with your nose. Some try to memorize which essential oil "belongs" to which note or are perplexed to read that different books put rose, for instance, as a heart note whereas other books signify rose as a base note. Concern yourself not with such parameters. Discover with your nose where rose goes. Observe the aroma—you will know where it flows and where it resonates on the scent scale. When creating with such lively plant matter that beholds diverse nuances of soil, harvest time, and distillation, allow for flexible minds and nostrils.

> *Tangerine seems to work okay for the top note. It aerates rather quickly, but it rides the jasmine and doesn't sink completely into it.*
>
> Tom Robbins[29]

Begin with an empty vessel. Let your nose dive into the unknown. Blend essential oils straight up, then dilute, or the other way around. Dilution widens and expands the weave. Concentrations are a tight knit that bequeaths. Add the essential oil nectar one by one, drop by drop, mixing, soma dripping, smelling each shift of intermingled drops. Mix your creation by rolling the capped bottle between the hands, infusing heat and energy. Record each drop for the re-creation of masterpieces and to dis-

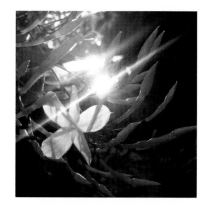

cover when your blend got too spicy or when it wholly harmonized with that last droplet of neroli. There will be communion and constant change as you blend, and as the oils blend over an hour, a dawn, or three moons.

While blending, a meditation may manifest in your mind. This is when your keen sense of smell and sensory translation come in. Blending silent stitches of simplicity, hear with your aromatic ear the drop as it splashes in the fragrant oceans. Listen to the scent. This constant communion of molecule meditation and the inner eye, above the olfactory bulb, may spark questions.

I think in synesthesia, so every aroma is a fantasia of color for me. Perfumes are painted in my mind's eye. What might you see? Colors? Shapes? Light? What is the movement of the blend? Narrow or sharp? Where does the breath journey in your body when you inhale the aroma? Are there spirals surging up and out?

Is the color cloudy? Do the pink petals need highlighting, the chamomile's blue hue and cardamom greens need widening? Would a drop of silver fir alight the interior? Would more lime heighten the rooted spikenard? Would a juicy jasmine note present a sensuality to mystify vet-iver's earthy vitality? Smell, inhale, add, adjust, and tune. Swiftly, slowly, and so on until the perfume is released, ready to have a unique union upon adornment. Uncontained, the whole aroma unfolds. Let your perfume bloom because it is the fragrance it loves.

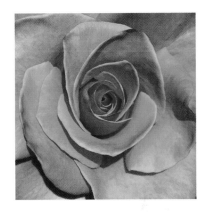

> *Why not laugh like a rose? Why not spread perfume?*
>
> Rumi[30]

UNDERARM CHARM

The scent of these arm-pits is an aroma finer than prayer.[31]

From the fragrance of flower phero-mones, we venture into the aromatic anemone of our armpits. Pheromone's etymology means "transfer of excite-ment," and these forms of hormones invisibly broadcast sexual signals. Our main transmitting messenger-molecules are the pheromones androstenol and androsterone excreted from our apo-crine glands and emitting from our armpits a musky aroma similar to that of the phytohormones found in sensual sandalwood oil.

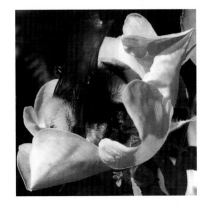

We have traveled from history's aro-matic renaissance to our current olfactory recession where we now mask our odors with an obsession for synthetic-scented confections—mere chimeras of past perfume preparations. Yet, real-to-the-feel aromatics still exist with botanicals beneficial to the bacteria of the rain forest in our pits. Why wouldn't one want the pheromones of plants to mix, meld, and enhance our aroma in lieu of synthetic aldehydes of androstenone packed in aluminum and petroleum oil?

Sweat the Small Stuff

Our "underarms are akin to lush rain forests brimming with diversity . . ."[32] Science has recently elevated the modest underarm to a unique and vital body microclimate that is part of the skin's microbiome. Its dark, warm dampness is the ideal environment for thousands of unique dermal bacteria, many of which are important for our health and immunity. Sweat is the body's precious and cooling dew of fun play, heart-pumping movement, and steamy soaks in the sauna. Some of the bacteria that thrive in the underarm feast on sweat, and one of the by-products of this banquet is our uniquely scented odor-print.

The Aphrodisiac in Your Armpit

Our sweat scent, our odor-print, is as original as our fingerprint, revealing our gender, immunity, fertility, health, and diet and diffusing our personal pheromone calling card. In the sixteenth century, long before the Age of Deodorant, people were intoxicated by the scent of a loved one moist with fresh sweat. Victorian women would hold peeled apples in their armpits until saturated with sweat, and then wrap ribbons around the apples and present them to their sweethearts to savor. Young gentlemen also learned to use their scent to attract young ladies by tucking kerchiefs in their armpits and waving these cloth scent-holders in the air near the ladies, releasing their pheromones to excite female interest.[33]

Whereas Napoleon Bonaparte begged his beloved Josephine not to bathe for three days so that he could revel in her natural aroma, the lovers' noses of today are led astray by "aromatic paranoia,"[34] conditioned by the cosmetics industry to prefer a sterilized and artificial scent over a natural scent.

> Smell is a potent wizard that transports us across thousands of miles and all the years we have lived . . . Even as I think of smells, my nose is full of scents that start awake sweet memories of summers gone and ripening fields far away.
>
> Helen Keller[35]

The Small Stuff

The armpit is an organ, cradling life-essential lymph nodes and glands. Unbefitting for an organ, the ingredients in deodorants and antiperspirants are largely formulated for corporate profit over consumer health. What's applied to the skin sinks in! In a telling article entitled "Underarm Cosmetics and Breast Cancer," the *Journal of Applied Toxicology* reported that there are "unexplained clinical observations showing a disproportionately high incidence of breast cancer in the upper outer quadrant of the breast, just the local area to which these cosmetics [deodorants/antiperspirants] are applied."[36]

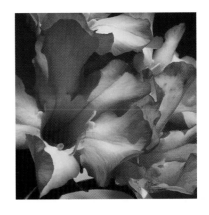

Before we spray, roll, and rub lotions and potions under our arms, perhaps we *should* sweat the small stuff by first considering the chemical substances that constitute antiperspirant deodorants. Here are the ingredients of a popular drugstore deodorant: Aluminum Zirconium Trichlorohydrex Gly, Talc, Mineral Oil, Cyclopentasiloxane, Stearyl Alcohol, C12-15 Alkyl Benzoate, PPG-14 Butyl Ether, Hydrogenated Castor Oil, Petrolatum, Phenyl Trimethicone, Cyclodextrin, Fragrance, Behenyl Alcohol.[37] How safe are these chemicals?

Touted as a safe alternative to antiperspirants, crystal deodorant stones have gained popularity over the last few years. Unbeknownst to many consumers, these crystal deodorants are made from alum, and the alum most widely used in the cosmetics industry is potassium aluminum sulfate. Aluminum, again!

Embrace the Sweetness of Your Sweat: Sweat, Smell, and Health

Sweat is a vital bodily process, and the quality of the odor of our sweat may be an indicator of health. The kidneys, liver, and gut are designed to eliminate toxins and waste products from the body. Sluggish digestion, improper hydration, as well as impaired kidney or liver function cause a backup of waste in the body that is then released in the sweat, giving it an unpleasant odor. A great first step to sweet-smelling sweat is to keep the digestive system cleared out by eating a colorful, organic whole-foods diet including probiotics and fermented food.

Also, unbalanced hormones stemming from issues with the adrenal glands may increase sweat and body odor. By passing on birth control pills and limiting your exposure to hormone-disrupting chemicals, your adrenal glands will be free to regulate the natural flow of hormones. Beware of birth control pills, because they influence a woman's olfactory system and alter preferences for mating partners. MHC genes are hidden in a man's natural odor, and usually women use these hidden scent treasures to pick partners whose MHC genes are different from their own. MHC genes are part of the immune system; so when a woman chooses a different set of genes, her children will have a more diverse MHC profile and strong immune systems. Moreover, women seem to be more sexually satisfied with MHC-dissimilar men. However, women on birth control pills tend to pick men who are MHC-similar. Scientists speculate that because the Pill causes hormonal shifts that resemble pregnancy, this urges women to surround themselves with nurturing family members, who would have similar MHC profiles.[38]

Deodorants to Odorants

Instead of masking odor or plugging sweat glands with antiperspirants, we can rely on nature's beautiful plant botanicals to charm, not harm, the underarm. Essential oils harmonize with our bodies, our sweat, our hormones, and our natural skin bacteria. Sandalwood essential oil, distilled from the inner bark of the sandalwood tree, is especially beautiful; it has an affinity for the armpit because it contains phytoandrogen, a substance similar to the androgen exuded by our armpits. Its warm scent smells beautiful on people; and unlike chemical-based, cancer-correlated deodorants, sandalwood oil contains alpha santalol and beta santalol, which make sandalwood a chemopreventive agent.[39]

Baking soda, a staple in many kitchens, is also a wonderful body freshener. Dust a clean armpit with baking soda, or tune in to your inner mixologist and make your own deodorants with the suggestions in Chapter Sixteen. Another simple solution, especially appealing for sun-lovers, is to sunbathe your pits. Sunshine is an effective bacteriostatic agent, so you can clean the armpits while raising your vitamin D intake. We can liberate our sweat from the "small stuff" and free our noses to enjoy the redolent odorants of exquisitely natural scents.

*And so he would now study perfumes, and the secrets of their manufac-
ture, distilling heavily-scented oils, and burning odorous gums from the
East. He saw that there was no mood of the mind that had not its coun-
terpart in the sensuous life, and set himself to discover their true rela-
tions, wondering what there was in frankincense that made one mystical,
and in ambergris that stirred one's passions, and in violets that woke the
memory of dead romances, and in musk that troubled the brain, and in
champak that stained the imagination; and seeking often to elaborate
a real psychology of perfumes, and to estimate the several influences
of sweet-smelling roots, and scented pollen-laden flower, of aromatic
balms, and of dark and fragrant woods, of spikenard that sickens, of hov-
enia that makes men mad, and of aloes that are said to be able to expel
melancholy from the soul.*

Oscar Wilde[40]

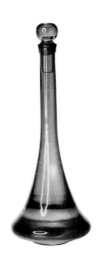

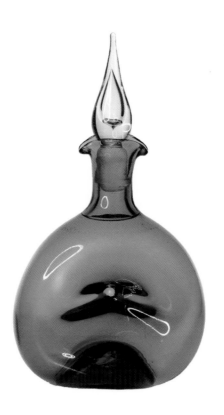

Chapter Thirteen

AROMATIC ALCHEMY FOR MODERNITY

By the time I was eighteen years old, aromatic essences brought a new dimension of delight to my life. I was bewildered by essences, by the sweet sweat of the elements. Essential oils drew me to their aromatic attention. It was an elation to be in the ambience of their aura, to create with the micro-world of a drop and transform it into a topical revelry or medicinal muse, and to paint perfumes from this palette of perfection. I was in earthly heaven. I searched and I divined for any ancient recipe I could find. In my university years, I collected every essential oil book and every rare copy of eighteenth-century perfume and alchemical-preparation books I could unearth. I had relatives in Europe comb through antique bookstores searching for treasures. When I read about rare oils, such as honey-scented immortelle, I had to find it to inhale. I was compelled to gather and to smell after reading about ancient unguents: Rhodium made of roses, Narcissinium made from narcissus, and balsamic Kyphi, which would "allay anxiety and brighten dreams."[1] I had to re-create these ancient opulent ointments to catch a whiff of what life was like. I was impelled to feel the fragrant textures that were plump with pigments and dripping with dense aromatics.

What was it about Kyphi that mystified a whole culture? What was it about these plant gems that carved new socioeconomic paths? What was the charm about combining aromatics with honey and wine?

So I gathered goods from far and wide. I melted and poured. I distilled and decanted. I mortared and pestled resins of frankincense and myrrh with galbanum's green notes and Douglas fir complete with Arabic gum to roll incense. I concocted honeyed perfumes and practical potions. I made aqua oleums and brewed medicinal balms of bergamot and ointments of osmanthus. If a plant was extinct, I searched for the modern equivalent, which led me to in-depth studies of botanical-constituent chemistry. The intimations of my spirit were stirred as I played with the poetry of plants past and present, and the ethers of my mind prayed to be infused with the scented stories written on the walls of the universe. I imagined the incensed hieroglyphs that have infused interstellar heavens, the lore and liniments of love wines, the tales of aromatic chrisms that have been consecrated, and the molecular mantras that mesmerized and tantalized the inner recesses of our minds.

One of the most fascinating figures in my studies was Avicenna, who is regarded as one of the most brilliant thinkers of all time. According to his autobiography, he studied mathematics and metaphysics as a boy, and by sixteen he began his exploration of medicine. By eighteen he was a full-fledged physician. He wrote more than 400 works, and about half of these are still in existence. He wrote poetry and materia medicas about the elements, astronomy, and more. Metaphysically, he wrote about beingness as an emanation and about untangling the differences between essence and existence. I was able to find copies of his *Canon of Medicine* and *The Book of Healing*, in which he described skilled massage techniques with aromatic oils and the virtues of hundreds of plants, including lavender and chamomile. Avicenna also invented the art of using steam distillation to capture the essence of plants as we know it today.

I consider him a founding father of cosmoetics and aroma-medicine. Through his wisdom we are further instilled with understanding that cosmetics are cosmic engagements with the elements that engage essence and existence. To have this poetic medicine man as the inventor of modern plant distillation gives depth to the metaphoric alchemy of distilling the human spirit. As humans ripen and strengthen our connection to the expanses of ether, we grow into deeper awareness that our bodies are "sacred garments"[2] for the animated élan of our souls.

Avicenna wrote much prose about roses, and he was the first to distill rosewater and rose essence from *Rosa centifolia*, which he used as a medicine in his pharmakon formulations. His distillation begins with the plant's earthly garments, the materia medica. Upon application of fire, the air element rises from the earth element, and the spirit of the plant separates from the plant dross. These airy distillate molecules become vapor and coalesce to the top of the alembic chamber, leaving all matter behind. Next, the cooling element of water invites the volatile vapors back into condensed form. The volatile vapors, having visited the spirit realm, now reconnect to life and are resurrected in liquid form. The result is the quintessence of the plant, the essential oil that embodies the captured volatile vibrations of plants. Yet bottles can barely contain them. Botanical-biotics evaporate; they escape into the air if left uncapped. Avicenna wrote, "It is in the nature of water to become transformed into earth through a predominating earthy virtue; it is in the nature of earth to become transformed into water through a predominating aqueous virtue."[3]

How did the rose ever open its heart and give to this world all its beauty? It felt the encouragement of light against its being.

Hafiz[4]

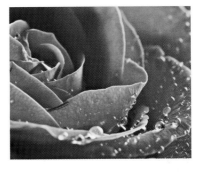

Historians tell us that perfumers and distillers had a great survival rate. Today, doctors would treat the bubonic plague with antibiotics, yet the fourteenth-century perfumers survived the plague and other diseases because they were protected by the antimicrobial plant molecules in essential oils.

Consecrated fragrant unguents were far from being perceived as a luxury or a product to cover up insecurity. It was a vital necessity in earlier eons, unlike our modern time that has relegated fragrance to the realm of masculine fantasy and feminine frivolity. The Dark Ages snuffed perfumed panacea preparations and medicants for the mind and the sensuality of the sense of smell. Although many monks and nuns, notably Saint Hildegard of Bingen, were adept botanists and herbal healers, some cultures under Christian influence experienced the church compounding this eclipse by condemning herbal healing arts as pagan pleasure. History then moved into the days of Descartes's dualism that divided the body-mind connection and considered the body a mere machine, and eventually this schism seeped its way into Western modern medicine and science.

When the age of Enlightenment blossomed with a renewed renaissance of nature's dignity and more holistic thinking, French philosopher Charles Fourier proposed that scent shaped human instinct and viewed "scent as fundamental to all existence."[5] Two centuries later, scientific research discovered that "aromatic molecules are one of the basic components of the interstellar space in which new stars are being constantly formed. This interstellar 'atmosphere' or gas is the almost direct source of the atoms of which we ourselves, along with the earth and the other planets, are made."[6]

Until the late 1800s, there was no division between plants, perfumes, and medicine. Medicine only came from plants. Botany was a branch of medicine! It wasn't until the early 1900s with the advent of synthetic chemicals that botanicals were divided off from pharmacology. This is when science started isolating active components of plants and then making synthetic mimics of them. It was then that plants lost their power, so to speak, and the pharmaceutical age was born.

The past is revisiting the present as medical research is beginning to look toward plant medicine again. The pharmaceutical industry is trying to figure out how they can piggyback synthetic drugs on essential oil molecules, because these oils are readily absorbed into the body and can quickly cross the blood–brain barrier. They offer a rapid delivery system, and because they do not linger in the body for long, they are also easy on the liver. Montaigne wisely reasoned, "Physicians might, I believe, extract greater utility from odours than they do, for I have often observed that they cause an alteration in me and work upon my spirits according to their several virtues . . ."[7]

Currently, there is a philosophical resurgence of the mind-body connection arising in part from scientific studies that have connected the gut microbiome via the super-sensory-highway of our vagus nerve as the key healer of anxiety and depression disorders. Further studies show that inhaling aromatic molecules of essential oils elevates emotions in the mental spheres by whispering to the hypothalamus to choreograph a cascade of positive neurotransmitters in the hormonal, nervous, and immune systems. For example, the psychological effect of essential oils on the nervous system in relationship to anxiety and depression was studied by Professor Paolo Rovesti of Milan University. He tested a variety of essential oils and their restorative effect on people with hysteria, anxiety, and nervous depression. He used both oral administration and inhalation. The most effective oils to alleviate anxiety were bergamot, lime, neroli, petitgrain, lavender, marjoram, violet leaf, rose, cypress, and opoponax. The oils he used for depression were lemon, orange, verbena, jasmine, ylang ylang, and sandalwood.[8]

Dr. Daniel Pénoël, a French physician proficient in medical aromatherapy, stated that "Aromatic medicine could eventually become the ecological medicine of the 21st century by balancing earth, water and atmospheric ecosystems."[9]

Essential oils protect our body, skin, and mouth much in the same way that they protect the plant against pathogens with their bacteriostatic nature. Antiquity appreciated medicinal plant virtues, and now we have gas chromatographs to map out how each essence is composed of hundreds of special substances that defy the development of bacterial resistance, encourage immunity, act as first-aid responders, and boost beauty by delivering nutrients and stimulating cells.

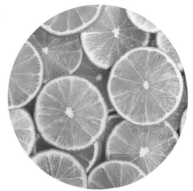

Often people think that they must imbibe an essential oil to gain benefits beyond the delight of the aroma. They think that the oils must be ingested to have a physiological effect in the body. Yet these majestic molecules can enter our beings and work their alchemy simply through inhalation.

Let's explore how essences are the perfect consecrating chrisms and botanical-biotics to attend to our bodies and mental ethers. When our inner and outer senses are drenched in the phenomena of the natural world, the natural elements are the sublime spirit food for our beings. Breathing is intertwined with smelling; the nose is a portal to the flow of known and unknown and unlocks an entrance into the brain, blood, and body. True fragrance offers a direct route to the frequencies of thoughts, and it has been used for eons as a way to open new doors of perception as aromatic molecules tickle the brain to release neurotransmitters. Volatile vibrations of odorous molecules float in the air; and when we inhale them, these molecules are swept up into the nostril, where odor molecules settle on the olfactory epithelia. This thin nasal skin contains olfactory sensory neurons that have more than twenty million odor receptors! Their journey from the olfactory epithelia to our brains is swift; the molecules pass through the cribriform plate into the olfactory cortex, which is connected to the limbic system, which influences emotions, and finally reach the hippocampus and amygdala. In the hippocampus, molecular-electrical impulses from the olfactory bulb activate hormonal activities, and neurotransmitters are released, including encephalin, endorphins, serotonin, and noradrenaline. These neurotransmitters are the lube of our internal lives. "Within the limbic system resides the regulatory mechanism of our highly explosive inner life, the secret core of our being. Here is the seat of our sexuality, the impulse of attraction and aversion, our motivation and our moods, our memory and creativity, as well as our autonomic nervous system."[10]

When consciousness rules breath, with inbreath we can smell all perfumes.[11]

Recipes for potent essences were inscribed on marble tablets in the Temple of Asclepius: "The best recipe for health is to apply sweet scents to the brain."

THE EASY ELEGANCE OF ESSENTIAL OILS

A single green sprouting thing would restore me . . .

Jane Kenyon[12]

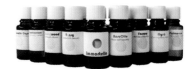

Essential oils are easy to use. Simply inhale or apply to the skin. Inhale from the bottle, a bath, a diffuser, a vapor pen, perfumes, a salt pipe, a nose-steam inhaler, housecleaning supplies, or a handkerchief. Apply neat (directly and undiluted), or use a diluted application in creams, oils, solid-perfume unguents, hair pomades, massage oils, or baths.

Diffuse the Situation

The scientific findings of forest bathing teach us that it is beneficial for people to spend time in nature. Fortunately, phytoncides and essential oils share a similar constituent—those precious terpenes. (Terpene is one of only two main components of essential oils; the other is phenylpropanoids.) Essential oils can provide forest therapy for us at home, every day, all year long regardless of the temperature or location. All essential oils are antibacterial, antimicrobial, and antifungal, and they all have a concentration of a terpene.

Forest bathe at home by filling it with these lovely, aromatic molecules by diffusing or steaming the particles into the air. Aromatic diffusers are artfully designed appliances that disperse a mist of oil into the air when combined with water. The particles of oil are so small that they stay airborne for about two hours.

Hospitals are beginning to use this scent technology to clear the air and keep staff happy. Vanderbilt University Medical Center's emergency department took the lead in forming an aromatherapy pilot program aimed at lowering the staff's stress, increasing energy levels, and minimizing the typical hospital smell. They began to diffuse oils throughout the department to naturally clean the air of microbes, bacteria, mold, and viruses and to fill their wing with refreshing and relaxing scents.[13] A survey answered by one hundred members of the hospital staff, both thirty

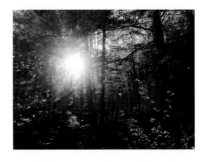

days before the program's launch and thirty days after, produced persuasive results: stress levels dropped to 3 percent, frustration dropped to 6 percent, and tiredness dropped to 13 percent after breathing diffused oils for a month.

Thrilled with how they felt at work, some of the hospital staff began diffusing oils at home, and the hospital administration is working through the protocol of diffusing oils in patient rooms to bolster patient health.[14]

Seven Methods of Inhaling Essential Oils

1. Shower: Add 2-3 drops of an essential oil to the bottom of the shower, and let the hot water disperse the aroma.

2. Aroma diffuser: Ultrasonic vibrations release microparticles of essential oils into the air.

3. Stove-top: Simmer a pot of water on the stove, and add a few drops of your preferred essential oil.

4. Fabric: Place a drop or two of an essential oil on a handkerchief, on your pillow at night, or on a cool, damp cloth, and drape the cloth over or near your face for a few minutes as you inhale.

5. Straight from the bottle, a salt pipe, or a vapor pen: Open the bottle, or inhale from the salt pipe or vapor pen, and take a whiff.

Steam Clean

Steam inhalation of essential oils is a more direct method of receiving the oils, and it gets the plant powers deep into the body. Simply bring a pot of water to boil, add a few drops of essential oil or a blend of oils, and lean over the steam with a towel draped over your head and shoulders to create a cloud of steam. Keep eyes closed, and breathe deeply through your nose and then your mouth for about ten minutes. You can also add a few drops of the oils to a hot bath or a steamy shower and take deep breaths. For a longer therapy session, especially to relieve congestion, run a steam vaporizer with a few drops of oil in a small room with the doors and windows closed.

To Dilute or Use Neat

Neat means "straight up" and undiluted. There are times when a little dab will do, and you will want to use a drop of undiluted essential oil. Examples of when you might want to use a drop neat are: zits, blemishes, cuts, scars, burns (peppermint and lavender), a mosquito bite, and as a perfume (a drop of jasmine or rose on your wrists, or hair). Otherwise, the plant potency of essential oils is best diluted in an organic, fresh-pressed carrier oil of jojoba, olive, coconut, cacao butter, rosehip, castor, tamanu, seabuckthorn, sandalwood nut, camellia, or red raspberry seed. (See the "Cosmoetic Materia Medica" in Chapter Fifteen for descriptions.) For liquid perfumes, use jojoba or organic vodka to dilute. Look for practical first-aid tips, blends for topical treatments, perfumes, dilution rates, and more in Chapter Sixteen.

Ingesting and the Culinary Use of Essential Oils

Across Europe and India and in many cultures throughout Asia, it is a popular and ancient practice to ingest essential oils and use them internally. Doctors and other medical practitioners in those countries often prescribe the ingestion of essential oils to heal or manage health issues and to bolster immunity. In the United States, as well as in most of North America, essential oils are less well known, so people shy away from that practice. Honestly, it is best to avoid eating (and applying) the low-quality, mass-produced essential oils that are sold by some health food stores and multilevel marketers.

Essential oils are under the purview of the FDA as food items, and it maintains mountains of regulations for the internal use of oils. Among those regulations, the FDA keeps a list of essential oils that are labeled Generally Recognized as Safe (GRAS). The GRAS label is granted to an essential oil by the FDA if it is "generally recognized, among qualified experts, as having been adequately shown to be safe under the conditions of its intended use. . . ."[15] The food and flavor industry adds the essential oils of bergamot, peppermint, and vanilla to boost the taste and aroma of juices, liqueurs, teas, candies, and many food items. The health-supplements industry uses the supercritical extracts of many herbs and plants in pills and capsules, including seabuckthorn berry, oregano, saw palmetto, and basil.

If you are going to ingest essential oils, it is important to plan for potency. Most really real, pure, and organic steam-distilled essential oils are safe to ingest (including some newer distillations left off the GRAS list), and many of them are distilled from common culinary items such as oranges, ginger, peppermint, cardamom, turmeric, rosemary, coffee, coriander, rose, chamomile, lemon, juniper berries, and many more. The key difference between eating the whole food and ingesting its essential oil is potency. Essential oils are powerfully potent, concentrated plant energy! For example, the aromatic molecules of sixty roses must be distilled to make one single drop of rose essential oil.

For clarity, let us compare this with coffee drinking. Drinking a cup of coffee is enjoyable. Drinking a pot of coffee is probably imprudent though. Similarly, imbibing a reasonable amount of an essential oil can be enjoyable, healthy, and safe, though guzzling a whole bottle is ill-considered. Wise use of oils follows the less-is-more principle, because the full botanical blessing is encompassed in just one drop. One single drop of oil is a dose or serving, and the daily allowance is 10 drops (0.5 ml) of an oil. It is also a best practice to mix the drop of essential oil with organic honey, olive oil, or coconut oil. When adding a drop of essential oil to a culinary creation, add one drop per portion and do so just before serving when possible.

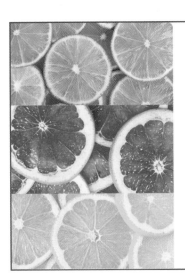

GRAS Essential Oils for Culinary Creations
If the essential oil is 100% authentic, pure and organic:

All Spice,	Fennel,	Nutmeg,
Angelica,	Frankincense,	Palmarosa,
Basil, Bergamot,	Grapefruit,	PaloSanot,
Blood Orange,	Geranium,	Peppermine,
Black Pepper,	Greenland Moss,	Petitgrain,
Black Cumin,	Hyssop,	Pine, Ravensara,
Cumin,	Immortelle,	Rose Otto,
Cardamom,	Juniper,	Rosemary, Sage,
Carrot Seed,	Lavender,	Seabuckthorn,
Chamoile,	Lemon,	Schizandra,
Cape Chamomile,	Lemongrass,	Spearmint,
German Chamomile,	Lime, Laurel,	Spruce, Tangerine,
Clary Sage,	Manuka,	Tea Tree,
Clove,	Marjoram,	Sweet Thyme,
Coffee Bean,	Mastic, Melissa,	Turmeric, Vanilla,
Coriander,	Musk Mallow,	Verbena, Yarrow,
Cypress,	Myrrh, Neroli,	Ylang
Eucalyptus,		

And, always dilute these 'hot' essential oils:
Cinnamon Bark, Oregano, Clove, Ginger, and Thyme

Let Your Nose and Intuition Be Your Guide

Adopting essential oils into daily life is easy. Be playful and curious, and have fun with these cherished treasures. As you welcome botanical elegance into your life, let your nose and your intuition guide you. Your nose knows what it likes and what is really real. When it comes to your health and your body, always be guided by the intelligence of your intuition. If your intuition inspires you to use essential oils and you feel that it will benefit your health, give it a try. The best essential oil to use is often the one you have on hand.

BATHING BEAUTY: SOAKING IT ALL IN

Bathing is always a beautiful moment for engaging with the element of water and refreshing our spirit and skin. Beyond soaking in the wisdom of water, baths are also a watery way to let the skin drink in the transdermal medicine of botanical-biotics, clays, apple cider vinegar, magnesium, vitamin C, iodine, baking soda, sea salt, and the finest frankincense followed by an anointing of botanical oils as a simple way to allow the water element to wash, refresh, and restore. (For descriptions of these beneficial bathing ingredients, see the "Cosmoetic Materia Medica" in Chapter Fifteen.)

As we move away from the days of soaking in synthetic suds, coal-tar derivatives, and chemical bath additives, we can keep bathing real to the feel and marinade our "moist envelope" in revitalizing remedies. Let your bath be your medicine. We can harness the power of transdermal absorption best in the bath. Our skin covers the entire surface area of the body, between 1 and 2 square meters (11–20 square feet), and every square centimeter has 40–70 hair follicles and 200–250 sweat ducts. At any one point, the skin is receiving about one-third of the circulating blood. This makes our skin an amazing absorptive canvas for quenching in the benefits of minerals and botanicals by bathing.

The unique properties of essential oils allow them to quickly and easily absorb deeply into the skin while boosting the vitality of our skin cells. Transdermal absorption of essential oil molecules is complex; yet simply put, their lipophilic components bypass the barrier properties of the skin and within minutes can be measured in blood circulation.

My esteemed bathing essential oil options are neroli, rose otto, frankincense, cardamom, marjoram, laurel, yarrow, bergamot, Douglas fir, chamomile, eucalyptus, and geranium.

Nature is the best physician.

Hippocrates[16]

Ancient Baths

The ancient Greeks and Romans thought highly of the skin; their legendary baths are monuments to the importance of skincare for good health. Bathing in these cultures was both medicinal and an important social, communal event.

Sweat baths were built in domed rooms heated by rocks in a fire. The rocks were lifted out of the fire to the middle of the room, and water was poured over them to create the steam. The Greeks and Romans were no strangers to the therapeutic use of botanical oils, and laurel leaves and needles from firs and junipers were placed on the hot rocks, or they received massages in the unctuarium chambers that supplied alabaster jars of aromatic unguents for healing and cleaning the skin.

The very first stop for a bather was the strigiling bath. A strigil is a curved, metal spoon-like tool that was coated in oil and brushed across every inch of skin to clean the skin and stimulate blood flow in preparation for the 100+ degrees Fahrenheit, 100 percent humidity hot sauna and bath. The bathing ritual continued with soaks in invigoratingly hot and frigid pools.

Hippocrates, the Father of Modern Medicine, is also the father of medicinal bathing. In *On Airs, Waters, and Places*, he wrote prolifically on the effects and benefits of different mineral and clay baths. When the body is immersed in the baths, the skin can absorb the precious minerals. The ancient Greeks used therapeutic baths employing clays, mud, salts, botanical oils, and herbal infusions.[17]

Bathing Tools

Gua sha and dry brushing can easily be used as present day techniques to attend to the skin's cleansing and resiliency. Dry brushing, a contemporary interpretation of strigiling, involves coating a brush with a drop of botanical oil and very gently brushing the skin, always moving in the direction of the heart. This simple and invigorating ritual before a bath or shower exfoliates the skin and supports a healthy overall immune response by stimulating the lymph system and

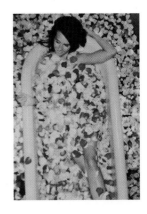

improving circulation. See Chapter Seventeen for more details on dry brushing and the lymph system.

Gua sha is the traditional Chinese therapy of skin scraping using smooth tools made of jade, polished wood, or ox horn.[18] Gua means "to rub" and *sha* is the reddening of the skin after the treatment. Gua sha relieves pain and stiffness, promotes mobility, conditions the skin, and improves normal blood circulation to the muscles and tissues being scraped.

Zhang Fengkui, a physician in the Ming dynasty, believed that illness enters the body through the mouth, nose, and skin pores and that the illness gets more and more dangerous the deeper in the body it goes. He proposed scraping the appropriate meridian point on the skin until it turned red. The skin of ill or injured areas of the body was repeatedly scraped and rubbed to stimulate blood circulation, enhance the qi, and invigorate the immune system. A hot water or steam bath followed the scraping. Through the scraping and then sweating, the toxins were eliminated and health returned.[19]

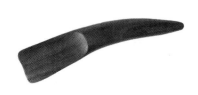

I like to use the gua sha skin tool by applying a botanical oil (such as one of the **Renegade Beauty Realms All Over Oils** in Chapter Sixteen) to my body after a quick hot shower or sauna. Then I run the wooden tool over my freshly oiled skin (similar to dry brushing but with a smooth tool) for a deeper clean. I then jump in the lake or back in the bath followed by another anointing of oil, which is lovely to do in the sun.

Air Baths

Surround your cells in airy atmospheres as you bare your skin to affair with fresh air. It is a super, simple endeavor, yet a revitalizer of nerves, skin, and spirit. "Air is considered by us as a *sine qua non* to restoration. It is so refreshing, so recuperative, so calculated to restore the body to healthful conditions, and so easily obtained, as to leave those who forbear to use it for the benefit of the sick without justification."[20]

Spring and fall have the perfect weather for this air feast. In the winter, pull up a chair and open the windows. In summer months, spritz bare skin with spring, frankincense, or rose waters for a refreshing tonic effect. As we are most often clothed, it is important to stimulate the skin's respiration system. Air bathing boosts the body's ability to shed metabolic waste, as the breeze stimulates the contracting and dilating of the skin's capillaries. Known as the "atmospheric cure," it was astutely noted that "one cannot take a sun-bath or light-bath without also receiving an air-bath, but the air-bath may be taken in one's own room, or in the darkness of night. It does not depend on the presence of light. It consists simply in exposing the nude body to the air."[21]

Earth Baths

Playing in the mud is fun! If your last memory of being covered in clay is several decades old, perhaps it is time to get muddy again! Clay bathing can be healthy and therapeutic due to the high mineral content of mud and the prolonged warmth it provides. Researchers have found that the application of warm mud—real mud—can improve skin problems, reduce inflammation, and ease burns and stings.

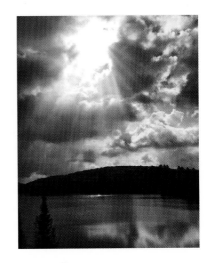

High-dose clay baths with two pounds of mud and an extended two-hour soak can be very beneficial for drawing toxins from the body, especially with the addition of the essential oils of coriander, chamomile, and marjoram.

Alternately, you can cake on the clay, lie on the earth, and bask in the sun. If you feel like staying dry, simply lie on the earth, ground into the healing pulse of the planet, and inhale all that the earth has to offer.

Forest Baths

Bathe yourself in the healing and uplifting essences of trees. Take a hike or add essential oils of black spruce, pine, cypress, juniper, eucalyptus, balsam, silver fir, and Douglas fir to your bath to transport yourself to a leisurely walk in the woods.

Hot-Spring Baths

Slipping into a hot spring is one of life's truly languid luxuries. Soaking in a mineral-rich hot spring, which is a natural pool of hot water heated by geothermal heat from the earth, is abundantly therapeutic. Whole vacations can be formed around soaking in springs, a popular pastime for therapeutic purposes as naturally warm and hot water can have a very high mineral content that itself is healing as well as boosting the water's buoyancy. Mimic mineral-rich hot springs at home, where you can create a cauldron of relaxation by adding magnesium, clay, Douglas fir, or pine essential oils to hot baths.

Moon Baths

Luminous moon rays reflect the light of the sun and shower it upon earth. Moon bathing in these reflected rays is a calming cosmic pursuit that offers infusions of gentle, yin energy to balance the yang energy of direct sun rays. It inspires relaxation, creativity, and intuition. Bright moon days, the period of waxing lunar days, are the optimal times for moon bathing. Anoint your brow and under your nostrils with frankincense. Relax, breathe deeply, and soak in the stars, trusting in life and knowing that we are also stardust.

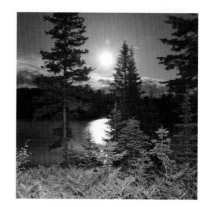

Medicine Baths

The foundation of a medicinal bath is the dynamic duo of magnesium and baking soda. Bathing in sodium bicarbonate is an excellent way to raise levels of bicarbonate in the body (bicarbonate is a biological component in the body), neutralize lactic acid in muscles, and boost alkalinity. When baking soda is combined with magnesium salts, we also absorb much-needed magnesium into our skin and cells.

Medicinal baths are replete with double doses (two to four cups) of magnesium and baking soda combined with 5 drops of an essential oil (depending on what emotional and health issues are being elevated), and 20 drops of Lugol's or nascent iodine as the base. To this, one can add sea salt, clay, or a Bubbly Bath Balm (see below).

Saunas

Sweating in a sauna is great for health. Traditional saunas use convection heat, and far-infrared saunas use infrared light to generate heat. As the temperature of your body increases, circulation in the skin goes up as blood vessels open up, and so blood pressure drops. The heat eases joint and muscle stiffness, and the body relaxes, so stress goes down. As our skin is our largest organ of elimination, saunas are an excellent way to sweat the small stuff, heavy metals and toxins, out.

Sitz Baths

Therapeutic sitz baths, also known as hip baths, are shallow baths where one is submerged in water up to hip level. This type of bathing was popularized in Europe as a therapeutic bath for discomfort and infections below the hips. It is beneficial for constipation, hemorrhoids, and fissures, as well as yeast, vaginal, urinary, penile, and prostate infections.

Sitz-bath ingredients for easing infections include baking soda, sea salt, apple cider vinegar, iodine, and the essential oils of frankincense, tea tree, and cypress.

Sunbaths

Baths of water are good, baths of air are better, baths of light are best.[22] Luxuriate in the warm rays of the sun. The sun blesses our skin with vitamin D, regulates our circadian rhythms, and stimulates production of sleep-inducing melanin. Oil up your body with botanicals, and let the sun shine in. See Chapter Seven to discover how to wisely imbibe the sun's warm wavelengths.

From this experience I emerged whole and clean, bitten to the bone by sun, washed pure by the icy sharpness of salt water, dried and bleached to the smooth tranquility that comes from dwelling among primal things.[23]

Water Baths

Popular in nineteenth-century Europe, water bathing was seen as curative, and spas that centered on water as a therapy (hydrotherapy) popularized sitz, epsom, mineral, and sulfur baths. This type of thermal healing was even prescribed by doctors at the time. The bath that was deemed to be the top tonic was the cold bath. Its virtues were extolled by Finnish naturopath Dr. Paavo Airola as stimulating to the glandular, immune,

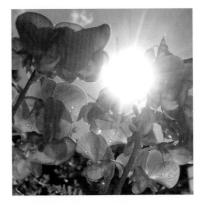

circulatory, and digestive systems as well as reawakening the flow of life force and increasing oxygen intake to the tissues.[24]

Cold baths and showers combined with breathing methods are currently taught by "The Iceman," Wim Hof, who encourages this therapy for people to build physical and emotional resilience. His methods successfully elevate mood, balance hormones, heal ailments, build strength, and improve sleep. You don't have to break the world record of standing in ice for more than an hour, or climbing Mount Everest in just shoes and shorts, like he did, yet you can partake in the Tummo-style breathing method that awakens inner warmth, and you can feel the power of a cold shower to get the benefit of this true tonic that revives body and spirit. Cool and cold water baths are exhilarating and stimulating. They can really get the heart racing! Cooler water can reduce skin inflammation and slightly lower body temperature.

Hot baths are muscle-relaxing, itch-reducing, and soul-soothing periods of privacy and introspection. Cold baths are inflammation reducing and a tonic to muscles and skin. Alternating between hot and cold water baths or showers is super invigorating to the circulatory and lymph systems.

Hot water raises the body temperature slightly and induces a healthy sweat. It is very relaxing and analgesic to sore, tired muscles and joints. Hot water can also speed up the healing of abscesses or skin irritation by bringing the infection to the skin's surface or diluting the toxin (such as poison ivy) via osmosis. "There must be quite a few things a hot bath won't cure, but I don't know many of them."[25]

The best is bathing in the fresh water of pure ponds, loquacious lakes, refreshing rivers, and in the expanse of the ocean. Going from sun, air, and earth baths into welcoming waters is luxurious. And, if you can add a warm-water source to that experience, such as a hot spring by a river, or a hot tub by a lake, and go back and forth between hot and cold, complete with dry brushing and body oiling, then that is a day in nature spa nirvana!

Thoreau basked in the spa of summer in Walden Pond: "I got up early and bathed in the pond; that was a religious exercise, and one of the best things that I did. They say that characters were engraven on the bathing tub of King Tchingthang to this effect: 'Renew thyself completely each day; do it again, and again, and forever again.' I can understand that. Morning brings back the heroic ages."[26] And I can understand that too: my favorite way to start the day is a sunbath while I drink in chlorophyll-infused spring water and work up a sweat, then a refreshing swim in the lake, followed by anointing opulent oils as I bask in the sun once again.

I find a bath meditative and usually prepare myself for the day in this manner.

Tom Ford[27]

Bubbly Bath Balms

Baking soda is an essential ingredient of any bathroom cabinet; and when it is mixed with vitamin C (ascorbic acid), fizzy bubbles of carbon dioxide are made. This fizz makes bath time fun, *and* these carbonated bubbles break down the sodium bicarbonate into tiny bubbles, which makes the CO_2 exponentially more bioavailable and permeable through cell membranes—and this is a good thing!

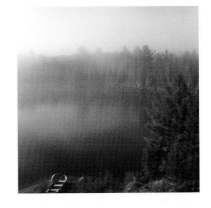

Bubbly CO_2 bathing was popularized in European water spas, as it is relaxing to blood pressure, improves blood flow, soothes kidneys, and shifts the body's pH to a more alkaline state.

FRANKINCENSE FIZZ FORTIFYING BATH BALMS

Therapeutic and strengthening for medicinal baths.

2 cups Baking Soda

20 drops Frankincense essential oil

10 drops Laurel essential oil

10 drops Blue Tansy essential oil

1 tablespoon Clay

1 tablespoon organic Jojoba, Olive, or Coconut oils

1 spritz bottle of pure water (any size will do)

Molds for the balms: muffin tins, silicone ice-cube trays, or chocolate molds[28]

BUBBLY BERGAMOT BLISS BATH BALMS

Bubbly bliss for children, before bedtime, and for relaxation.

  1 cup Vitamin C (ascorbic acid)

  2 cups Baking Soda

  20 drops Bergamot essential oil

  10 drops Ylang essential oil

  10 drops Lavender essential oil

  1 tablespoon organic Jojoba, Olive, or Coconut oils

  1 spritz bottle of pure water (any size will do)

  Molds for the balms: muffin tins, silicone ice-cube trays, or chocolate molds

MIXING INSTRUCTIONS

Thoroughly mix together baking soda and ascorbic acid in a bowl.

Add the essential oils to the tablespoon of carrier oil. Add this combo to the bowl, and mix together quickly before the mixture starts to fizz.

Spray water onto the mixture a mist at a time and continue mixing. Achieve a consistency where the combination is still crumbly yet able to hold its shape when pressed into the palm of your hand. Pack the mix firmly into the molds.

Allow the balms to dry for a couple of hours in a warm, dry place, away from sunlight.

Enjoy within a month for a full fizz effect. They will not go rancid, only lose their fizz.

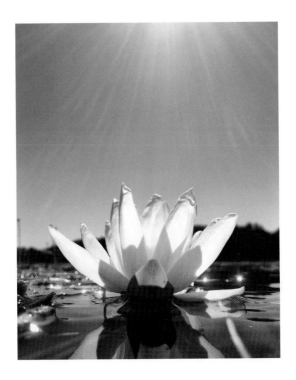

Those virgin lilies, all the night
Bathing their beauties in the lake,
That they may rise more fresh and bright,
When their beloved sun's awake.[29]

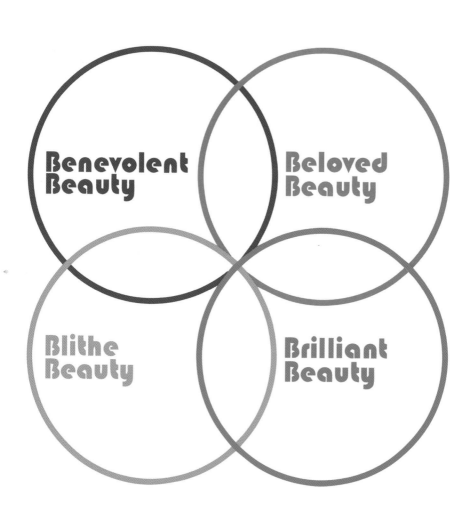

Chapter Fourteen

THE RENEGADE BEAUTY REALMS

Renegade Beauty Realms are unique spheres that invite you into effortless *elationship* with your skin and bare the essence of your innate beauty. Each sphere describes how the skin engages with the elements and unveils the botanicals that bring balance to *your* moist envelope.

Our journey through the realms includes a tour of synthetic formulations, to a fresh new world of innovative blueprints in beauty products and staples to stock in your Renegade Beauty Apothecary. Chapter Fifteen, "Renegade Beauty Secrets," is a carefully curated list and description of botanical oils for a well-appointed apothecary. Chapter Sixteen, "Renegade Beauty Recipes," shares simple DIY formulas to lovingly attend to your body from head to toe. Chapter Seventeen, "Renegade Beauty Solutions," is your go-to guide for wholesome and whole-body self-care strategies. Chapter Eighteen, "Being Beauty," offers you a glowing invocation to feel beautiful in the skin you are in.

SKIN TYPE HYPE AND RENEGADE REALMS

Modern-day skincare regimes can feel like a confession of the skin's transgression: hormonal skin around the chin, an oily T-zone, sensitive skin, or acne-prone skin. Skin type hype promises that every pore will be restored to the mecca of normal by careful compliance with set products and multistep programs.

Bottles of chemical cleansers, harsh exfoliators, drying alcoholic toners, microbiome-disturbing moisturizers, and solvent masks labeled for skin types clutter many bathrooms. These twice-a-day, multistep skincare regimes are heavily marketed, highly synthetic, and hyped on the false premise of skin type. Perhaps you may have noticed that regardless of how closely you follow the prescribed regimen, your skin less than flowers into balanced, healthy skin.

If you feel some insecurity or dissatisfaction about your skin, know that industrialized cosmetics use classifications to market to your worries. Dermatology, the science of skin, has no standard objective measure of "skin type." Skin type classifications (dry, normal, sensitive, combination, oily, and acne-prone) are mere constructs of cosmetics manufacturers. They are marketing tactics, an advertiser's dream of industrialized hygiene, to sell products—products that often cause the issues they claim to resolve.

You do not need to identify, categorize, or label your skin type. Bust free from all that renders skin sensitive and unstable: aggressive, synthetic skincare products, out-of-balance hormones, deficient nutrition, and inefficient digestion. Beautiful skin is the perfect poise of what you put on it and what you put in you. Once you are feeding the internal and the external with fulsome foods and liquids with life force, your skin will strengthen and glow with resilience and radiance.

Busting through skin type hype and rigid skincare regimes, the Renegade Beauty Realms explore a new paradigm of engaging with botanicals for beauty care and replenishing our beings with our self-renewing systems. Beauty culminates in the millions of tiny cells and bacteria in our bodies, and these Renegade Beauty Realms are your invitation to imbibe the elemental libations of cellular rejuvenation.

FROM FORMULAIC FORMULAS TO RENEGADE BEAUTY BLUEPRINTS

"100 percent natural" can be 100 percent unnatural.[1] "100 percent pure" is a hollow term devoid of meaning.[2] "Certified organic" skincare only has to be 70 percent organic.[3] Methylparaben in organic skincare? No problem! Therapeutic grade,[4] noncomedogenic,[5] and hypoallergenic[6] are the meaningless mantras of branding. So what constitutes the insides of the bottles upon bottles that promise the fountain of youth? There are four main categories of ingredients that are used in modern bodycare manufacturing: preservatives, emulsifiers, surfactants, and emollients.

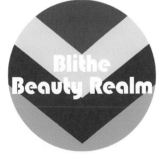

This realm belongs to the resiliency of water. Clear, cool, and refreshing like diving into a lake, feeling snow, and sipping spring water. Blithe Beauty botanicals bestow comforting calm on red, reactive, itchy skin bringing to balance irritation and inflammation.
"Beauty is a light in the heart."
Khalil Glbran

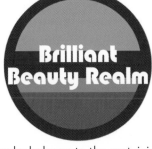

This realm belongs to the sustaining soil of the earth element. Revivifying and resetting like lying on the earth and forest bathing in the fall. Brilliant Beauty botanicals profoundly purify pores and clarify complexions.
"If you have good thoughts they will shine out of your face like sunbeams and you will always look lovely." Roald Dahl

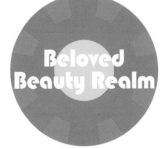

This realm belongs to the wise wavelengths of the sun's replenishing solar rays. Regenerative and restoring like rejoicing in summer's sunshine. Beloved Beauty botanicals beckon to the innate wisdom of the skin, defying dryness and reigniting rosy blooms in venerable skin.
"What was said to the rose that made it open was sold to me here in my chest." Rumi

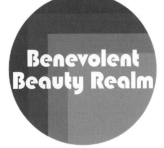

This realm belongs to the gentle grace of airy atmospheres. Smoothing, sealing, and healing like a balmy, spring breeze. Benevolent Beauty botanicals harmonize hyperpigmentation, soothe sensitivity, and even skin tone.
"For in the dew of little things the heart finds its morning and is refreshed." Khalil Glbran

Preservatives extend the shelf life of water-based products and oxidative ingredients by exterminating bacteria in the bottle as well as the beneficial bacteria of our biome. Synthetic preservatives range from parabens to isopropyl alcohols and can alter the pH of skin. They are severely drying, disrupt the endocrine system, mutate microbes, and disturb the beneficial bacteria's food supply.

Synthetic emulsifiers join emollients (oils) to aqueous solutions (water). Ranging from propylene glycol to polysorbates, these chemicals leave an invisible residue that irritates the balance of the stratum corneum, acid mantle, and hydro-lipid barrier along with disturbing the microbiome. Sudsy surfactants (anionic, cationic, amphoteric, and nonionic), from sodium lauryl sulfates to cocamide DEA, have been scientifically stated to insert microscopic particles into pores[7] and agitate the acid mantle. As a surfactants' role is to break down oils and fats, you can imagine what long-term use of chemical surfactants does to aggravate our skin's sebum and dry out our hydro-lipid layer, hence the need for humectants and emollients. . . . Emollients, from petroleum to polymers to silicone to soy, add in moisture, yet this range of lubrication imbalances our skin's flora-nation, causes inflammation, blocks respiration, and plugs pores.

Learn to recognize the counterfeit coins
That may buy you just a moment of pleasure,
But then drag you down for days

Hafiz[8]

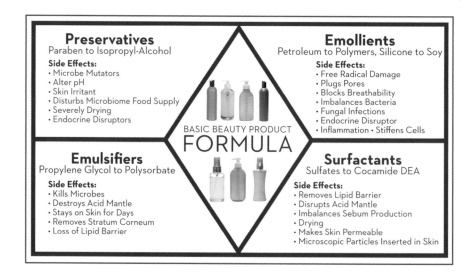

Preservatives
Paraben to Isopropyl-Alcohol
Side Effects:
• Microbe Mutators
• Alter pH
• Skin Irritant
• Disturbs Microbiome Food Supply
• Severely Drying
• Endocrine Disruptors

Emollients
Petroleum to Polymers, Silicone to Soy
Side Effects:
• Free Radical Damage
• Plugs Pores
• Blocks Breathability
• Imbalances Bacteria
• Fungal Infections
• Endocrine Disruptor
• Inflammation • Stiffens Cells

BASIC BEAUTY PRODUCT
FORMULA

Emulsifiers
Propylene Glycol to Polysorbate
Side Effects:
• Kills Microbes
• Destroys Acid Mantle
• Stays on Skin for Days
• Removes Stratum Corneum
• Loss of Lipid Barrier

Surfactants
Sulfates to Cocamide DEA
Side Effects:
• Removes Lipid Barrier
• Disrupts Acid Mantle
• Imbalances Sebum Production
• Drying
• Makes Skin Permeable
• Microscopic Particles Inserted in Skin

The penetration of chemicals we commonly use creates a vicious cycle of dermal dysbiosis and premature aging that is difficult to escape. Although there are thousands upon thousands of synthetic skincare chemicals that can concoct a product, my purpose is to simplify the structure into the four main chemical groups that are fused into bottles of beauty products.[9] My aim is to elucidate how we can easily replace the "need" to care for our skin with caustic chemicals with a garden of life-enhancing balancing botanicals. We can create cosmic cosmetics, or cosmoetics, for the pleasure of beautifying. Now more than ever, we can luxuriate in the ancient art of applying to our skin the plant essences that were once so precious that many were revered more than gold. Thanks to dedicated distillers who capture the essence of these unguents and boost availability, we have access to a bevy of botanicals that we can use, guided by our modern knowledge of skin science.

Every object, every being,
is a jar full of delight.

Be a connoisseur,
and taste with caution.

Any wine will get you high.
Judge like a king, and choose the purest,

the ones unadulterated with fear,
or some urgency about "what's needed."

Rumi[10]

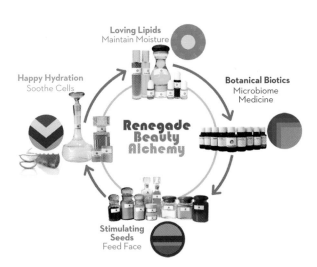

Loving Lipids
Maintain Moisture

Happy Hydration
Soothe Cells

Botanical Biotics
Microbiome
Medicine

Renegade
Beauty
Alchemy

Stimulating
Seeds
Feed Face

RENEGADE BEAUTY BLUEPRINTS

Elements and botanicals define Renegade Beauty Blueprints because, quite simply, our skin is alive! For an ingredient palette of perfection, these fundamental four formula factors of happy hydration, loving lipids, stimulating seeds, and botanical-biotics fuse new and ancient wisdom to reveal your best skin ever. Easily mix, moisturize, mask, and remedy by combining together ingredients from two, three, or four of these categories to nourish skin. Or begin with recipes from Chapter Sixteen, which has an array of formula suggestions.

Happy hydration begins with spring water (or filtered water), aqueous extracts of rose and frankincense hydrosols, apple cider vinegar, and fresh aloe's generous gel, which is 99 percent water. These topical toners renew and restore the top layers of the skin without disturbing the makeup of the microbiome, stiffening cells, or stripping away the stratum corneum. Pure sources of harmonious hydration quench, cleanse, and soothe cells in sync with our bodies of water.

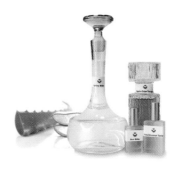

Loving lipids lubricate with cold-pressed plant oils of jojoba, coconut, camellia, tamanu, rosehips, raspberry seed, and sandalwood nut oils to maintain moisture in an array of magnificent ways. In fat-bearing botanicals, plant tissues are bestowed with select cells that produce opulent oils classified as triglycerides. These sumptuous secretions work synergistically with our skin's sebum and cells and contain nourishing lipids full of vitamins, pigments, phytosterols, ceramides, and beneficial, microbicidal fatty acids that are essential to the integrity of the skin's natural defense system. Besides the

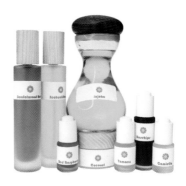

moisture manna these emollients provide, they also enhance the penetration of botanical-biotics, delivering layers of lively liquid to the care of the microbiome and membranes.

Botanical-biotics bring in the alchemy of active essential oils and extracts to muse medicine upon the microbiome and skin. Specialized plant cells, ducts, and glands store these aromatic essences that are excreted from roots, fruits, sap, seeds, flowers, and tree bark, wood, and leaves. These molecular metabolites, pressed and steamed from cells within the plant's epidermis, are excellent for

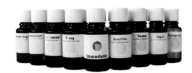

stimulating skincare as they work symbiotically with our cells and body's ecology. These essences ally with our bodies, turning on electrons, protective genes, and anti-inflammatory proteins; stimulating circulation; feeding immunity; and keeping collagen healthy. These concentrated quintessences make perfectly potent and effective targeted treatments along with galvanizing the delivery of loving lipids and stimulating seeds to the skin.

Stimulating seeds of probiotics, honey, clay, charcoal, iodine, baking soda, sea salt, powdered vitamin C, and crushed herbs of rosehip and rosemary feed the face and body transdermally. Besides the ability of these sustaining substances to gently cleanse pores, effectively exfoliate, absorb impurities, and balance the

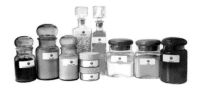

biome, these nutrients also provide pigments, minerals, enzymes, and vitamins to feed beneficial bacteria and skin cells. Spa your skin with these mineral-rich materials that are easy to activate with water, lipids, and/or essential oils to make masks to massage on the face, body, and scalp and to spot-treat imbalanced areas.

When your skin is symptom-free, balanced, and feeling lovely, all of the glorious realms and all botanical libations are open to explore. All the Renegade Beauty Recipes for skincare are active with antiaging allies, brimming with botanicals to balance, and ripe with loving lipids to replenish.

RENEGADE BEAUTY REALMS CHART

This list is a lexicon of affinities associated with each Renegade Beauty Realm. The words on this chart are not intended to treat, diagnose, or advise on any condition. It is a guide that might inspire intuition, understanding, and awareness about the skin.

Renegade Beauty Realms	Blithe Beauty	Benevolent Beauty
Chart of Skin Affinities	Resilient	Grace
	"Beauty is a light in the heart" Khalil Gibran	"For in the dew of little things the heart finds its morning and is refreshed." Khalil Gibran
Beauty Realm Benefits	Soothes + Sutures Calming + Cooling Seals Skin - Anti-inflammatory Anti-Itch + Disinfectant Calming Analgesic	Smoothens + Seals Cell Regenerating Evens Skin Tone - Antiseptic Circulatory + Cytophylatic Balancing Tonic
Skin Indications	Weepy, Irritated, Reactive, Red, Inflamed	Blemishes, Melasma, Uneven, Sensitive
Skin Symptoms	Eczema, psoriasis, dandruff, rash, dermatitis, bites, burns, polyps, herpes, hives, shingles, sunburn, weepy pores, rough texture, itchy	Hyperpigmentation, Scars, Skin Tags, cuperose, broken capillaries, Milia, fine lines, open pores, uneven tone, whiteheads, fine lines
Skin Role	Gatekeeper	Hydrolipid Barrier
Epidermis Strata	Stratum Spinosum	Stratum Granulosm
Epidermis Cells	Langerhans Cells	Merkel Cells
Microbiome Community	Firmicutes	Proteobacteria
Colonized By	Streptococcus aureus, Malaezia	Corynebacterium, Malaezia
Microbiome Reaction	Viral; Flares result from plummets in microbial diversity	Bacterial Imbalance in the deeper skin strata
Probiotic	Lactobacillus plantarum	Lactobacillus acidophilus
Classic Dermotolgy Recommendations	Systemic Antibiotics, Corticosteroids	Hydroquinone, Retinoids
Fat-Soluble Vitamin	K2	E
Mineral	Magnesium	Sulfur/Silica
Triggers	Dairy	Sugar
Skin Stressor	Inflammation	Glycation
Body System	Immune	Nerve & Cirulatory
TCM	Heat	Wind
Elements	Water	Ether
Plant Constituents	Terpenes, Esters, Sesquiterpene Hydrocarbons	Aldehydes, Lactones, Esters
Essential Oils	Frankincense, Peppermint, Sandalwood, Cypress, Blue Tansy, Yarrow, Cape Chamomile, German Chamomiles	Rose Otto, Immortelle, Cape Chamomile, Frankincense, Cypress, Lavender, Sweet Thyme, Sandalwood
Botanical Lipids	Jojoba + Tamanu Oils	Jojoba + Sandalwood Nut Oils
Feeling	Energized + Focused	Joy + Engaged

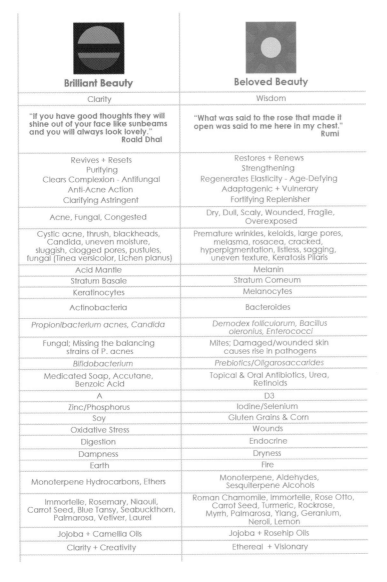

Brilliant Beauty	Beloved Beauty
Clarity	Wisdom
"If you have good thoughts they will shine out of your face like sunbeams and you will always look lovely." Roald Dhal	"What was said to the rose that made it open was said to me here in my chest." Rumi
Revives + Resets Purifying Clears Complexion - Antifungal Anti-Acne Action Clarifying Astringent	Restores + Renews Strengthening Regenerates Elasticity - Age-Defying Adaptagenic + Vulnerary Fortifying Replenisher
Acne, Fungal, Congested	Dry, Dull, Scaly, Wounded, Fragile, Overexposed
Cystic acne, thrush, blackheads, Candida, uneven moisture, sluggish, clogged pores, pustules, fungal (Tinea versicolor, Lichen planus)	Premature wrinkles, keloids, large pores, melasma, rosacea, cracked, hyperpigmentation, listless, sagging, uneven texture, Keratosis Pilaris
Acid Mantle	Melanin
Stratum Basale	Stratum Corneum
Keratinocytes	Melanocytes
Actinobacteria	Bacteroides
Propionibacterium acnes, Candida	Demodex folliculorum, Bacillus oleronius, Enterococci
Fungal; Missing the balancing strains of P. acnes	Mites; Damaged/wounded skin causes rise in pathogens
Bifidobacterium	Prebiotics/Oligarosaccarides
Medicated Soap, Accutane, Benzoic Acid	Topical & Oral Antibiotics, Urea, Retinoids
A	D3
Zinc/Phosphorus	Iodine/Selenium
Soy	Gluten Grains & Corn
Oxidative Stress	Wounds
Digestion	Endocrine
Dampness	Dryness
Earth	Fire
Monoterpene Hydrocarbons, Ethers	Monoterpene, Aldehydes, Sesquiterpene Alcohols
Immortelle, Rosemary, Niaouli, Carrot Seed, Blue Tansy, Seabuckthorn, Palmarosa, Vetiver, Laurel	Roman Chamomile, Immortelle, Rose Otto, Carrot Seed, Turmeric, Rockrose, Myrrh, Palmarosa, Ylang, Geranium, Neroli, Lemon
Jojoba + Camellia Oils	Jojoba + Rosehip Oils
Clarity + Creativity	Ethereal + Visionary

Affinity Defintions for the Renegade Beauty Realms Chart

Beauty Realm	The benefits of the botanicals assigned to the job of balancing symptoms
Benefits	The specific ways this realm helps the skin
Skin Indications	Traits or signs of skin issues
Skin Symptoms	Manifestation of imbalance
Skin Role	Skin area that may need harmonizing in this realm
Epidermis Strata	Skin layer affected
Epidermis Cells	Type of skin cells affected
Microbiome Community	We can arrest the affliction, repair our skin, and maintain a microbiome of bustling bacteria by following this simple formula: Stop, Seal, and Seed
Colonized By	The imbalanced bacterial colonies
Microbiome Reaction	When the microbiome is disturbed through diet, commerical products, and chemicals it reacts and this can show up in the skin in this way.
Probiotic	Seed the skin, gut, and mouth
Classic Dermotolgy Recommendations	Common pharmacological treatments for this issue
Fat-Soluble Vitamin	The possible vitamin deficiency associated with this skin issue
Mineral	The possible mineral deficiency associated with this skin issue
Triggers	Foods that may trigger the skin to react
Skin Stressor	How the skin responds to the above dietary stressors
Body System	Possible body system under stress that may show up as skin issue
TCM	Traditional Chinese Medicine
Elements	Ayurvedic philosophy
Plant Constituents	Chemical constituents of essential oils that activate healing of these issues
Essential Oils	Botanical-biotic suggestions for each realm
Botanical Lipids	The elegant emollient suggestions to lubricate skin layers for each realm
Feeling	The good feelings associated with each realm

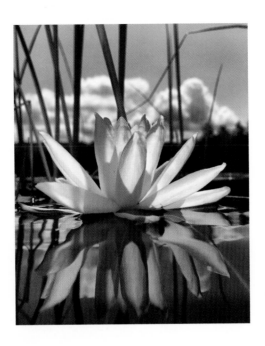

there is no mark against you.

your being is a holy beauty.

you.
are a holy beauty.

—Nayyirah Waheed

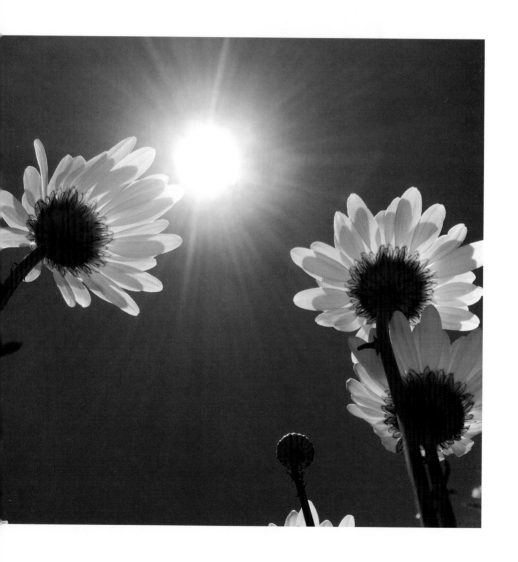

Chapter Fifteen

RENEGADE BEAUTY SECRETS

Tap into the stream of well-being and receive the whispers of nature's secrets that are revealed to us through our senses. When mesmerizing molecules coalesce with our bodies, these vast intricate strands of nature's telegrams allow us to feel the finery of knowing that not only are we from the same source that spirals the sun's rays every single day, we are also an extension of that source. Adoring our pores with the prose of plants tunes us in to the song of nature's open secret.

Make acquaintance with the powers of rose flowers, frankincense, peppermint, myrrh, and more. Every essential oil has a verse in the language of the lymph, in the melody of the endocrine, in the balance of the biome, and in the song of the skin. Benevolently, botanicals attend to the body's reception: renewing molecules of perception, boosting immunity, and inspiring purity in every pore. Each dewy drop is a secret agent of anti-inflammatory, antimicrobial, and antiviral activity; each drop is a healing infinity. Each plant secretion seeds a unique expression of realms upon realms being quenched and drenched by diverse rain and soil. Each plant's exuberance is astonishingly rare in texture, fragrance, and cadence; and when botanicals from the land interact with our glands, grace our face, muse our minds, liberate our lungs, and orchestrate our cells, we are united with beauty.

This is Renegade Beauty: releasing ourselves from skin scrutiny, being benevolent with our bodies, and regaling in radiant health by nourishing every cell with gifts from the earth and engaging with the ether of the elements.

Dwell on the beauty of life. Watch the stars, and see yourself running with them.[1]

COSMOETIC CABINET

Stocking the Aromatic Apothecary

Here you will find the fundamental ingredients to stock your cosmoetic cabinet so that you have on hand the botanical boons, aromatic assets, and medicinal materials to expand your Renegade Beauty. Simply start with a few staples from each category so that you can attend to your skin with simplicity and sometimes spa-like luxury as you soak in these serene substances from your self-care apothecary.

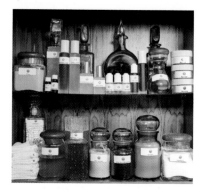

> Doctors and chemists will be surprised at the wide range of odoriferous substances which may be used medicinally, and at the great variety of their chemical functions. Besides the antiseptic and antimicrobial properties of which it is currently made, the essential oils are also antitoxic and antiviral; they have a powerful energizing effect and possess an undeniable cicatrizing property. In the future their role will be even greater.
>
> R. M. Gattefossé[2]

COSMOETIC MATERIA MEDICA[3]

Loving Lipids

Elegant emollients to lubricate epidermal layers and restore the hydro-lipid barrier, these natural nectars pressed from plants deliver delicious moisture to clarify and penetrate pores with adoring oils opulent in beautifying benefits.

JOJOBA OIL (SIMMONDSIA CHINENSIS)

Wholesome jojoba is the foundational lipid of all the Renegade Beauty Realms and is also the desert's answer to dry, brittle skin and hair. Dwelling among sandstorms and cacti, jojoba emerges as an ebullient, emollient oasis. As this strong shrub bakes underneath the desert sun, pearls of liquid gold germinate inside jojoba seeds. These seeds burst forth a golden oil that is cold-pressed to deliver a lipid that is super similar to our skin's natural sebum. Sinking effortlessly into skin, it transfers phytonutrients to the tissues' deepest layers, helping skin retain moisture and replenish elasticity. Brilliantly beneficial to skin with its abundance of phenolic

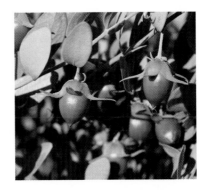

compounds, nutrients, and vitamin E tocopherols, jojoba lubricates like oil, yet it is actually a liquid plant wax, so it will not go rancid, which effectively eliminates free radicals from your skincare. Incredibly rich and silky, jojoba provides long-lasting skin-conditioning effects. It is a great carrier for essential oils and herbal infusions.

Organic jojoba oil has traditionally been used to moisturize skin and hair, stimulate hair growth, unclog blocked follicles, clear acne, reduce the appearance of wrinkles, and treat dandruff. Jojoba regulates skin oil production, making it especially beneficial for people with acne. It offers bountiful beauty benefits for skin, hair, and nails. It can be used as a moisturizer, cleanser, shaving lotion, aftershave, body oil, makeup remover, scar treatment, stretch-mark minimizer, cuticle moisturizer, hair conditioner, sunburn soother, and dry-scalp buster.

Camellia Oil (*Camellia japonica*)

Cherished camellia oil comes from the Japanese winter-blooming flower, *tsubaki,* known as the "rose of winter." Camellia's succulent seeds are cold-pressed to reveal an elegant elixir of endless moisture. Skin relishes in its easily absorbed deep infusion of omega-9, palmitic fatty acids, antioxidants, nourishing polyphenols, vitamins A and D, selenium, and high amounts

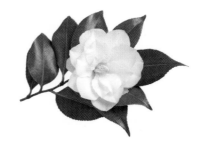

of alpha-tocopherol, a strain of vitamin E that synergizes with the skin's natural sebum. Camellia replenishes lipids, regulates sebaceous secretions, and purifies pores. Thirsty winter skin is reborn with this effective emollient that revives elasticity and reduces dry lines. It is also a time-tested treasure of Japanese geishas, who traditionally used the oil to keep their long tresses shiny and soft, to remove makeup, and to moisturize skin, hair, and nails.

ROSEHIP OIL (*ROSA RUBIGINOSA*)

Replenishing rosehip oil is cold-pressed from the crimson-colored fruit of the rose plant that appears on the stem after the flowers. Both the fruit and the seeds are brimming with vitamins C and E, antioxidants, retinol-A, essential fatty acids, and antimicrobials that have been soothing skin since ancient days. Native Americans, Mayans, and Egyptians all used rosehips to lubricate dry skin, relieve itchy skin, relax wrinkles, soften scars, shrink pores, and remedy acne. Rosehips also contain elasticity-boosting lycopene to rejuvenate skin that has suffered burns, eczema, psoriasis, and rosacea.

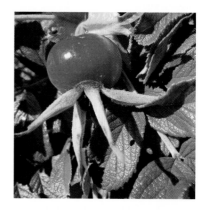

SANDALWOOD NUT OIL (*SANTALUM SPICATUM*)

Soothing, smoothing sandalwood nut oil is one of the most luscious lipids I have ever applied to my skin. This opulent oil is freshly pressed through the process of supercritical extraction from sandalwood nuts grown in the wilds of Western Australia. An ancient emollient and anti-inflammatory agent, sandalwood nut oil has been a staple of indigenous Australian life and is still used today by modern-day indigenous communities. For centuries, indigenous Australians used the oil from sandalwood nuts to soften their hair, skin, and scalp. It is also used to prevent the signs of aging, to moisturize facial skin, and to protect skin from the drying desert environment. Sandalwood nuts were crushed and made into poultices, then placed on the facial skin to form a mask. These masks were used to make the skin smoother, softer, and tauter. Sandalwood nuts or "seeds" were also consumed to soothe stiff joints.

The molecular composition of sandalwood nut oil is mainly longer-chain fatty acids, including oleic acid (50 percent) and ximenynic acid (30–35 percent).[4] These lush lipids help to preserve the integrity of skin cell walls, support cell restructuring, strengthen cell membranes, and make rapid cellular renewal possible. Thanks to the presence of these lipids, sandalwood nut oil can be used to improve the functionality of sebaceous tissues, prevent collagen loss, strengthen the skin's

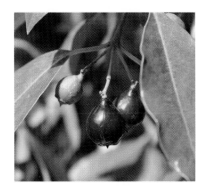

extracellular matrix, improve the elasticity of skin, and tighten sagging skin. The high levels of ximenynic acid make it a naturally occurring skin protectant, stimulant, and anti-inflammatory agent. Ximenynic acid is said to prevent the breakdown of collagen, which may lead to improved elasticity of the skin. The strong microvascular constricting action that increases blood circulation to the skin has been shown to reduce cellulite, regulate sebum production, and prevent hair loss.

Ximenynic acid is also used to inhibit inflammation of the skin, joints, and internal organs. It does this by binding to inflammation-causing enzymes in the body, thus preventing the inflammation process before it begins. Without inflammation, the skin is free to heal itself from the inside out, thus reducing the appearance of lines and wrinkles. This luscious anti-inflammatory lipid also makes this oil an overall skin protectant that soothes tense muscles, joint pain, bruises, lesions, and burns.

Seabuckthorn Berry Oil (*Hippophae rhamnoides*)

Super seabuckthorn berry is a supercritical extract that is potently packed with heavenly healing properties of both fatty acids and aromatic oil. This bright-orange berry oil descends deep into the lipid layers of the skin, diminishing imbalances from the inside out. Perfectly poised in omega-3, -6, -7, and -9 fatty acids, this vital extract captures more than 190 bioactive substances from the edible berry. A single drop of this ample oil contains 190 different bioactive compounds, which work together to reduce inflammation, redness, and water loss in every skin cell. Plush in precious vitamins C, E, A, B1, B2, and B12, antioxidants, forty-one carotenoids including beta carotene, and seventeen phytosterols known to reduce redness and protect collagen fibers and cell membranes.

Seabuckthorn synergizes with skin by supporting cell-tissue regeneration by extraordinarily accelerating wound, scar, and burn healing, along with soothing acne, eczema, scar tissue, and stretch marks. It remedies skin exposed to radiation; Russian cosmonauts used it for radiation burns in outer space. "After the disaster at the nuclear plant in Chernobyl, Seabuckthorn oil was used to treat the radiation burns of people exposed. Seabuckthorn is used in hair products to prevent baldness and stimulate hair growth."[5] Besides softening skin, these extraordinary anti-inflammatory plant properties revitalize connective tissue, offering photoprotective properties that make it a natural sunscreen that harmonizes our skin both before and after enjoying the sun.

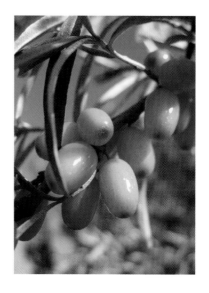

Tamanu Oil (*Calophyllum inophyllum*)

Tropical tamanu oil is an ancient South Pacific skin secret, now revealed. Used for centuries by the native peoples of Southeast Asia and Polynesia, tamanu is a veritable dream-cream for skin that is dry, damaged, burned, scarred, or simply in need of some serious TLC.

Tamanu oil is cold-pressed from the kernels of the fruit of the *Calophyllum inophyllum* tree native to Polynesia. The kernels themselves do not produce oil until after they are dried in the sun for at least one month, at which time they produce a sticky-sweet oil that is a nourishing nectar for the skin. In Fiji, native people have been using tamanu oil for centuries to heal burns and wounds, fade scars, and treat painful skin and nerve conditions like skin ulcers, sciatica, shingles, rheumatism, and leprosy. "People on the coasts of the Indian Ocean use *calophyllum* oil as a panacea. It finds its main application as an immune-modulating component in skin-care products which benefit from its phagocytosis-stimulating qualities . . . This oil is recommended in cases of skin conditions accompanied by a build-up of pus."[6]

This organic oil is more than just a carrier oil, as it contains both fatty and aromatic oils and is replete with nourishing compounds, including lipids, fatty acids, and anti-inflammatory agents. The main lipids present in tamanu oil are glycolipids that fortify healthy skin cells, phospholipids that strengthen skin cells and increase flexibility, and neutral lipids that enhance the formation of healthy membranes. Tamanu also contains high levels of calophyllic acid, an essential fatty acid that has been shown to fight bacteria, reduce inflammation, and even inhibit *Staphylococcus aureus*. Known for its stunning capacity to heal the skin, tamanu also evens skin tone and encourages the acceleration of new skin cells that form

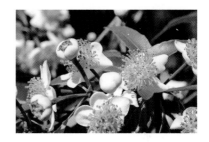

new tissue. This cicatrizing catalyst is significant in its ability to reduce redness, diminish melasma, remedy rashes, and soothe itchy and irritated skin. Oxidative stress will recess as tamanu contains beta-glucan, which provides botanical protection to the top layer (the stratum corneum) of the skin's thin epithelium. Tamanu's rich lipid profile delivers deep moisture into the skin's layers to heal scars, burns, and wounds from the inside out. When further enhanced with the power of essential oils, all of these beneficial compounds come together to create one of the most nourishing, nutrient-rich carrier oils on the planet.

Additional Loving Lipids

Cacao Butter (*Theobroma cacao*)

Creamy cacao butter, a magnificent moisturizer of Mesoamerica for eons, imparts a delicious chocolate aroma and is deeply hydrating. This emollient extraordinaire is pressed from chocolate beans and contains fabulous fatty acids. Always buy organic, raw cacao butter to ensure that valuable nutrients and antioxidants are not lost to high-temperature manufacturing processes. Although solid at room temperature, this buttery sweetness glides seamlessly on the skin.

CASTOR OIL *(RICINUS COMMUNIS)*

Commendable castor oil is cold-pressed from seeds of a plant that grows wild in tropical and Mediterranean climates. This very viscous and lubricative oil was turned into healing unguents and ointments by the early cultures of Egypt, India, Japan, China, and Persia. Castor oil is a triglyceride lipid composed of unique fatty acids, 90 percent of which are rare ricinoleic acids. The oil also contains esters that soothe skin. Ricinoleic acids, the main remedying component of castor oil, are antifungal and antiviral and have a decongestant and detoxifying effect on the skin and lymphatic system.

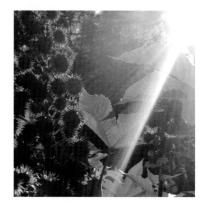

A classic constipation remedy, this purgative oil can cleanse the digestive tract and is considered a safe internal remedy for constipation in small doses. Avoid castor oil internally when pregnant, and always buy organic.

Skin-salving topical use of castor oil includes applications of castor oil packs and applying it directly to the skin. Massage castor oil into skin by mixing with marjoram, juniper, tamanu, or peppermint essential oils to soothe muscle and joint pain, including osteoarthritis. Effective as an antifungal, castor oil is known to clear common skin conditions like ringworm, jock itch (tinea cruris), and athlete's foot. Add a few drops of **Brilliant Beauty Spot Treatment** to castor oil, apply onto the affected area before bedtime, and let the oil soak in overnight. Repeat until skin is clear. Healthy hair growth is stimulated when castor oil is applied to the scalp, eyelashes, and eyebrows.

Castor oil packs are applied to encourage lymphatic circulation in these areas: the abdomen, breasts, uterus, liver, thymus gland, thyroid gland, and sore muscles and joints. The idea is to keep castor oil on a piece of cloth on the skin for at least an hour with a heat source to stimulate lymph and liver function. A study found that castor oil packs produced a temporary increase in the number of immune-boosting T-11 cells and lymphocytes.[7] Castor oil packs can help improve liver detoxification, improve lymphatic circulation, and reduce inflammation.

How to Make a Castor Oil Pack

1. Create the time and space to relax for at least an hour.

2. Supplies: mason jar, organic castor oil, cotton flannel, a thicker towel or plastic protective barrier to cover the cotton flannel, and a hot water bottle or an infrared heating pad. Castor oil does stain, so set up the area with older towels or wear older clothes.

3. Cut the cloth into three strips in the size to suit the area of the body you are covering. Hours before, soak the flannel by putting the fabric in the mason jar with castor oil, and shake every so often to cover all areas of the cloth.

4. Place the soaked cloth over the area to treat. Cover with the plastic or protective barrier, and apply the heat source. Relax for an hour. Wash the fabric in natural laundry soap with baking soda to remove the castor oil. Put clean flannel strips back in the mason jar and store in the fridge.

COCONUT OIL (COCOS NUCIFERA)

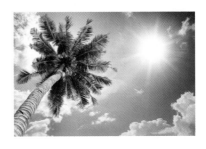

Creamy coconut is a deeply penetrating moisturizer that protects each cell. Cold-pressed, virgin coconut oil is chock-full of lubricating healthy fats called medium-chain fatty acids (MCFAs, also known as medium-chain triglycerides or MCTs), which include unique caprylic, lauric, and capric fatty acids that are effective anti-microbial, antibacterial, and antifungal agents. It is solid at room temperature yet melts on contact and soothingly soaks into skin. From head to toe, coconut has copious benefits to the skin as moisturizer, makeup remover, toothpaste, suntan harmonizer, lip balm, lubricant, oral oil pulling, aftershave, beard and hair pomade, cuticle oil, and stretch-mark soother. Although this wonder oil is a beauty, for a very small percentage of people, facial skin can react, so do a patch test before applying it to your face.

Coconut's antifungal lipids also benefit skin fungal infections, and it makes a good carrier-oil option for cold sore spot treatment with essential oils. Lauric acid in the oil is effective at penetrating the cell-receptor site of the virus in this skin condition and inhibits the virus from replicating, leading to a swifter solution for cold sores. Always buy virgin, organic, cold-pressed, unrefined coconut oil.

Coconut MCT Oil (Cocos nucifera)

Organic, unrefined coconut naturally contains both medium-chain triglycerides (MCTs) and long-chain triglycerides (LCTs). The MCTs, including caproic, caprylic, and capric acids, are extracted to create a concentrated oil with all the beneficial compounds of coconut oil. It takes about 20 tablespoons of ordinary coconut oil to make 1 tablespoon of a coconut-oil-based MCT oil. Unlike coconut oil, MCT oil remains a liquid at any temperature. MCT oil abounds with beneficial nutrients for the mouth, body, and brain. When selecting an MCT oil, look for signs of potency and purity. Many coconut oils are refined and heavily processed, which can leave behind solvents and oxidized fat. Look for a nutraceutical-quality MCT to find the purest oil with the longest shelf life. Read the labels and choose one with the highest amounts of C6 (caproic), C8 (caprylic), and C10 (capric) fatty acids.

Olive Oil (Olea europaea)

Liquid gold to the ancient Greeks, extra-virgin olive oil is a staple in most kitchen pantries today. Early Mediterranean cultures knew of its culinary and skincare attributes and used it in cooking, for making soaps, and to moisturize and heal disrupted skin. In *The Hippocratic Corpus*, Hippocrates recorded more than sixty olive oil ointments to treat topical skin disorders. Back in the day, olive oil was abundantly applied to the skin and then removed with a strigil, a metal spoon-like tool that scraped the oil across every inch of skin to cleanse and exfoliate prior to a hot bath.

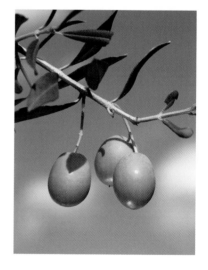

Our ancient ancestors believed that olive oil's life-giving longevity was due to an olive tree's thousand-year lifespan and that the fruit and oil were gifts of life from the tree. Legendary for living past 100 years, Greek philosopher Democritus attributed his health to bathing his insides in honey, and his exterior in olive oil.[8] Supercentenarian Jeanne

Louise Calment, who lived till 122, claimed that daily doses of olive oil supplied to her skin boosted her longevity.[9]

Olive oil is opulent in essential amino acids, squalene, flavonoids, anti-inflammatory polyphenols of oleocanthal, vital antioxidants, and vitamins A, K, C, and E. Many olive oils are really oil blends, and companies are not required to divulge all the oils inside the bottle on the label. Finding really, really real olive oil can be challenging. For a thorough education in the virtues of olive oil and to find a source of pure oil near you, check out the website Truth in Olive Oil.

RED RASPBERRY SEED OIL (*RUBUS IDAEUS*)

Ravishing red raspberry seed oil is a cold-pressed plant oil rich in essential fatty acids (linoleic, alpha-linolenic, and oleic acids), vitamin A, carotenoids, and antioxidant activity, including tocopherols and tocotrienols. The tocopherols are primarily gamma- and alpha-tocopherols, which contribute to this oil's excellent free-radical ion-scavenging capability and lipid support. It is super soothing to skin lesions, rashes, rosacea, and eczema because this beautifying oil is anti-inflammatory, antibacterial, and antiviral and includes ellagic acid, which is anticarcinogenic and antimutagenic.

According to a laboratory study, raw red raspberry seed oil may have potential use as a broad-range sun protectant.[10] Under a spectrometer, raspberry seed oil absorbed both UVB and UVC rays and scattered UVA rays. The study found the oil to have a sun protection quality equal to that of titanium dioxide and may provide protection similar to SPF-25. Although plant oils offer qualities of harmonizing our skin to the sun's rays, always test what works best for your skin and time in the sun, as everyone's skin and melanin levels vary.

Botanical-Biotics

"For in the dew of little things the heart finds its morning and is refreshed."[11] Dewy drops of essential oils each have a unique ambrosial aroma and are all antifungal, antiviral, and anti-inflammatory to varying degrees. These ethereal essences have the plant intelligence to be buddies with beneficial bacteria, kin for your skin, elegant inspirers of immunity, and orators of oral care. These nourishing nectars with gifted molecules mix with the mind and emotions to clarify, edify, and uplift—what an amazing offering for a cosmoetic ingredient.

BLUE TANSY (*TANACETUM ANNUUM*)

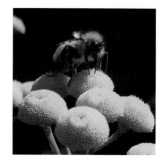

Beautiful blue tansy is a blue bundle of medicinal power and is incredibly soothing and calming to the skin and the spirit. This azure oil abundant in the botanical compound azulene, which is a soothing sesquiterpene, provides calming and cooling phytochemical constituents that are an anti-inflammatory dream. "This class of compounds inhibits transcription factor, NF-kappa beta, which plays an important role in the cascade of events mediating inflammation. *Tanacetum annuum* apparently works at an early stage of the inflammation cascade, preventing the synthesis of the proteins that would transmit inflammation."[12] Ease inflammatory flare-ups on the skin, soothe sunburns, heal damaged or broken skin, alleviate itching, help hives, remedy rashes, and drench dry skin. Blue tansy is a supreme skin soother. Apply to skin that needs deep relaxing. Dilute with jojoba to make calming serums that can be applied to red, irritated, inflamed, blemished skin, and allow the epidermis to drink in the true blue tonic. This fragrant oil ameliorates allergies, reduces swelling, and serenely sedates, all wrapped up in drops of a vibrant blue hue. Respiratory imbalances are reassured when using this oil as an inhalant, with a diffuser, a salt pipe, or a simple handkerchief.

CAPE CHAMOMILE (*ERIOCEPHALUS PUNCTULATUS*)

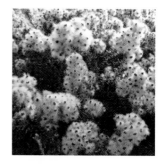

Captivating cape chamomile's essence calms minds, clears skin, and comforts adrenals. This uplifting essential oil exudes a beautiful, fine fruity-floral fragrance that is one of my favorite aromas. Cape chamomile has a high content of rare, nourishing ester and azulene compounds that impart a teal-blue hue and potent anti-inflammatory, antispasmodic, and antiseptic actions to soothe all manner of skin imbalances and muscle twitches. This rejuvenating remedy regulates sebum and sedates skin infections, rashes, acne blemishes, rosacea, eczema, and dermatitis.

CARROT SEED (*DAUCUS CAROTA*)

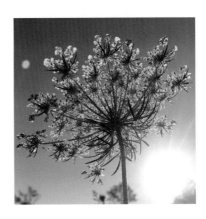

Wild carrot, also called Queen Anne's lace, alights skin, liver, and face with the grace of sesquiterpenes known for their highly regenerative actions. Calming carrot seed's essence is a mildly sweet and inspiring woodsy aroma distilled from the seeds of the wild flowering plants. Traditionally known for its extraordinary abilities to revive liver and skin cells, carrot seed has also been used as a deluxe digestive tonic. This effective skin elixir enhances elasticity and brings balance to both oily and dry skin, revives dry, pallid, and acneic skin tissue, displaying "a distinct revitalizing effect on skin suffering from lack of tone."[13]

CHAMOMILE (*ANTHEMIS NOBILIS*)

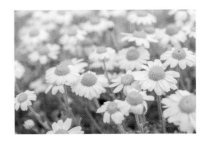

Comforting chamomile essential oil is steam-distilled from the delicate diminutive petals of French chamomile flowers. This flower, famed for its calming caress, is also known as Roman chamomile. Its gentle grace was revered by the ancient Egyptians, the Moors, and the Saxons as a sacred elixir worthy of the angels. Cheering chamomile offers us its sweet honey-hay-floral, hypnotic fruit-scented powers of sedation: pacifying apprehension, softening tension, and nestling nerves. This essence is rich in easing esters, making it the gentlest go-to oil to soothe unruly skin conditions and to serenely enter into alpha brainwaves of relaxation.

This ethereal aroma is also an endowed antispasmodic that relaxes muscles, minds, and inflamed skin. Mix with jojoba and beeswax to create calm massaging balms for babies and moms. Slip into skincare serums to heal and seal scars, flakiness, melasma, and rosacea. Apply neat to a myriad of tissue issues, like acne, bites, bruises, blemishes, and cuts. Inhale via a bottle, diffuser, or salt pipe for a soothing experience of serenity. It's beautiful in baths before bedtime. Culinary creations yield to chamomile's dainty divinations, and a drop of this easing essence added to honey and warm water before resting your head in bed is a peaceful way to end the day.

CYPRESS (*CUPRESSUS SEMPERVIRENS*)

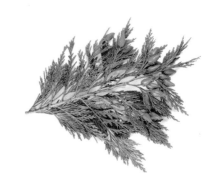

Splendid cypress essential oil is extracted from the mighty needles of the majestic evergreen tree that stretches proudly toward the heavens as it watches over centuries of existence. The essence of cypress is as healing as it is refreshing, and it has been used to bring comfort in times of sorrow for thousands of years. Strengthening cypress oil is a cooling, fortifying tonic and astringent. The antiseptic and hemostatic properties of cypress make it a wonderful treatment for wounds, while its sudorific properties encourage the skin to release pent-up toxins. Cypress is stellar for stimulating the lymph system. Dr. Kurt Schnaubelt wrote that it "helps to prevent the spread of varicose veins, hemorrhoids, and edema, especially of the lower limbs."[14] Cypress clears congestion, heals skin conditions like hemorrhoids and cellulite, lowers blood pressure, lifts the spirits, balances excess oil on the skin, soothes dandruff, makes a deft deodorant, and repels insects.

FRANKINCENSE (*BOSWELLIA CARTERII*)

The quintessential essence for cultivating reverence is frankincense. Liquid pearls from the tree of life, frankincense is distilled from the resinous sap of the tree. Anointed and inhaled in spiritual ceremonies for thousands of years, this fine, fragrant oil nestles the nerves, deepens breathing during meditation, and increases the intuition of our inner guidance. Holding the wisdom of the ages, frankincense is a formidable anti-inflammatory essence that soothes scars, smoothes uneven skin, and diminishes melasma. Sacred frankincense is beautifully balsamic in nature, giving it the unparalleled power to heal wounds, fade scars, treat wrinkles, and reduce inflammation. This oil is an awesome astringent that has been used for thousands of years to nourish dry skin and ease signs of aging.

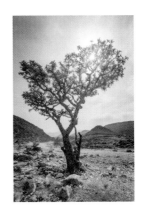

Geranium *(Pelargonium graveolens)*

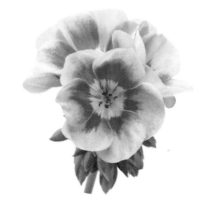

Generous geranium essence bursts forth a fresh green, sweet-scented rosy radiance. The very best is distilled from organic petals in Madagascar. This soothing and revitalizing essence encourages emotional and physical adaptability, longevity, and balance. Geranium gives skin a gorgeous natural glow by stimulating blood circulation and assisting the release of toxins. It reduces the appearance of stretch marks and tightens skin that has become loose. Geranium drives moisture into thirsty skin, and brings balance to the sebum of the acne-prone. By arousing the circulatory system, varicose veins, spider veins, broken capillaries, traumatized tissues, cellulite, and sluggish lymph systems all benefit from geranium's circulation-generation and fluid-decongesting properties.

Heralded as a female tonic, it balances menstrual cycles and adrenal dysregulation. Geranium indicates effectiveness as an adrenocortical restorative remedy.[15] A "light adrenal gland stimulant and hormonal normalizer, geranium is a balancing agent for many conditions. Just sniffing the fragrance can regulate blood pressure by a few points . . . In one study it killed all bacteria tested, including Salmonella and Staphylococcus and in another, it inhibited all fungi being tested."[16]

German Chamomile (*Matricaria chamomilla*)

Beloved blue chamomile essence is distilled from flowers grown in Germany and harvested in the early-morning hours for the most potent extract. High quantities of chamazulene impart this distillation with a deep oceanic blue color, and compelling cooling and calming properties especially suited for skincare. With its inky blue hue, German chamomile contains constituents of sesquiterpenes (azulene) and sesquiterpenols (alpha-bisabolol), making this oil an anti-inflammatory extraordinaire. Soothe nervous tension, rashes, acne, eczema, psoriasis, itchiness, inflammation, and irritation with this precious plant's opulent blue offering.

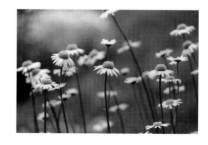

Immortelle (*Helichrysum italicum*)

Everlasting immortelle is a stellar cell-stimulating, scar-healing, and skin-protecting essence that shines divine for all kinds of skincare. This fragrant-floral oil is wild crafted on the island of Corsica, where the flowers can prosper with ocean breezes and sunshine. In the rocky Corsican cliffs, the flowers grow at an altitude of 4,000 feet.

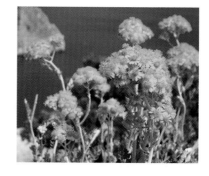

Immortelle aids in cell regeneration and is used to relieve topical pain, to stimulate liver function, and as a skin tonic for acne, wrinkles, cuts, postsurgical wounds, bruises, and burns. A stimulant and protective agent, immortelle defends the skin against damaging free radicals while fading scars, stretch marks, and melasma. "Helichrysum essential oil is extremely useful after surgery for the reduction of hematomas, improving healing, preventing cheloid [keloid] scars, reducing lymphatic edemas following cleaning or dissecting of lymph nodes and preventing fibrous bands following abdominal surgeries."[17] This multifaceted gem of an oil has many emotional benefits as well. I have experienced breathtaking emotional levity simply by inhaling this honey-scented elixir known to metabolize emotions and make transcendent understanding possible.

LAUREL (*LAURUS NOBILIS*)

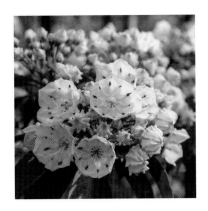

Lovely laurel is revered for its ability to vivify the psychic mind. This stimulating essence increases perception and fosters elevated states of clarity and peace. In ancient Greece, many wreaths were made with laurel's wither-free leaves; and poets, philosophers, victors, emperors, and athletes were crowned with laurel. At the Temple of Apollo at Delphi, priestesses chewed and incensed laurel leaves in the evening to increase intuitive insight, induce dreams of divination, and receive clairvoyant contributions to the Delphic Oracle. This divine distillation is your ally in resurrecting relaxed respiration, reviving the lymph, renewing skin, and diving deep into dreamland.

The regenerative, restorative virtues of laurel oil are revealed when considering the tree's symbol of resurrection, because the tree immediately regenerates itself after sustaining damage. Laurel is one of the "most effective all-round strengthening and preventive oils. It has superior expectorant, mucolytic, viricide, and antifungal properties. It is much milder than clove oil and may be applied more liberally."[18] Mix into massage oils for lymphatic circulation, apply on the chest to invigorate, include in skin serums to clear acne and blemishes, and rub on the soles of the feet for an immune-boosting treat. Laurel loves the lungs when inhaled from a salt pipe, bottle, or diffuser. It is a masterful oil for meditation, mental focus, creative inspiration, and intuition. Sprinkle on pillows for divining dreams. It is a refreshing note in hair tonics and colognes for its herbaceous, balsamic fougère. Use this happy household cleaner to cleanse, disinfect, and infuse spring freshness into the air.

LAVENDER (*LAVANDULA ANGUSTIFOLIA*)

Languid lavender is famed for its ability to soothe body and mind. It is a popular plant for treating insomnia, stress, and anxiety, yet it is also a powerful remedy for treating physical imbalances. This gentle-yet-powerful skin tonic is restorative and healing. Its anti-inflammatory action makes it perfect for cuts, burns, and wounds, while its stimulating effect inspires the skin cells, acne, and scars to heal more quickly. Lavender's abundant anti-bacterial properties prevent cuts, scrapes, and insect bites from becoming infected. "Current science tells us that each component in lavender has its own range of pleiotropic effects. Linalool, a main component of lavender, simultaneously inhibits HMG CoA reductase (anti-tumor, antifungal), and reduces spasms. It is anticonvulsant and modifies autonomic nervous system activity. The effects of linalool are then layered with at least an equal number of physiological effects of linalyl acetate, another main component . . . This list could be continued almost indefinitely, given that over

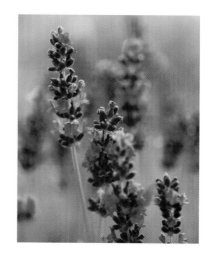

1,200 components have been identified in lavender essential oil."[19] The lovely scent of lavender caresses the senses, letting nervous tension go and lessening mental restlessness. Lavender is a lullaby that dispels depression, furthers focus, soothes stress, and increases lymph flow.

Lemon (*Citrus limon*)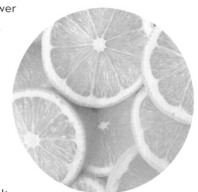

Lovely, lively lemon essence is a revitalizing elixir of delectable delight. Extracted from the rinds of thousands of lemon peels, each drop contains within it the power to elevate mood and invigorate the senses. In the same way, it revitalizes the skin and boosts the immune system. This sunny citrus essence is a delicious-smelling detoxifier that supports the nervous system while uplifting the most import-ant sense of all—our sense of humor!

The botanical components of citral and limonene contribute to the oil's fresh scent and act as a skin-cell regenerator. It balances sebum and is beneficial in skin serums for acne, dull complexions, cellulite, and varicose veins. "Recently, lemon-peel oil has received renewed public interest through the discovery of the anti-tumor effects of limonene. For use in aromatherapy, lemon oil should be obtained exclusively from organically grown fruits . . . Lemon oil has anti-infectious and antiviral activity. It can be used as a component of blends aimed at liver regeneration and detoxification."[20]

Myrrh (Commiphora myrrha)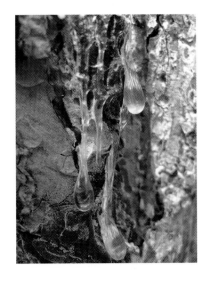

Magnificent myrrh essence contains the same otherworldly aroma and healing properties that made it a favorite of so many ancient civilizations. In Heliopolis, Egypt's city built in honor of the sun god Ra, worshippers burned incense morning, noon, and night to track the sun's path. Myrrh incense was burned at high noon.[21] Ancient Egyptians used myrrh oil to embalm and as a beauty unguent, detoxifying agent, and fragrant perfume. Myrrh is famous as one of the three precious gifts given at the birth of Jesus by the three wise men. It was considered sacred in biblical times. They anointed altars with this potent sap as the epitome of purity.

A gift of myrrh resin would have been a special gift indeed. Historically, all manner of physical ailments were topically addressed with mixtures of this precious oil, including respiratory ailments like bronchitis and laryngitis, skin conditions like eczema and dry skin, digestive imbalances, and oral conditions like mouth ulcers, gum disease, and bad breath. Myrrh has been used for more than 3,800 years as a powerful plant of restoration for skincare. With high levels of soothing sesquiterpenes, myrrh is an optimal oil for oral health, wrinkles, wounds, keloids, burns, rosacea, melasma, and dry, dull, uneven skin. This opulent oleoresin is beautiful in sunbathing oils, and displays promising chemopreventive properties, as it induces healthy cellular apoptosis.

Myrrh also bears an expansive heating and drying nature that warms the heart center, mollifies nervous tension, and balances the brain's cerebral spheres. "Myrrh has a very profound effect on a person's entire being by re-equilibrating the psycho-neuro-endocrine-immunological systems."[22]

NEROLI (CITRUS AURANTIUM)

Blissful neroli blossoms are harvested from heaven-scented orange groves where the delicate blooms of the orange tree offer their ambrosial nectar. Neroli is one of the most exquisite essential oils; it emanates a euphoric aroma reminiscent of an Elysian orchard. It is named after a seventeenth-century Italian princess who perfumed her clothing and baths with the essence of orange. This fragrant floral will bathe your being in luminous luxury.

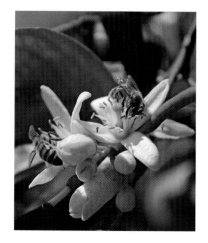

Ethereal and effectively astringent, neroli oil fades fine lines, scars, and stretch marks. It improves skin's elasticity, strengthens fragile skin, and balances overproductive oil glands. Neroli is anti-inflammatory and antibacterial, and helps to reduce pore size and prevent water loss in skin cells. Its constituents include linalool and limonene. It also includes a youth hormone called ocimene that may contribute to its effectiveness in preventing stretch marks.[23] With its aroma unleashed, neroli awakens the senses, calms frazzled nerves with its tranquil neurotonic properties, soothes insomnia, appeases postpartum depression, and "one drop dabbed anywhere, such as the sternum area, will ease anxiety."[24]

NIAOULI (MELALEUCA QUINQUENERVIA)

Numinous niaouli essential oil is the lively, luminous cousin of tea tree. If you find tea tree a bit pungent or medicinal smelling, niaouli's reviving essence offers extra disinfecting power[25] wrapped in a warmer, sweeter, more camphorous scent. Sometimes referred to as five-veined paperbark oil, or MQV (a nickname based on the Latin name), niaouli plays a prominent role in one's aromatherapy arsenal.

Niaouli clears nasal passages; and during epidemics, niaouli-soaked handkerchiefs were breathed into to prevent the spread of germs and disease.[26] MQV as an antihistamine is used to clear chest congestion, purify the air, alleviate allergies, and focus the mind. Brimming with effective antiseptic and antibacterial properties, niaouli has the ability to tighten tissues and is quite helpful for blemishes and acne issues too. Just as tea tree oil is known for clearing acne

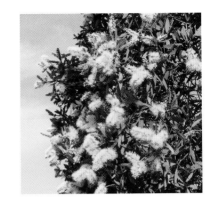

and fighting bacteria on the skin, niaouli offers similar benefits for sensitive skin. Skin ulcers, hemorrhoids, oral problems, dermatitis rashes, fungal rashes, lesions, insect bites, wounds, and boils can all be treated with niaouli's astringent tonic.

PALMAROSA (CYMBOPOGON MARTINII)

Pleasant palmarosa is distilled from a tropical, fragrant grass, resulting in an aromatic oil that smells like a lemony geranium rose and is simply splendid for the nose! This formidable skin rejuvenator rich in mighty monoterpenols, emollient esters, loving linalool, and generous geraniols regulates sebaceous glands and encourages healthy skin cells. Palmarosa stimulates skin cells and has a reputation for regulating skin imbalances like cystic acne and

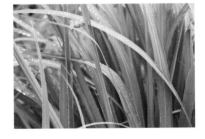

irritating dryness. Palmarosa balances oil production in all skin types, making oily skin less oily and dry skin less dry. Containing potent antimicrobial and antifungal properties, palmarosa is a popular treatment for athlete's foot and other fungal infections or rashes. Spider veins also benefit from an application of palmarosa. This oil is known for helping all body systems work together more efficiently.

Palmarosa is also a tonic to tummies experiencing digestive dampness and weakness via its anti-inflammatory actions. Emerging as an important restorative remedy to the gut and oral ecology, palmarosa "acts as a restorative to the microflora with both prebiotic-like and detoxicant action. These twin actions are able to both support healthy commensals and eliminate pathogenic strains in the gut, thereby addressing today's average state of intestinal dysbiosis in a truly comprehensive way."[27]

Peppermint (*Mentha piperita*)

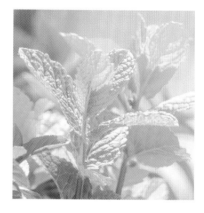

Bursting with minty freshness and powerful plant properties, peppermint's cooling qualities are key in this essential oil's ability to pacify throbs, reduce redness, and tranquilize itchiness. All the rage in Europe by the end of the nineteenth century, peppermint was and is much more than a mere breath freshener; it is known to ease headaches, clear the sinuses, improve digestion, and be victorious against a variety of viruses. "Mint" derives from the Latin *mente*, meaning "thought," as our antiquity ancestors considered it a boost for the brain. Peppermint feels cooling and nice like ice; and it is therefore one of those essential essential oils that belongs in every first-aid and travel kit. Peppermint's potent antibacterial, antiviral, and anti-inflammatory properties soothe pain, itching, and irritation, so it is a great oil to treat rashes, insect bites, and blemishes. Peppermint oil is fiercely antifungal, making it a fantastic remedy for fungal infections of the skin and nails. Its antiseptic benefits stimulate and revitalize dull skin and bring balance to oily skin.

Rockrose (*Cistus landiferus*)

Replenishing rockrose is neither a rock nor a rose; it is a Mediterranean wildflower that resembles wild roses. Rockrose may very well have been the "rose of Sharon" mentioned in the Bible's Song of Solomon, and it has remained incredibly popular in Spain and east India, where it is included in pure amber perfumes. This essential oil elixir awakens the senses with its warm, balsamic, herbaceous-amber fragrance, emanating an aroma that will deeply touch your spirit.

Rockrose's affinity for skincare was recognized by ancient Egyptians who mixed it into beauty creams. It was a key ingredient in the unguents and ointments for skin imbalances due to its drying, antiseptic, cell-rejuvenating nature. Mature, scarred, congested, and sunburned skin will relish the oil's tonifying, healing, and moisturizing properties. Dr. Kurt Schnaubelt writes of this herbal essence, "The oil of rockrose is produced in hot, sun-drenched regions. It is used in aromamedicine for its astringent and tightening qualities. Rockrose is the fastest-acting oil to stop bleeding from open wounds."[28]

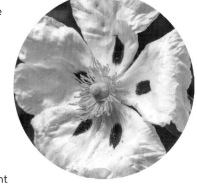

ROSEMARY (*ROSMARINUS OFFICINALIS*)

Rousing rosemary is an herbaceous revive-alive-verve tonic with a refreshing, penetrating aroma. Think of rosemary as the feisty friend that stimulates sluggishness out of its stagnancy, helping lymph, liver, digestive, immune, and skin systems thrive with renewed freshness. Rosemary enhances the skin's metabolism and is particularly suited to skin, hair, and cuticle care with its antiseptic, cleansing, cell-rejuvenating, acne-clearing, and skin-stimulating qualities. Rosemary oil is filled with antioxidants and bioactive compounds that are cell protective, including carnosic acid, camphor, and rosmaridiphenol. Clarifying to congestion as an effective mucolytic and antiviral expectorant, rosemary's reviving aroma is also mentally restorative, helping to increase focus and dispel confusion. Additionally, rosemary releases emotional stagnation, revving emotions to move from apathy into renewed confidence and motivation.

Rose Otto (*Rosa damascena*)

Regal rose otto is a steam-distilled divination from the Valley of Roses in Bulgaria and has been an integral ingredient in skincare preparations for centuries. Poets, writers, and mystics have extolled the heartwarming effects of rose otto, which opens the heart to love. This amorous oil encourages trust, elevates moods, and helps ease heartbreak. Beyond its angelic aroma and healing vibrations, rose otto is the most precious, sought-after, and medicinally potent oil of any rose variety. Divine grace for beauty and face, radiant rose revives every filament of our being with its elegant essence. It takes sixty roses to make one drop of rose otto essential oil! The "otto" in rose otto refers to it being a steam distillation. This is the only type of rose essence one wants to use in skincare. All other rose oils are absolutes, and those are best for perfumes and blends. Soothing to the heart and smoothing to wrinkles, it is a key ally in skin rejuvenation, inviting balance and healing to all skin conditions. The most medicinal and superlative for skincare, rose otto adds resiliency and elasticity to the connective tissue in the skin. It is a vulnerary, meaning that it speeds up the healing of tissues with its opulent antiseptic properties.

> I ask the rose, Where did you get
>   such skin?
> She laughs. How could she answer?
> She is drunk, but not enough to
>   say secrets.
>
> Rumi

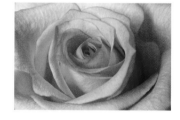

Sandalwood (*Santalum album*)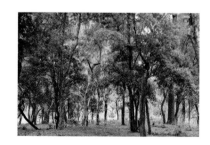

Heaven-scented sandalwood essence is distilled from the heartwood of the aromatic tree. Sandalwood suffuses with magnificent moisture and antimicrobial powers. Sensual sandalwood oil is a staple of natural hair and skin care since antiquity. This ancient aphrodisiac also contains a botanical pheromone similar to androsterone, the underarm pheromone secretion that acts as a sexual signal. This makes it a dashing deodorant that is super effective by simply applying a drop to each armpit. This serene oil contains alpha santalol and beta santalol, which have been studied to show that these monoterpene compounds inhibit abnormal cell growth,[29] making sandalwood a steadfast serum for toning, regulating, and moisturizing the skin. In another study, sandalwood was applied topically for twenty weeks and decreased the incidence of skin papillomas and induced healthy apoptosis, suggesting that sandalwood is chemopreventive[30] Soothing sandalwood, sacred for thousands of years, hastens skin repair, fades melasma, and reduces scarring.

Sweet Thyme (*Thymus vulgaris ct. linalool*)

Salving sweet thyme is as strong as it is soft. This special variety of thyme is a favorite of mine and the ancient Greeks. This perfectly potent medicinal plant is steam-distilled from the dried leaves and flowers of the *Thymus vulgaris* ct. *linalool* herb. It offers a warm, buttery aroma that is incredibly gentle yet incredibly effective at attending to ailments. Also known as sweet thyme, thyme linalool (differing wholly from the "nature-identical" isolate linalool) stimulates and energizes the body and mind while being mild enough to treat very young children and the elderly. It is a treasured ingredient for oral-care and skincare serums, gently rebalancing and removing impurities of the mouth and skin pores. This gentle yet potent antiseptic essence is an anti-infectious and antimicrobial ally for the skin, soothing and clarifying sebaceous glands, blemishes, acne, fungal rashes, clogged pores, and *Candida*. "In this oil the mildness of linalool and linalyl acetate is combined with the strong antiseptic action of thyme. It is excellent for impurities of the skin. Its gentleness and antimicrobial effects have made it an aromatherapy classic overnight. It is a pleasant tonic for nervous exhaustion, and is irreplaceable in skincare."[31]

Turmeric (*Curcuma longa*)

Treasured turmeric essential extract is herbal nourishment of golden goodness for skin, stomachs, mouths, and throats. Through supercritical extraction, all of turmeric's lipophilic (oil-loving) compounds are captured from the plant's roots. This special extraction process captures much more of the aromatic volatile oils, lipids, and pigments than a typical powdered herb does. Its nour- 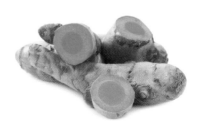 ishing qualities contain antiseptic and antimicrobial properties that turn away pathogenic bacteria and fungi, helping the gut's garden and oral oasis maintain their homeostasis. Turmeric oil essence is rich in antioxidants and potent anti-inflammatory properties that activate more than a dozen protective anti-inflammatory proteins in the skin cells. When the natural cell-protective mechanism is activated with turmeric phytonutrients, the response is said to be far superior to the protective action of antioxidants alone. One of the most incredible properties of turmeric is that its phytonutrients attract electrons. These electrophiles prevent the oxidation of lipids, which in turn results in protected skin cells and radiance!

Vetiver (*Chrysopogon zizanioides*)

Vivacious vetiver is distilled from the pungent roots of a very aromatic trop- ical grass. The goodness of this oil is grounding and calming for the skin and spirit, anointing the roots of each skin layer as the rain anoints the grass. Vetiver is a marvelous moisturizer that helps skin maintain its youthful plump- ness while soothing tired tissues, soft- ening scars and stretch marks, and balancing sebum production. Adapto- genic in nature, vetiver oil is a powerful antifungal, a circulatory stimulant, and an immunostimulant that strengthens

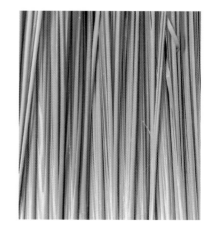

connective tissues, stimulates stagnant lymph systems, and tends to balance the skin's biome. "Very few remedies, aromatic or otherwise, exert the same depth of restorative action as vetiver, repairing as it does the body's four core systems, the nervous, the endocrine, gastrointestinal and immune."[32]

YARROW (*ACHILLEA MILLEFOLIUM*)

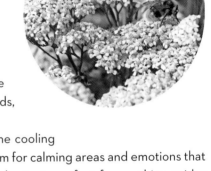

Yielding yarrow essence is a botanical blessing steam-distilled from the flowering tops of wild yarrow. Extensively used by Native Americans in herbal medicine applications, yarrow was consumed to lower fevers and to cure the symptoms of colds and respiratory infections. Chewing the roots, leaves, and petals of this plant helped ease digestion, and the mashed pulp of yarrow was an effective treatment for bruises, scrapes, cuts, wounds, and insect bites.

Ample in sesquiterpenes thanks to the cooling compound chamazulene, yarrow is a dream for calming areas and emotions that have become inflamed. Yarrow is a vascular tonic perfect for soothing spider veins, blemishes, and rashes. Sluggish lymph systems adore yarrow, and lungs love yarrow in the salt pipe. Combine with peppermint for any area that needs styptic "botanical ice"—for anything that itches it sure is nice!

This tried-and-true blue oil is so potent, legend has it that Achilles doused himself in yarrow oil in order to protect himself from his enemies' arrows. The only part of his body not protected by yarrow was . . . his Achilles' heel! Hence the Latin genus name *Achillea*, and *millefolium* means "a thousand leaves."

YLANG YLANG (*CANANGA ODORATA*)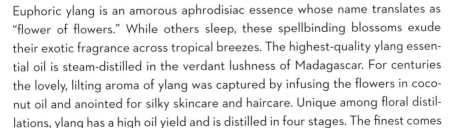

Euphoric ylang is an amorous aphrodisiac essence whose name translates as "flower of flowers." While others sleep, these spellbinding blossoms exude their exotic fragrance across tropical breezes. The highest-quality ylang essential oil is steam-distilled in the verdant lushness of Madagascar. For centuries the lovely, lilting aroma of ylang was captured by infusing the flowers in coconut oil and anointed for silky skincare and haircare. Unique among floral distillations, ylang has a high oil yield and is distilled in four stages. The finest comes from the first part of the distillation, known as "extra" or "superior." The first distillation is the cream of the crop with the most ethereal aroma from the peak amount of aromatic and skin-healing ester compounds. The subsequent distillations are classified as first, second, and third, and these are the more commonly available distillations. Therapeutically, ylang has qualities that synergize the dual actions of regulating and relaxing body systems.

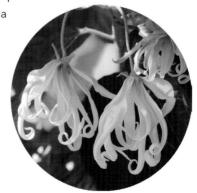

The superior distillation of ylang is super sensual and sublime for skincare, as it is a cell regenerator and regulates oil production in both the skin and the scalp. Ylang yields skin-softening, facial-muscle-relaxing, skin-tone-balancing, and hair-strengthening qualities. The molecules of this fine floral fragrance stimulate the brain to release relaxing, euphoric endorphins, easing anxiety and stress. The heady, serenely sweet aroma heightens the senses to receive life's beauty.

Additional Essential Oil Ingredients for Formulating, Diffusing, Inhaling, and Elevating Emotion

Bergamot (Citrus bergamia)

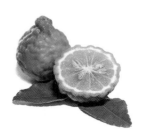

Blissful bergamot is filled with sunny floral-fruit cheer. Renowned for its ability to incite feelings of happiness, this citrus oil is distilled from the fruit of the *Citrus bergamia* tree, which blossoms during the inviting Italian winter. The aroma of bergamot is familiar to many as the scent of Earl Grey tea.

This exquisite essence is soothing to scars, stretch marks, and eczema, and doubles as a digestive aid. Its true power lies in its unparalleled ability to dispel depression and ease anxiety by inviting feelings of radiant relief as bergamot balances the brain's hypothalamus. These psychological effects of bergamot were studied by Paoli Rovesti at the University of Milan, who conducted research at psychiatric clinics. He described the aroma of bergamot as having the capacity to relieve fear and calm anxiety. Rovesti claimed it is "the most valuable oil at the aromatherapist's disposal."[33] He also recommended bergamot for people who desired to quit smoking, as it is relaxing and eases stress and nervousness.

Bergamot essential oil has also performed brilliantly when scrutinized by Western medical studies. In one test, bergamot was proved to reduce damage to human stem cells, while another study showed bergamot to be effective at reducing lung inflammation in people suffering from cystic fibrosis.[34,35]

As with many citrus oils, bergamot is photosensitizing, so it is important to not apply it undiluted to the skin and then expose the skin directly to sunlight. It is not photosensitizing when diluted to 1 percent or less in a blend with a carrier oil, such as jojoba, coconut, or olive oil, so it is safe to use in a bodycare blend and then go out in the sun.

Black Spruce (*Picea mariana*)

Strengthening-spruce essential oil is wild crafted and steam-distilled deep in the heart of the Canadian wilderness. This refreshing oil is stimulating and invigorating, and may ease fatigue and rev the adrenal glands. Spruce oil is milder and gentler than other evergreen oils, and is traditionally used as a decongestant. Enjoy an inviting fragrance of evergreen, freshly fallen snow, and sweet wood as you clarify your lungs and ease tension in your body.

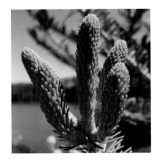

Blood Orange (*Citrus sinensis*)

Buoyant blood orange essential oil is happy, harmonious, bright-light aroma that inspires joy wherever it goes! Warm feelings of love and laughter appear as moodiness and anxiety disappear. Blood orange has been historically used to relax frazzled nerves, improve the condition of skin, and cleanse the lymphatic system.

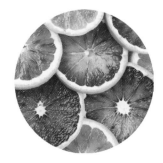

Eucalyptus (*Eucalyptus globulus*)

Expectorant extraordinaire, eucalyptus expands inhalations and exhalations with its clearing camphorous aroma. Decades upon decades, this deluxe decongestant has helped humans breathe by cleansing and clearing spaces, places, and faces.

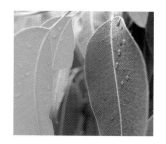

Ginger Root (*Zingiber officinale*)

Spicy and enlivening, ginger root essential oil packs an herbaceous punch! A supercritical extract from organic ginger grown in Madagascar adds a warming zing in your throat so you feel ready to sing! As one of the most popular spices in the world, ginger's effective qualities have been proved by their extensive use in ancient Indian and Chinese cultures.

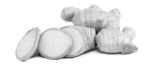

Grapefruit (*Citrus paradisi*)

Feel good with gleeful grapefruit! This circulation-stimulating citrus with an affinity for the lymph system gets your qi going in the morning. Refresh your senses with this sunny citrus essence that lifts the spirits, and disharmony is nothing more than a distant memory.

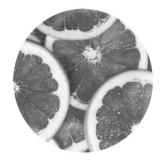

Inula (*Inula graveolens*)

This rare essence is revered as the mightiest mucolytic in the aromatherapy arsenal. This gem is excellent at eliminating phlegm and aerating airways. Composed of clarifying and calming esters (50 percent bornyl acetate) and sesquiterpene lactones, inula oil moves mucus to ease belabored breathing.

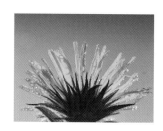

MARJORAM (*ORIGANUM MAJORANA*)

Marjoram has been used to purify body, mind, and spirit since biblical times. It was used by the Greeks and Romans to invoke states of enlightened peace. Steam-distilled to capture the medicinal powers of this fragrant herb, marjoram soothes and stabilizes while protecting the body and mind from the stressful effects of external environmental stimuli. Extreme emotions, sleeplessness, and tension are all brought back into balance with the calming power of marjoram.

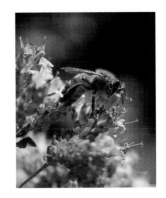

OREGANO (*ORIGANUM VULGARE*)

Opulent oregano is a classic botanical-biotic heal-all that illuminates immunity, eliminates invaders, and calls clarity. It is considered a culinary and a "hot" oil and must be diluted before use.

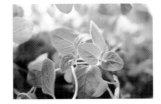

SCHIZANDRA BERRY (*SCHIZANDRA SPENANTHERA*)

Sumptuous schizandra berry extract is distilled from the berries of the Indonesian schizandra shrub. These berries are a staple in Traditional Chinese Medicine, and have been used for thousands of years to boost the body's qi and raise the body's stress threshold. Known as *wu wei zi* in Chinese, this "five-flavor fruit" contains a complex palette of flavors that are bitter, salty, spicy, sweet, and sour. Schizandra oil is a supercritical extraction and contains all of the lipophilic components for even more aromatherapeutic benefits than it has flavors!

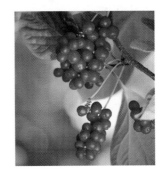

Tea Tree (*Melaleuca alternifolia*)

Touted as a medical miracle, tea tree essence is an antiseptic extraordinaire that heals, soothes, and cleans cuts, wounds, and inflamed skin. This Australian treasure is steam-distilled, exuding a fresh camphorous scent. It has been used by indigenous Aborigines for centuries. In ancient Australia, tea tree leaves were crushed and inhaled as a cold and cough remedy. Leaves were 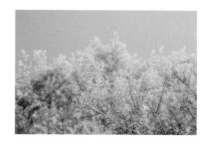 also steeped to make a pungent liquid that was applied to skin infections and open wounds and was used as a medicinal elixir to heal sore throats and internal imbalances. Tea tree essential oil is an ancient answer to first-aid needs. Whether one has been bitten by hungry mosquitoes during a camping trip or one needs a quick way to clean a cut, tea tree oil is a time-tested and handy heal-all. Today, tea tree essential oil is used to treat acne, eczema, dandruff, coughs, yeast infections, burns, cuts, lice, sunburns, sinus infections, and chest congestion.

Tea tree teems with antiviral, antifungal, and antibacterial properties, making it perfect for periodontal care. It is a "therapeutic agent in chronic gingivitis and periodontitis, conditions that have both bacterial and inflammatory components."[36]

Happy Hydration

Quench and cleanse epidermal layers with these sources of hydration that harmonize the skin's cells and biome with true tonics to tonify and clarify.

Aloe Vera (*Aloe barbadensis*)

Amazing aloe is a familiar botanical gem from the desert. It was called the "plant of immortality" by the ancient Egyptians. It is 99 percent water and contains seventy-five beneficial compounds, including amino acids, vitamins, enzymes, minerals, sugars, and salicylic acid. Aloe contains seven of the essential amino acids required by humans for optimal health. Applied topically to the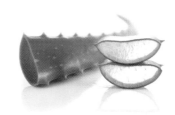

skin, the amino acids soften rough and hardened skin cells for softer, smoother skin. The zinc in the aloe gel acts as a gentle astringent. As a potent healer, it increases collagen creation and accelerates wound healing and strength.

Aloe is protective against radiation and sunburn damage to the skin. When aloe is applied topically, an antioxidant protein called metallothionein is generated in the skin. Metallothionein scavenges free radicals and, because it is rich in cysteine, a glutathione precursor, it prevents the oxidation of superoxide dismutase (SOD) and glutathione in the skin.[37]

Skip the bottled gels—they have been heavily processed, they may have hidden preservatives, and purity may have been compromised in the process. Aloe is an easy plant to grow; put a plant on your bathroom counter for quick access. Just break open a leaf and squeeze out the juice whenever you want. It can be used on the skin, in the hair, in the mouth, and as a carrier.

APPLE CIDER VINEGAR (ACETIC ACID)

Activating apple cider vinegar, made by fermenting the juice of apples, has been an apothecary staple for thousands of years. Benefits abound with internal use of ACV, and it is exceptionally therapeutic when used topically. Chock-full of nutrients, ACV contains lactic, citric, and malic acids as well as vitamins A, B1, B2, B6, C, and E. It also has calcium, potassium, pectin, mineral salt, and amino acids that the skin can absorb transdermally. *Always* dilute by 50 percent to use topically for first aid, skincare, and haircare.

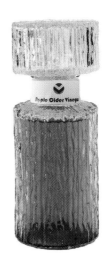

Apple cider vinegar excels as a bath and clay-mask additive, skin toner, sunburn soother, milia minimizer, and wound cleaner. With a pH similar to that of the acid mantle, ACV can restore the skin, especially after years of using sudsy cleansers that are too alkaline for the acid mantle and lipid layers. Used along with jojoba oil to cleanse, astringent ACV clears surfactants that have lodged themselves into the stratum corneum. Naturally containing alpha hydroxy acids, this liquid exfoliant will gently freshen skin, even tone, and moderate melasma. Blemishes and acne benefit from the malic acid's antibacterial effects.

It is lovely for locks as a hair rinse and soothing to dry, itchy scalps with dandruff. Super shininess is the result when used as a hair rinse. Herbs, such as rosemary, nettles, horsetail, and oat straw, can be added to full-strength ACV and strained out after one moon cycle for an additional boon to this already-amazing fermented tonic.

Frankincense Hydrosol (Boswellia carterii)

Refreshing frankincense hydrosol is a skin-quenching tonic that drenches pores with its cherished humectant and healing qualities. Frankincense water, as it is also known, is the medicinal water containing microsoluble constituents from the distillation of frankincense tears. Fundamentally, it is an aqueous version of the aromatic essential oil. It is a face tonic with a fine fragrance and ethereal effectiveness especially suited to evening skin tone, improving elasticity, and assisting skin in retaining moisture.

Turn caring for your skin into a mediation with this medicinal mist that may be used to revitalize skin after cleansing or shaving, and to revive the spirit any time of day.

Rose Hydrosol (Rosa damascena)

Resilient rosewater prepares the pores to receive the hydration they adore. Rose hydrosol, also referred to as rosewater, is culled from the first round of steam-distilled rose petals of *Rosa damascena* in the production of rose otto essential oil. The best rose hydrosol comes from the primary distillation and never, ever has any additional water or alcohol added. As rose petals dance in a fountain of dew during distillation, microsoluble components of the essential oil impart the hydrosol with the memory of roses, along with releasing beneficial water-soluble constituents for sublime skincare. Rose hydrosol is mildly astringent and acts as a hydrating humectant that lifts the spirits and soothes thirsty skin. A single spritz of pure rosewater infuses your skin with profound beauty that has been prized through millennia. Cleopatra was an avid fan of rosewater's refreshing dew; she sipped it, bathed in it, and soaked her sails in this regal water. Rumi waxed poetically,

> If a beetle moves toward rosewater, it proves
> that the solution is diluted. Beetles
> love dung, not rose essence.[38]

Analysis of organic rose hydrosol reveals beneficial esters, aldehydes, sesquiterpenol, geraniol, citronellol, and linalool that create a cordial that is antifungal, anti-infectious, anti-inflammatory, antispasmodic, antiviral, bactericidal, balancing, calming, cicatrizant, and circulatory.[39]

Awaken and renew the respiration of the skin with rosewater's unique hydration. Mist face before and after cleansing with oil. It may also be enjoyed throughout the day when you need a little revivifying, during flights to hydrate skin, as a delightful aftershave, or as a gentle makeup remover.

WATER

Pure water is key to nourish and finely tune each tiny skin pore. Every pore is like a little door into your being and bloodstream, and it needs to be nourished with untainted, mineral-rich water. First and foremost, if municipal tap water is what comes out of your faucets, invest in a water filter—either a simple shower filter or a whole-home water filter. It is amazing what skin conditions clear up once chlorine, fluoride, and the cocktail of unknown tap-contaminants are removed from what should be life-giving water. Another option, especially when traveling, is to buy a glass bottle of spring water and use it exclusively for washing your face. Pour straight from the bottle onto your cloth for oil cleansing, and make a mister to spritz skin with dewy

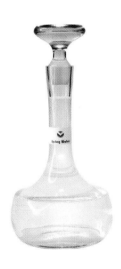

droplets. When I travel, I bring a wrench and a showerhead filter that I can easily affix to existing plumbing. If I cannot change the filter, I will wash and rinse with a cloth and spring water.

Skin cells thrive on spring water that holds the memory and minerals of its vortexed voyage through the purifying filter of sands and stones as it bubbles up to the earth's surface. This is the aqua vitae that will vivify your visage.

All water has a perfect memory and is forever trying to get back to where it was.

Toni Morrison

Stimulating Seeds

Think of these good-natured nourishments as caring condiments to boost the biome's beneficial bacteria, soothe sebum, purify pores, strengthen the stratum corneum, and support the skin's cells. This is the spa-like manna to maintain the skin's mantle.

ACTIVATED CHARCOAL

This cleansing carbon acts like a magnet to toxins. Exceptional for skin and oral care, it is also administered in hospital emergency rooms to expel alcohol and drug poisons. Its beneficial binding action makes it a formidable cosmoetic cleanser as it binds to toxins. This black powder clarifies blackheads and purifies pores by pulling out undesirable microparticles and surfactants to help tighten pores. It is great as an on-the-spot mini-mask when mixed with **Brilliant Beauty Spot Treatment.** It works as a first-aid remedy when mixed with clay and peppermint oil. Activated charcoal may also be combined with baking soda as a tooth polish and to remove chemical buildup on the hair and scalp for deeply cleaned and volumized hair.

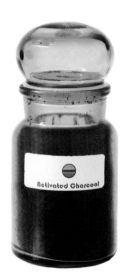

Baking Soda (Sodium Bicarbonate)

Beneficial baking soda is a naturally occurring alkali substance produced by our bodies and also found in the earth in the form of mineral deposits and dissolved in mineral springs. Beyond its green-cleaning capacity to scrub tubs and lift stains from laundry, baking soda also befits the body.

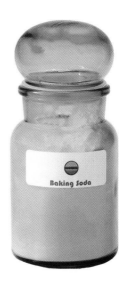

Taken internally, baking soda is an excellent buffering agent to help the kidneys mop up heavy metals and neutralize toxins. Boost your body's bicarbonate reserves and alkalinity with a pinch of powder in a glass of water first thing in the morning. Bathing in baking soda, especially with magnesium salts and droplets of essential oils like lavender or chamomile, relaxes muscles and mind before bed. Dusting armpits with baking soda works as a deodorant. Shampooing with it lifts surfactants from the scalp, and for a dry shampoo, sprinkle it on the hair and massage into the scalp. Add a dash to your cleansing oil and cloth for a mild exfoliant, too.

Baking soda also shines as a toothpaste. It is an effective tooth-cleaning polish, and its alkaline action helps to eliminate biofilms, reduces oral acidity levels, neutralizes pathogens, and naturally whitens teeth. It is significantly less abrasive than the cleaning agents of chalk and silica that are used in commercial toothpastes. Paul H. Keyes, DDS, clinical investigator at the National Institute of Dental Research, advised regular brushing with sea salt and/or baking soda, as it prevents all destructive periodontal disease.[40]

Clays

Whether one uses bentonite, pyrophyllite, illite, rhassoul, fuller's earth, or kaolin, these multitasking mineral-rich mud masks have adorned skin since ancient eras. Our ancestors discerned that dirt does the body good! While each type of clay has unique properties, they all essentially function as magnetic magic that detoxifies microparticles from the door of every pore. Internally, clays also draw out undesirables from the digestive tract. When clay is mixed with water, molecules get electrically charged, resulting in pore-tightening, acne-clearing, fungal-removing, melasma-diminishing, complexion-smoothing, and impurity-absorbing perfection. Clays can be drying, so it's best to play around with adding honey or jojoba for a soothing spa treatment. They are also an effective tooth polish and can be added to oil-pulling formulas. They are nourishing and cleansing to the hair and scalp when mixed with oil before shampooing, and are dutiful when brushed in as a dry shampoo. I love using clay as a bandage for small cuts, scrapes, and wounds.

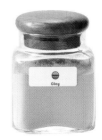

HONEY

> One only begins to understand the life of the bees when one knows that the bee lives in an atmosphere completely pervaded by love.[41]

Healing honey is an ambrosial blessing created by the grand design of glorious honeybees. These passionate pollinators are elemental to Gaia's garden, yet the current use of GMOs and poisonous pesticides (especially neonicotinoids) is challenging the global immune system of the hive's intelligence, setting this insect tribe's path to colony collapse

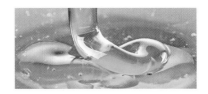

disorder. Now more than ever, it is time to celebrate the gifts of bees by supporting organic beekeepers who ethically harvest honey, propolis, pollen, and beeswax so that healthy populations proliferate. We envision an abundance of bees flitting about fields of flowers making their miraculous magic.

Honey, illustrious for its sweet nectar, is also a Herculean skin healer. It has been a timeless treasure used by ancient cultures in making curing compounds for skin and respiratory infections, burns, sore throats, and digestive disorders. Therapeutic use of honey fell by the wayside with the advent of antibiotics, even though hundreds of honey articles can be found in medical journals and peer-reviewed scientific studies. Now that antibiotic resistance is a real deal, honey is in full study once again as researchers rediscover that it is effective against at least sixty types of resistant pathogens and their biofilms, including *Pseudomonas aeruginosa, Streptococcus pyogenes, Escherichia coli,* and MRSA (methicillin-resistant *Staphylococcus aureus*).[42]

Seek raw, organic honey from local beekeepers, and avoid "Grade A" honey from supermarkets, as this is just expensive high-fructose corn syrup. Another outrageous travesty of commercial honey is that hives are drained of all their honey, which is replaced with high-fructose corn syrup to feed the hive! Processing honey with heat destroys valuable vitamins, minerals, enzymes, and glucose oxidase. The glucose oxidase is an essential aspect of honey's healing; when it comes into contact with body fluids like saliva or the exudates produced by a skin wound, the glucose oxidase releases healing hydrogen peroxide, which is antibacterial and antiviral.

Adding the botanical-biotics of essential oils to raw honey multiplies its power and makes for potent blends that can be applied to wounds[43] and facial masks to even skin tone, energize the acid mantle, soothe the stratum corneum, soften scars, ease acne pitting, and speed up the healing of cesarean sections.[44]

BEESWAX

Brilliant beeswax is another blessing from the bee-hive. Agile as architects, bees create homes that consist of hexagon-shaped honeycombs that are made of beautiful beeswax. The wax is secreted by special glands on the worker bees and is used for honey storage and pupal protection inside the hive. The wax from organic happy honeybees shields the skin by forming a breathable antibac-terial layer[45] that seals the skin's succulence and heals dry, chapped skin and lips. Differing deeply from pore-clogging petroleum-based paraben waxes, beeswax is biologically brimming with vitamin A, esters, and fatty acids that lock in mois-ture as a hydrating humectant. Beeswax is key for

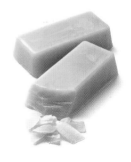

making cosmoetic balms and unique perfume unguents. This anti-inflammatory waxy wonder is perfect for lip balms, diaper-rash ointments, and anti-itch balms, as it soothes irritated skin and prevents bacterial and fungal growth.

Iodine

Indispensable iodine is an electron-rich, essential mineral and potent ancestral antioxidant that is needed by every cell, every organ, and every tissue in the body. Topically, iodine may be used for wounds, bedsores, keloid formations, and scars. It stimulates healthy hair growth and helps to repair the intracellular matrix of connective tissue too. Iodine supplementation can be accomplished orally and via transdermal absorption. Skin experiments by an oncologist found that transdermal application of iodine is helpful for moles, skin fungal infections, and lesions. His instructions are to paint a 7 percent iodine solution on the area ten to twenty times twice a day for five days and then once a day for another ten days.[46] When a scab forms, keep painting it with iodine, under it and above it; never pick the scab but allow it to lift out of the dermis and fall away naturally. If you would like to try this, consider talking with a holistic health care professional for assistance.

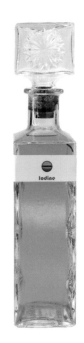

Magnesium Salts and Epsom Salts (Magnesium Chloride or Magnesium Sulfate)

These magnesium miracles are bathing beauties. Magnesium salt is made from seawater, and soaking in seawater salt boosts the body's magnesium stores. Epsom salts are also a form of magnesium that helps soothe joints and calm nerves. Both types are superb muscle and mind relaxants. Magnesium is essential to mitochondrial function, and daily baths with these amazing additives assist in alleviating pain, insomnia, some skin conditions, and restless legs syndrome.

PROBIOTICS (*LACTOBACILLI, OF L. FERMENTUM, L. PLANTARUM, L. CASEI, L. REUTERI, AND L. RHAMNOSUS, AND BIFIDOBACTERIUM*)

Multiply microbes in the skin and body's bacterial bank account by ingesting and applying probiotics. The topical application of probiotics rebuilds microbial diversity that has been depleted by common skincare chemicals, balances the biome of the epidermal layers, boosts the skin's innate immunity, strengthens the stratum corneum and lipid layers, nourishes and maintains the acid mantle, increases natural ceramide and lipid production, harmonizes the skin to receive the sun's rays, balances the sebaceous glands, alleviates fungal and bacterial rashes, assists in healing scars and wounds, and supports collagen synthesis.[47] With all these benefits, methods to deliver probiotics to the dermis are in scientific and medical development. Yet, we don't have to wait! Simply open a probiotic capsule, add it to a wholesome skin serum or honey mask, and apply. Replenish with bacteria-friendly botanicals so that you can meet the life of your skin and revel in the perfection you were born with.

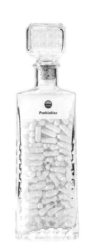

ROSEHIPS (*ROSA RUBIGINOSA*)

Rosehips powder is brimming with nourishing vitamins C, A, and E, calcium and iron, bioflavonoids, selenium, manganese, and B complex vitamins. It is also abundant in antioxidants: carotenoids, flavonoids, and polyphenols. Favorable fruit acids and rare rose pectin make this a mildly astringent, gelatinous powder that is an excellent emollient-exfoliant that makes a fortifying facial mask.

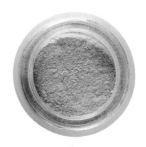

ROSEMARY (*ROSMARINUS OFFICINALIS*)

Rosemary powder resets skin with its antiseptic and antimicrobial properties that bring balance to blemishes, acne, eczema, and sebum. Use with **Brilliant Beauty Spot Treatment** to make mini-masks for acne and blemishes, as an all-over mask

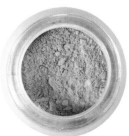

with clay, as a gentle exfoliator with jojoba, or as a tooth powder with sea salt and baking soda.

Sea Salt (Sodium Chloride)

Oceanic salt is an alkaline ally for our skin, as our bodies contain the same concentration of minerals as seawater. Sea salt is plentiful in minerals that are essential to intracellular communication: magnesium, calcium, sodium, potassium, and trace minerals. It is an essential apothecary item, as it can be used as a stimulating scalp scrub before shampooing, as a body scrub, a smooth-

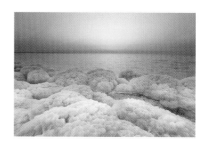

ing mask mixed with honey, a mouthwash, a talented toothpaste, a deodorant, a nourishing salt soak for baths, and a cleansing and nifty nail-brightening soak.

Salt sole water is also a mineral tonic that can be made by dissolving sea salt in spring water: fill a 16-ounce mason jar with 4 ounces of sea salt, cover with a nonmetal lid, and let the salt dissolve overnight. Decant and stir with nonmetal utensils. Add a teaspoon of salt sole to drinking water (for the trace minerals), and dilute further with water to use as a mouthwash and as a misting spritz for a sebum-balancing tonic. It can also be used as a **Beach Breeze Hair Spray.**

Vitamin C (L-Ascorbic Acid)

Vital vitamin C is an essential nutrient for the body, and it is also effective topically. When sourcing this supplemental powder, always procure corn-free, no-GMO vitamin C. This potent antioxidant can be added to serums, masks, and toners to strengthen skin, smooth skin texture, even skin tone, and speed up wound healing. This form of vitamin C is water-soluble and can easily be added to a spritz bottle to mist onto skin. For a really neat, waterproof sunburn-prevention protocol, mix pure vitamin C powder in a 10 percent solution with water

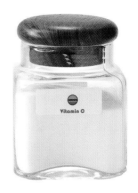

and lightly mist onto exposed skin, allowing it to soak in, and spray once again before sun exposure.

Tools and Miscellanea

Organic cotton rounds, face cloths, gua sha skin tool, salt pipe, aroma diffuser, jade roller, small mixing bowl, blending brush, and empty glass bottles and jars.

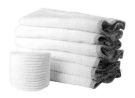

Quite simply, one could go to a health food store and gather bulk baking soda, sea salt, a liter of apple cider vinegar, olive oil, and spring water to take care of skin and teeth and be far better off than spending a dime on drugstore-variety chemical-laden skincare.

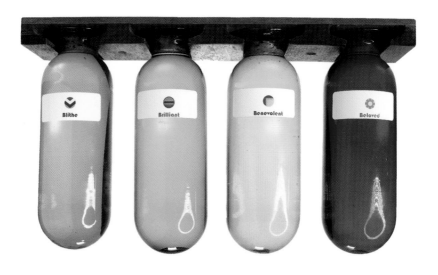

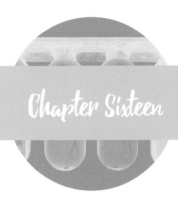

Chapter Sixteen

RENEGADE BEAUTY
RECIPES

Now is the time for you to know that all you do is sacred . . . Now is the time for you to deeply understand the impossibility that there is anything but grace.[1]

"When Nature begins to reveal her open secret . . ."[2] Ablutions in beauty are a sacred communion, from playing with plant matter, to friendship with each anointment and gesture that graces your being. The fairest flower blossoms in you. Groom each petal. Yield to the perfume that abounds around, and from, you. Nourish all the senses that have been parched for your essence. Gifts from the land bring a wild reception to be your finest bathing attendants. Essences and aqua oleums, stirred and applied, are the fragrant, moist blessing that is a divine body dressing. Loving sips for the skin, the dews of plant wisdom flower your face. The sun, the moon, the wind, the rain, the soil, the trees, the lakes, and the leaves are all here to bathe in, on, and around you.

Attention is the embodiment of ablutions, summoning every body filament alive: the wholly pleasure of whole, of washing water over emotion, of anointing flower oils to flesh, of nourishing tongue and belly. Attention is the alchemy of awareness.

Follow the clues: the wisdom on, in, and around the body. These are the rocks to be unearthed, the wilderness to be wandered and wondered: brought into the sun, into the light of awareness.

For where attention is,
Beauty follows,
Beauty flowers.

These Renegade Beauty Recipes are keys to the living library of beautifying with botanicals. Every bottle brimming with botanicals is a hidden gem desiring to be known and shown to your skin. Gleefully, a plant's quintessence entwines with your essence to be the healing helix it dreamed to divine: a precious mixture of cosmic-cellular chime. Essence upon essence upon your essence. The possibilities—the play—are endless. This plant-extract poetry may be anointed, inhaled, sipped, and stirred: moisturizers with myrrh, baths with blue tansy, inhalations of immortelle, palmarosa perfumes, cypress toning mists, sandalwood serums, chamomile creams, and lavender linen dreams. These tips and tricks are honed from formulating with botanicals and my decades of desire to simplify, purify, and create more ease and effortlessness in ablutions.

This is your plant kin. Dive in!

Beauty was not simply something to behold; it was something one could do.

Toni Morrison[3]

BEAUTIFUL BODYCARE

Blithe Beauty All Over Oil

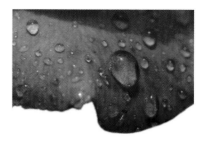

Calming and cooling for washing and moisturizing face and body with a focus on skin flare-ups.

60 ml Jojoba

1 ml Frankincense

1 ml Peppermint

1 ml Blue Tansy

Blithe Beauty Splendid Serum

Calming and cooling emollient for face and special areas of cellulite, burns, rashes, and flare-ups.

30 ml Jojoba

5 ml Tamanu

1 ml Frankincense

10 drops Yarrow

10 drops Sandalwood

10 drops Peppermint

Blithe Beauty Spot Treatment

Targeted treatment for acne, bumps, blemishes, flare-ups, cuts, anti-itch, and first aid.

3 ml Frankincense

1 ml Peppermint

1 ml Blue Tansy

1 ml German Chamomile

Benevolent Beauty All Over Oil

Smoothing and soothing for washing and moisturizing face and body with a focus on sensitive skin and melasma.

60 ml Jojoba

1 ml Lavender

1 ml Sandalwood

1 ml Sweet Thyme

Benevolent Beauty Splendid Serum

Smoothing and soothing emollient for face and special areas of stretch marks, blemishes, scars, and melasma.

30 ml Jojoba

5 ml Sandalwood Nut Oil

1 ml Lavender

10 drops Rose Otto

10 drops Sandalwood

10 drops Immortelle

Benevolent Beauty Spot Treatment

Targeted treatment for acne, bumps, blemishes, melasma, and scars

3 ml Lavender

1 ml Immortelle

1 ml Rose Otto

1 ml Frankincense

Brilliant Beauty All Over Oil

Smoothing and soothing for washing and moisturizing face and body with a focus on acne.

60 ml Jojoba

1 ml Rosemary

1 ml Carrot Seed

1 ml Palmarosa

Brilliant Beauty Splendid Serum

Smoothing and soothing emollient for face and special areas of acne and stretch marks.

25 ml Jojoba

5 ml Camellia Oil

5 ml Seabuckthorn Berry Oil

10 drops Vetiver

10 drops Laurel

10 drops Carrot Seed

10 drops Sweet Thyme

Brilliant Beauty Spot Treatment

Targeted treatment for acne, bumps, blemishes, and fungal flare-ups.

2 ml Rosemary

2 ml Niaouli

1 ml Immortelle *AKA Helichryum*

1 ml Sweet Thyme

Beloved Beauty All Over Oil

Smoothing and soothing for washing and moisturizing face and body with a special focus on rosacea and dry skin.

60 ml Jojoba

1 ml Chamomile

1 ml Carrot Seed

1 ml Ylang

1 ml Lemon

Beloved Beauty Splendid Serum

Smoothing and soothing emollient for face and special areas of scars, melasma, and rosacea.

30 ml Jojoba

5 ml Rosehips

10 drops Rose Otto

10 drops Rockrose

10 drops Geranium

10 drops Immortelle

Beloved Beauty Spot Treatment

Targeted treatment for melasma, bumps, blemishes, and scars.

2 ml Immortelle

1 ml Rose Otto

1 ml Carrot Seed

1 ml Myrrh

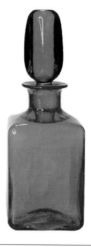

Dilution Made Easy

1% dilution =
7–10 drops of essential oil
+ 2 tablespoons of carrier oil

2% dilution =
14–20 drops of essential oils
+ 2 tablespoons of carrier

2 tablespoons = 1 oz = 30 ml
20 drops = 1 ml

Grapefruit Glow Body Scrub

Combine ingredients in a jar and mix together.

Apply with hands or a cloth before a bath, shower, or dip in a lake.

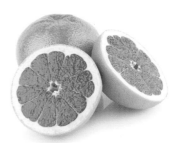

4 tablespoons finely ground Sea Salt

1 tablespoon Baking Soda

60 ml Jojoba

1 ml Grapefruit

1 ml Vetiver

10 drops Laurel

10 drops Carrot Seed

Astringent Face Tonic

Make fresh each day or store in the fridge.

Can be spritzed on skin or poured on a cloth for washing face.

30 ml Apple Cider Vinegar

30 ml Water

10 ml Rosewater (optional)

5 drops Immortelle, Lavender, Frankincense, or Niaouli

Calm Balm

Calming, cooling, and anti-itch for inflamed, irritated, and tender tissues. This can be used on everything from sinus stuffiness to rashes and cuts to hemorrhoids.

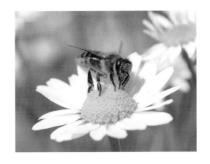

Melt beeswax in a bain-marie (double boiler). When melted, add jojoba and heat until liquid again. Add essential oils last. Stir together, pour into jars, and let cool overnight.

25 ml Beeswax

70 ml Jojoba

5 ml Peppermint

2 ml Blue Tansy

1 ml Yarrow

1 ml Frankincense

3 Probiotic capsules (optional)

Everything Balm

Soothing, smoothing balm for healing and sealing. This can be used for everything from dry elbows to a hair pomade.

Melt beeswax in a bain-marie (double boiler). When melted, add jojoba and heat until liquid again. Add essential oils last. Stir together, pour into jars, and let cool overnight.

25 ml Beeswax

70 ml Jojoba

2 ml Chamomile

2 ml Lavender

2 ml Sandalwood

2 ml Geranium

1 ml Sweet Thyme

Happy Honey Mask

Mix and jar full amount, or whip up a smaller batch on the spot.

30 ml Honey

5 drops Immortelle

5 drops Sweet Thyme

Skin Seed Mask

Combine, and add the apple cider vinegar/water combo until desired consistency. Apply and leave on for an hour if possible.

- 5 ml Activated Charcoal
- 10 ml Clay
- 3 Probiotic capsules
- 5 ml Rosehips powder
- 5 ml Honey
- 20 ml Apple Cider Vinegar : Water (50:50)
- 2 drops Carrot Seed
- 2 drops Frankincense
- 1 drop Sweet Thyme

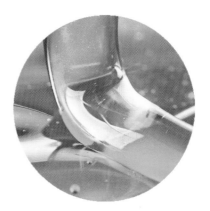

Pore Clarifying Mask

Mix in a jar. To use, put some in the palm of your hand or mix in a bowl, adding water until a spreadable consistency. Leave on for at least a few minutes, or longer for a spa treatment. It may also be used as a cleansing face wash.

- 15 ml Clay
- 5 ml Rosemary powder
- 5 ml Activated Charcoal
- 5 ml Jojoba
- 2 drops Carrot Seed
- 2 drops Niaouli
- 2 drops Rosemary

Pore Calming Mask

Mix in a jar. To use, put some in the palm of your hand or mix in a bowl, adding water until a spreadable consistency. Leave on for at least a few minutes, or longer for a spa treatment. It may also be used as a face wash.

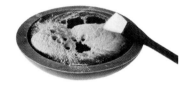

15 ml Clay

15 ml Rosehips powder

10 ml Honey

5 ml Rosehips Oil

5 drops Blue Tansy

3 drops Immortelle

3 drops Chamomile

Sunbather Bronzer

This sunbathing beauty will extend time in the sun and bring on a golden tan. It is by no means a sunblock; I think of it as a "sun harmonizer." For some it will extend their time in the sun by ten minutes and for others an hour. It all depends on the amount of melanin in your skin, the season, and the geographic location.

60 ml Jojoba

20 ml Coconut Oil (melt in jar in warm water to liquefy before blending)

3 ml Seabuckthorn Berry

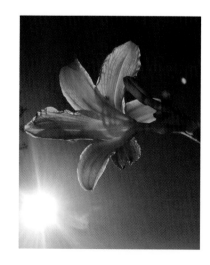

20 ml Red Raspberry Seed Oil

3 ml Tamanu

1 ml Frankincense

1 ml Sandalwood

1 ml Carrot Seed

1 ml Immortelle

10 drops Geranium

Botanical-Biotic Suppositories

Suppositories are a soothing way to use botanicals. They can be used as a soothing type of serum for yoni tissue repair and lubrication or as a good way to absorb botanical medicine for imbalances, from yeast infections to hemorrhoids. Even though inserting an anal suppository seems far away from the lungs, using botanicals in this way is also effective for healing the lungs to clear up congestion.

> *The suggestion of essential oil suppositories originates from French-style aromatherapy, which has found them to be highly effective in the treatment of serious acute and chronic bronchitis. The French literature on medical aromatherapy is full of suggestions for suppository formulas for a wide variety of conditions . . . this method delivers essential oils directly to the lung tissues . . . they reach the lower bronchial capillaries in their original lipophilic and volatile state, still capable of eliminating pathogenic microorganisms and dissolving and expectorating mucus.*[4]

Melt cacao butter slowly in a double boiler. Add coconut oil until liquid. Add essential oils. Let it almost solidify and then roll into the appropriate size, or while still liquid pour into very small chocolate silicone molds and pop in the fridge to cure.

Base:

20 ml Cacao Butter

10 ml Coconut Oil

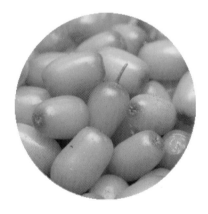

Medicinal:

1 ml Laurel

1 ml Chamomile

1 ml Frankincense

Tissue Soothing:

1 ml Seabuckthorn

1 ml Immortelle

10 drops Rose Otto

10 drops Ylang

Headache Help

Apply this concentrated chrism by the drop to temples, neck, and brow. It soothes muscle tension too.

15 ml Jojoba

10 ml Peppermint

1 ml Blue Tansy

1 ml Marjoram

Marjoram Moontime Blend

This concentrated chrism can be applied to the belly and lower back during moon cycles.

Also lovely to use with the Maya Abdominal Therapy massage technique (see "Menstruation" in Chapter Seventeen for more).

30 ml Jojoba

5 ml Marjoram

3 ml Geranium

10 drops Rose Otto

10 drops Frankincense

EYES

Beautiful Brow + Lash Blend

Apply to eyebrows and eyelashes at night to encourage growth and strength.

30 ml Castor Oil

5 drops Myrrh

5 drops Lemon

Cleopatra Charcoal Mascara

  1 teaspoon Activated Charcoal

  1 teaspoon Beeswax

  1 teaspoon Castor Oil

  1 teaspoon Coconut Oil

  3 drops Frankincense

  3 drops Myrrh

  2 empty mascara containers[5]

If it is warm where you live or you would like more of a "waterproof" mascara, edge up the beeswax.

In a bain-marie (double boiler), melt beeswax in a glass jar. When melted, add coconut, castor, activated charcoal, and lastly the essential oils. Stir until evenly blended.

Pour melted and blended ingredients into a small pastry bag or small plastic bag. Cut a small hole in the corner of the bag once filled. Insert bag tip into mascara bottle. Press mascara very slowly into the tube (it's easier with a helper) until it is all in. Cap, and you are ready to go.

NOSE AND EARS

Sinus Soother

The concentrated chrism may be applied by the drop around sinuses and congested areas.
Leave out the jojoba to enjoy in a diffuser or salt pipe.

  20 ml Jojoba

  1 ml Eucalyptus

  1 ml Rosemary

  1 ml Black Spruce

  10 drops Peppermint

  10 drops Inula

Dear Ear Oil

Combine and massage around ear area with lymphatic massage strokes on the surrounding neck area.

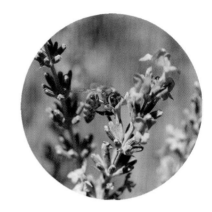

30 ml Jojoba

1 ml Frankincense

1 ml Lavender

1 ml Eucalyptus

Luxor Nose Balm

This probiotic nose balm tends to the inner sanctum of your nasal microbiome. Perfect for jet-sets, polyps, dry winter noses, or simply tending to your nasal garden.

Melt beeswax in a bain-marie (double boiler). When melted, add jojoba and heat until liquid again. Add essential oils last. Stir together, pour into jars, and let cool overnight.

10 ml Beeswax

30 ml Jojoba

10 drops Frankincense

10 drops Eucalyptus

10 drops Rosemary

10 drops Blue Tansy

2 Probiotic capsules

HANDS

Lemon + Baking Soda Nail Brightening Soak

Soaking nails in lemon, tea tree, and baking soda diminishes yellowing and staining, while sea salt softens cuticles and strengthens nails.

Mix ingredients in a small bowl of water. Swish together, soak nails for ten minutes, and then scrub nails. Moisturize cuticles with **Everything Balm** or one of the **Renegade Beauty Realms All Over Oils.** For stronger purification and to enhance the whiteness of nail tips, add a drop of tea tree under each nail if your nails are longer.

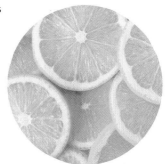

- 5 ml Sea Salt
- 5 ml Baking Soda
- 60 ml water
- 5 drops Lemon
- 3 drops Tea Tree

Tea Tree Hand Sanitizer

Fill a small spritz bottle with 3 parts organic vodka with 1 part of any of these essential oils: Tea Tree, Eucalyptus, Lavender, or Frankincense.

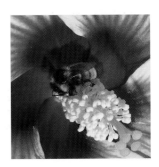

PITS

Delightful Deodorant

Combine in a lidded glass container and let solidify at room temperature.

- 60 ml Baking Soda
- 30 ml Coconut Oil (liquefied)
- 30 drops one or a combination of these essential oils: Sandalwood, Frankincense, Lavender, Cape Chamomile, Rosemary, Palmarosa, Sweet Thyme, or Black Spruce

Frankincense Friendly Flora Deodorant

Melt cacao butter, coconut oil, and beeswax over low heat. Stir in the baking soda and essential oils. Let the mixture cool until thickened yet not hard, and add the probiotic powder. Stir well. Pour into a glass jar to harden. You need only one or two swipes.

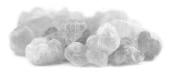

35 ml Cacao Butter

10 ml Coconut Oil

5 ml Beeswax

10 ml Baking Soda

20 drops Frankincense

10 drops Vetiver

2 capsules powdered Probiotics

Or simply apply a drop of sandalwood to each armpit.

PERFUME

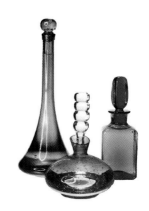

Molecularly mesmerize and elegantly enchant your aura with the aromatic ambrosia of essential oils. In ancient Greece, if you were passing someone and you thought that they smelled lovely, you would say that they smelled "like thyme breath," which meant that the person smelled like the sweet fragrance of thyme. From the root word "thyme" we also have the word "thymiatechny." It is a real word! It means the art of using plants or the art of using perfumes as your medicine.

So let perfume be your medicine with the easy elegance of essential oils.

Single Notes: Many distillations are simply divine on their own as perfume. Anoint these aromas by the drop (or dilute with a dab of jojoba) on pulse points, neck, and hair. Prolong your perfumed aura by placing a drop or two in your hair. The scent lasts longer because, unlike skin, hair does not absorb essential oils.

Jasmine, Sandalwood, Vetiver, Rose, Vanilla, Petitgrain, Ylang, Neroli, and the rarer absolutes of Orange Blossom, Hyacinth, Gardenia Tiare, Tuberose, Champa Blossoms, Osmanthus, Jonquil, Narcissus, Carnation, and Labdanum

Perfect Pairs: Double your perfume pleasure by combining these pairs, which can be bottled 50:50 with jojoba (or organic vodka for atomizers) for a perfume. A concentration of 30:70 will create more of an eau de cologne ratio.

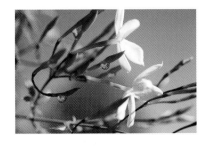

Vetiver + Rose

Sandalwood + Jasmine

Patchouli + Vanilla

Spikenard + Ylang

Vanilla + Neroli

Vetiver + Douglas Fir

Jasmine + Ylang

Signature Scent: Create sensual signature scents with these engaging aromas. Dilute into 30 ml of organic vodka or jojoba (beyond jojoba's healing qualities, it is an optimal oil for perfumery as it never goes rancid, keeping your precious perfumes perfect). As these aromas age, their scents will coalesce in the bottle, and the aromas will pleasantly ripen. See more tips on blending perfumes in Chapter Twelve.

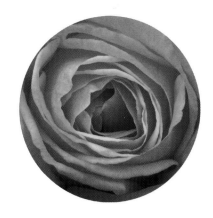

Flower of Flowers

2 ml Jasmine

1 ml Ylang

1 ml Patchouli

2 ml Blood Orange

Earth Mirth

2 ml Vetiver

1 ml Douglas Fir

1 ml Sandalwood

1 ml Lemon

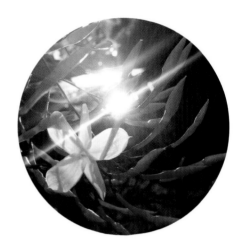

Citrus Synergy

1 ml Blood Orange

1 ml Lemon

1 ml Grapefruit

3 ml Sandalwood

1 ml Vetiver

Verdant Vanilla

2 ml Vetiver

1 ml Vanilla

2 ml Lemon

10 drops Cardamom

HEALTHY HAIRCARE

The No-Shampoo Method

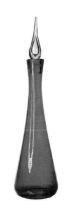

Most days, rinsing your hair with pure water and massaging your scalp with your fingertips are all your hair needs to be clean. If you have been a heavy user of hair products, you may experience a few days of oiliness as your scalp recalibrates. A headband or ponytail may get you through those days. If your hair is damaged and dry, after rinsing your hair with water rub a very small dab of **Everything Balm,** jojoba, or coconut oil through damp hair, concentrating on the damaged areas. It is best to do this at night so the oils can really sink in deep.

The no-poo method of cleansing hair is perfect for washing away the buildup of polymers and surfactants that strip away healthy oils from the scalp and hair. This simple method helps hair when transitioning to healthier shampoos and when moving toward washing hair less frequently. See "Haircare" in Chapter Seventeen for more.

Baking soda can be used in this method. Simply dissolve 15 ml of baking soda into warm water. Apply the solution to the scalp and gently massage in, much like you would use shampoo yet without the suds. Then rinse with the Happy Hair Rinse.

Happy Hair Rinse

Mix fresh and pour onto hair after showering.

- 1 cup Apple Cider Vinegar
- 1 cup Water
- 5 drops Frankincense or Lavender

Apple cider vinegar helps close the hair cuticles so that each strand is smoother, and smoother hair is shinier. As a rinse, it will remove buildup from other hair products.

Sandalwood Scalp Oil

Combine oils and massage into scalp before shampooing.

Hopefully you can create times to leave this treatment on overnight.

40 ml Jojoba

5 ml Tamanu

1 ml Sandalwood

10 drops Vetiver

10 drops Black Spruce

10 drops Geranium

1 ml Peppermint (optional for itchy scalps)

Beach Breeze Hair Spray

If you like the tousled look inspired by hair dried in oceanic breezes, this easy formula will help you get the look.

Dissolve the sea salt into warm water and add the essential oils. Using your fingers, work a little bit of this mixture through dry hair, scrunch with your fingers, and let it air dry.

10 ml Sea Salt

240 ml Warm Water

12 drops of one or two of these essences: Ylang, Jasmine, Rose Otto, Frankincense, Sandalwood, Vetiver, Rosemary, Chamomile, or Palmarosa

10 drops Jojoba (optional for dry hair)

Happy Hair Dry Shampoo

Mix, jar, and apply a dash to your scalp and part lines to extend times between washings.

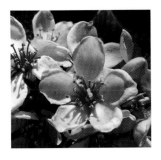

> 30 ml Baking Soda
>
> 10 ml Rosemary or Rosehips powder
>
> 10 drops Chamomile
>
> 10 drops Ylang
>
> 2 Probiotic capsules

OPTIMAL ORAL CARE

Eight Steps to Successful Self-Dentistry

1. Start with the **Minty Mouthwash.**
2. Scrape the tongue two or three times.
3. Brushing the Gums: Use a soft, dry toothbrush and apply a drop of **Peppy Tooth Serum.**
4. Polishing the Teeth: Use a dry round-headed electric toothbrush with **Peppy Toothpaste** or simply with baking soda.
5. Clean the gum lines with a Sulcabrush or a rubber-tipped gum tool.
6. Floss! Apply one drop of **Peppy Tooth Serum** along the floss.
7. Saltwater rinse or oil pull.
8. Use an oral irrigator or a blunt-tipped syringe with the **Minty Mouthwash** to rinse the gum pockets, and take extra care with any receding gums.

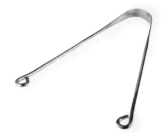

Peppy Toothpaste

Liquefy coconut oil in a double boiler and add in the other ingredients.

Mix together, pour into jars (a different jar for each person in the family), and pop in the fridge to solidify.

Once solidified, it can be kept out of the fridge.

30 ml Coconut Oil

20 ml Baking Soda

20 drops Peppermint

10 drops Myrrh

10 drops Sweet Thyme

Peppy Tooth Serum

This concentrated chrism is to be used sparingly by the drop to deeply clean between teeth with floss, in a blunt-tipped syringe for cleaning the gum line, and dabbed on cankers or mas-saged onto gums for extra care. This mix is therapeutically concentrated, so do a patch test before using.

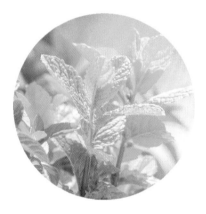

20 ml MCT Oil

5 ml Frankincense

5 ml Peppermint

1 ml Sweet Thyme

3 drops Oregano

Minty Mouthwash

Make a strong saltwater rinse by dissolving salt in warm water. You want it to taste as salty as the ocean. Baking soda is also a good rinse. Saliva is similar biochemically to baking soda, and baking soda is also alkaline, which is exactly what the saliva needs. Adding frankincense and peppermint boosts botanical-biotic action. Shake before use.

10 ml Sea Salt or Baking Soda

500 ml Water

2 drops Frankincense

2 drops Peppermint

AROMATIC AIR-CARE

Bye-Bye Bugs Insect Repellant

Add this concentrate to a spritz bottle or to body oil at 5-7 percent.

2 ml Eucalyptus

1 ml Peppermint

5 ml Geranium

2 ml Cedar

Lavender Linen Spray

Lovely spritzed on linens for an aromatic lullaby.

Combine ingredients in a glass spray bottle. Leave out the water, and this concentrate can be used for bedtime baths, diffused, or inhaled with a salt pipe.

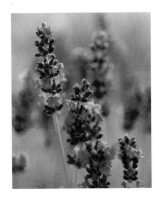

50 ml Water

5 ml Lavender

10 drops Marjoram

10 drops Sweet Thyme

10 drops Grapefruit

Immune-Boosting Spray

This may be used to clean surfaces, spritz pillows, and refresh rooms and cars.

Combine ingredients in a glass spray bottle. Leave out the water, and this concentrate can also be diffused or used in a salt pipe.

50 ml Water

4 ml Eucalyptus

2 ml Black Spruce

1 ml Rosemary

1 ml Lemon

RENEGADE BEAUTY: BEST ABLUTIONS

1. Engage with the elements. Let nature be your finest beauty attendant.

2. Maintain a bustling microbiome of beneficial bacteria.

3. Appreciate your body and beauty in this moment. Appreciate all the beautiful life-affirming actions your body accomplishes every day.

4. Keep it real to the feel. Let everything artificial, unessential, contrived, and synthetic fall away.

5. Digest the best. Eat fresh, organic, colorful, wholesome, fulsome foods and drink pure water.

6. Easily Beautiful: Activate the innate intelligence of the body to rejuvenate and replenish.

7. Brush Up: Stimulate the skin and lymph system with dry brushing.

8. Let perfume be your medicine. Bless and refresh your beauty with botanicals.

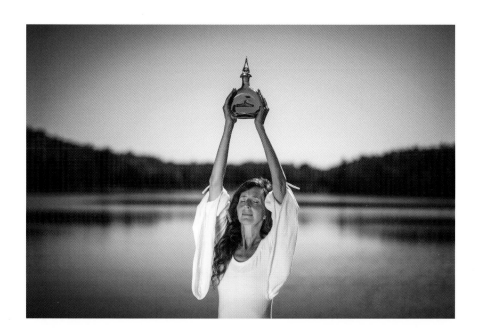

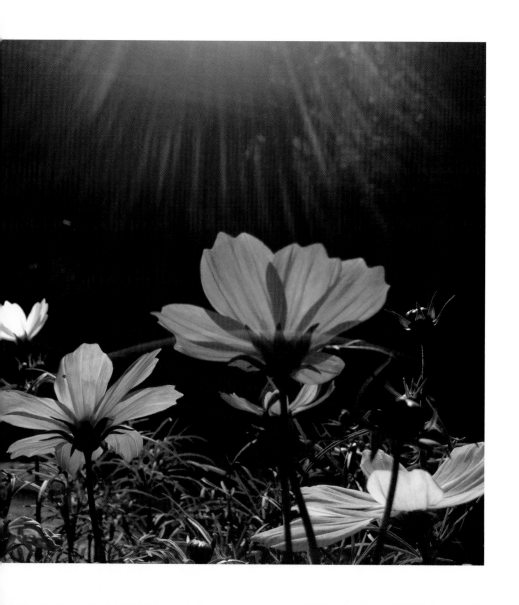

Chapter Seventeen

RENEGADE BEAUTY SOLUTIONS

In this chapter, I offer protocols on specific skin, health, and beauty issues that focus on radiance from the inside out and further explore the gut–beauty connection. These are suggestions based on my own experience, paths that professionals have used to improve health and well-being, and data from scientific research. Use your intuition to guide your decisions, and revel in responsibility for your own radiant health. Life continually shows us that we cannot always control each and every condition, yet we can relax in the infinite knowledge that there is always a solution.

Words in **purple** refer to solutions you can read more about in this chapter. Words in **green** refer to DIY recipes for botanicals to use topically to treat or ease specific issues found in Chapter Sixteen.

The art of healing comes from nature, not from the physician. Therefore the physician must start from nature, with an open mind.

Paracelsus[1]

If we're going to heal, let it be glorious.

Beyoncé[2]

ACNE

Acne occurrence is a skin signal suggesting hormonal imbalances and digestive dysbiosis. These internal issues arise with: excess hormones from accumulation of xenoestrogens and birth control pills, overproduction of hormones like cortisol that creates a disarraying domino effect on the endocrine system, toxin stimulation of hormone production, and inefficiencies in hormone elimination cycles due to a sluggish liver and lymph system.

Digestive congestion clogs elimination cycles too, as it slows the processing of hormonal secretions being released through the liver's filtration system. A hormonal logjam in the liver causes the manifestation of hormonal acne, much to the chagrin of the chin and jawline.

Little blemishes that blossom overnight are small signals of a toxin's trespass; no big deal, maybe just something off kilter with a meal, or a quick cascade of adrenal stress. Simply apply a dab of **Brilliant or Benevolent Beauty Spot Treatment** to the blemish; if it is a wet or weepy blemish, leave it to air dry with the Spot Treatment. If the blemish is dry, seal in the Spot Treatment with one of the **Renegade Beauty Splendid Serums** or **Calm Balm.** To begin, a quick oil cleanse with one of the **Renegade Beauty Realms All Over Oils** and a cloth will dust off any flaky skin, and then you are ready to greet the day; if possible, let the blemish air dry and feel the kiss of sunshine too.

Chemical acne is caused by the cyclical loop of pores reacting to caustic topical products touted to solve acne that toss the skin into a tailspin as it attempts to recalibrate from the alcohols, antibiotics, azelaic acids, benzoyl peroxides, petroleum, retinoids, and salicylic acids that disrupt the ecology of each pore. Let go of these lacerating lotions and stop the suds to avoid the soapy surfactants that disrupt sebum. Sometimes there is a detox phase when switching to more soothing systems, as the microbiome, hydro-lipid barrier, and stratum corneum recalibrate.

Food for Thought: Soy is such a harbinger of acne, and it triggers the deeper development of systemic cystic acne. Avoid all forms of unfermented soy, as it stimulates estrogen production and disrupts the endocrine system. A diet of cruciferous veggies and supplements of diindolylmethane (DIM), iodine, and indole-3-carbinol clear excess estrogen. Boosting your gut microbial population is a good first step in healing your skin.

Balance with Botanicals: Even though many aspects of acne are systemic, it is amazing to see acne clear up by simply switching what is being applied to the skin. Settle overactive sebaceous glands by washing your face with jojoba oil, a liquid plant wax that is perfect for the task because it is symbiotic with our sebum. No more nitpicking pores! Jojoba unplugs pores by dissolving oxidized sebum. Botanicals from the Brilliant Beauty Realm will effectively eradicate acne. They may be used to spot-treat with a drop applied to acne and/or added to jojoba for cleansing and moisturizing. See Chapter Sixteen for acne care: **Brilliant Beauty All Over Oil** to cleanse, **Brilliant Beauty Spot Treatment, Astringent Face Tonic,** and **Pore Clarifying Mask.**

Super Supplements: probiotics and prebiotics, psyllium, aloe, and triphala; and see **Hormones** for hormone-harmonizing herbs.

ADRENALS

The adrenal glands produce the hormones cortisol, DHEA, and aldosterone. They regulate blood pressure, metabolism, energy production, stress responses, and the creation of androgens and estrogens. Adrenal insufficiency, or Addison's disease, is a serious medical condition in which the adrenal glands are damaged and can't produce enough cortisol. It is diagnosed with blood and saliva tests. Symptoms include fatigue, nausea, depression, low blood pressure, weakness, weight loss, low appetite, headaches, and craving salty foods.

Adrenal fatigue is not yet a recognized medical condition, yet it sure makes you feel crummy. It occurs when the adrenal glands are overworked due to ongoing stressful life conditions and burnout. The symptoms are fatigue, irritability, changes in appetite, and craving salty foods. **Meditation,** movement, good **Sleep,** and a healthy diet can help your body more efficiently manage stress.

Many people have found that adding a pinch of good-quality sea salt to their water first thing in the morning helps to boost adrenal health.

Dive Deeper: Heal digestion and leaky guts. Read: *Salt Your Way to Health* by Dr. David Brownstein; and *The Adrenal Thyroid Revolution* by Dr. Aviva Romm.

AGING AND WRINKLES

Prematurely aging skin, fine lines, dark spots, and wrinkles are frequently blamed on the sun, though we are learning that aging is sped up by hormonal shifts, synthetic skincare that disrupts the beauty of the biome, malnutrition from processed foods with rancid PUFA (polyunsaturated fatty acids) oils, and meals bereft of minerals and high in sugars that lead to glycation.

If you don't have wrinkles, you haven't laughed enough.

Phyllis Diller[3]

Change Your Thoughts: Tune in to your worthiness and wisdom, and let go of linear paradigms of time. Enjoy your flowering like a fine wine. Champion the sage of your age with the enthusiasm of an eight-year-old (remember when you joyfully expressed your age in years and months)! This moment is your present gift: an eternal open-ended reality, always fresh, never the same. This is the beauty of time: it is alive! Live in the blossoming, the ever-arriving, presence. Life, beauty, tranquility, and simplicity do not depend on time. The idea of linear time, hence linear age, limits life. Birth, then a slow habitual journey to death, is the line. It is not the end of the body that causes aging, but living in the constraints of conflict, worry, and doubt that condition the mind to contract in conclusion, dulling its extraordinary capacity to be young. Want to reverse the signs of aging? Abandon the cage of age. Life source spirals as the seasons: live in this flowering moment.

I tell myself that I must see something in the mirror besides my wrinkled veneer if I am to have any calm; that I will have to make my peace with the loss of smooth skin, and find satisfaction in the gaining of something to take its place. Something, yes, that should always have been me. Or something that has always been in me but has never seen the light of day.

Peggy Freydberg[4]

Food for Thought: Keep blood sugar balanced to prevent **Glycation** and inflammation. Avoid inflammatory foods: rancid processed polyunsaturated vegetable oils (differing from cold-pressed plant oils), processed foods, simple carbohydrates, and sugars. To boost collagen production, be sure to include plenty of amino acids in the diet. There is also organic collagen that you can add to smoothies and drinks. Include antioxidant, rainbow-rich foods and lots of healthy fats!

Balance with Botanicals: From the Beloved Beauty Realm, these oils inhibit the negative enzymes elastase and *collagenase* that erode the skin's elasticity: Roman chamomile, immortelle, rose otto, carrot seed, turmeric, rockrose, myrrh, palmarosa, ylang.

AIR TRAVEL

Also see **Nose Health** and **Dryness.**

Traveling by plane can definitely be challenging in such close quarters, especially with the current "flu of the day" scares—someone sneezes and you try not to breathe for a minute to avoid inhaling their germs. Don't let germs put a damper on your travel plans; essential oils make great co-pilots, as they are all antibacterial and antiviral. I bring a little forest of oils with me when I travel. My travel kit includes a bottle of frankincense oil, a bottle of **Tea Tree Hand Sanitizer,** and an **Everything Balm.** (Remember that the bottles must be 2 ounces or smaller to make it through airport security.) The tea tree oil can be used to clean hands and protect the ears by applying a tiny bit in there. Anoint the inside of the nose with the balm to keep the lining of the nose moist and, as you breathe in the possibly germy air in the plane, the air gets filtered through the essential oils as it travels through the nose. I also use a cotton mask, which looks like a surgical mask, and apply essential oils of black spruce, eucalyptus, and frankincense to the interior. This creates a humid microclimate of perfectly pure air. I also always pack my salt pipe. I like to clean the tray table and arm-rests with a little bit of **Tea Tree Hand Sanitizer.**

Dive Deeper: Look into the HumanCharger, a light device that helps one adjust to time zones; and charcoal air filters that fit inside the nose. Pack a tincture bottle of dandelion to release any water retention, and extra probiotics to boost the immune system.

AROMA DIFFUSION

Aroma diffusers mist molecules of essential oils to add aromatic ambience and microscopic medicine to care for the air in bedrooms, living rooms, studios, and offices. Most diffusers are ultrasonic and humidify the air too. Simply combine the essential oils you want to diffuse in water, and inhale the airy elixir of molecules that cleanse, purify, and refresh any atmosphere. Pure, organic essential oils micro-misted into the air enter the bloodstream through the nose and lungs and seed their pure plant potency

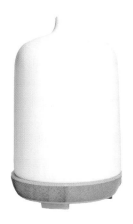

into every cell. Within minutes, nerves settle, feelings uplift, breathing deepens, and clarity and creativity flow.

Apothecary: neroli, blood orange, grapefruit, black spruce, frankincense, chamomile, laurel, lavender, geranium, ylang, inula

BIRTH CONTROL

Hormone-based birth control—including vaginal rings, patches, Pills, and hormone-releasing IUDs—comes with side effects that range from unpleasant to risky. The manufacturers' black box warnings include: blood clots, stroke, heart disease, skin pigmentation, spotting, and bigger fibroids. Women who use hormone-based contraception regularly complain of weight gain, acne, bloating, migraines, back pain, and decreased sex drive. The most common complaint and reason why women stop taking the Pill is depression.[5] Research in 2012 found that the use of oral, vaginal, and skin-patch contraception reduced insulin sensitivity and induced chronic inflammation.[6] Further research that year published in Contraception reported that low-dose Pills may be a potential risk factor for cardiovascular disease, and the study stated that supplemental vitamins E and C may be needed to downgrade the risk.[7] Oddly, newer versions of birth control (patches, vaginal rings, and Pills with drospirenone) appear to increase the risk of cardiac events and blood clots. Why the clots? Oral estrogen stimulates the liver, where blood-clotting factors are made. Hormone-based contraception is especially dangerous for women over forty and women who smoke. Women over forty are more susceptible to heart and lung issues and blood clots, and one study found that women over forty are at higher risk for glaucoma if they use the Pill for three years or more.[8]

Copper IUDs also have issues. Some women have had powerfully negative responses to the copper in the copper-covered IUDs: cramping, anemia, heavy bleeding, bleeding between periods, vaginitis, backaches, pain, hair loss, cystic acne, increased estrogen, and even panic attacks. Some women discover that they are allergic to copper or that their bodies are absorbing the copper and that they have reached toxic levels. The medical community and IUD manufacturers reject that the copper can cause psychological, physical, and hormonal imbalances, though scientific research on copper toxicity is "surprisingly sparse."[9]

Restore Your Body after Birth Control: Weaning your body off the Pill and IUDs may go smoothly, or you may experience some negative side effects. There are steps you can take to help restore your body. Good nutrition is always a great place to start. Bioflavonoids, B vitamins, and healthy fats are building blocks for natural hormone production. Cruciferous vegetables are great sources of plant compounds that help the body keep hormones well balanced. During digestion, indole-3-carbinol is converted to diindolylmethane (DIM), which is an amazing cancer fighter and hormone metabolizer. DIM is available as a supplement; be sure to eat the whole cruciferous plant to get all the fiber, vitamin C, and phytochemicals that work synergistically with the DIM to keep your body healthy. Maca is a popular Peruvian food celebrated for invigorating libido. It is also a hormone adaptogen that will improve hormonal balance. Milk thistle and dandelion tinctures help support the liver as your body detoxes the synthetic hormones. It may be a good idea to have heavy-metal testing and a hormone panel run with a health practitioner well trained in hormone balancing.

Fertile Alternatives: There are alternative methods of managing fertility, and a few of them help you get more in tune with your body's ebb and flow. The Billings Ovulation Method[10] involves recording the quantity and consistency of vaginal mucus to track ovulation, and Lunar Nourishment offers lunar-cycle ovulation training. The Fertility Awareness Method[11] uses your resting temperature along with menstruation days to track fertility.

Intrauterine neem for women and oral neem for men is an ancient and current birth control method in India. It is an effective (and temporary) safe spermicide.[12] There have been many scientific studies on its efficacy and safety, yet most were on animals or insects; there are two with male subjects. Neem's effect as birth control was tested with twenty members of the Indian Army. Daily oral doses of several drops of neem seed oil in gelatin capsules were given to married soldiers. The effect took six weeks to become 100 percent effective, and it remained effective during the entire year of the trial and was reversed six weeks after the subjects stopped taking the capsules. During this time, none of the wives became pregnant, and the men experienced no side effects and maintained their virility.[13] Another test for long-term male birth control injected a very minute amount of neem oil into the vas deferens, providing up to eight months of birth control. The test revealed that the birth control effect may come from an increased ability of immune response in the lymph nodes. The men experienced zero side effects and no change in sperm production.[14]

If you are interested in using neem oil for birth control, it would be wise to work alongside a naturopath or a professional trained in its use. And of course, there are always condoms—though hold off on synthetic lubes and spermicides please! See Chapter Ten for more information.

Was it entirely paranoid to suspect that all those stoppers, thingamajigs, and substances devised to prevent conception were intended not to liberate womankind from the biological and social penalties imposed on her natural passions but, rather, at the insidious design of capitalistic puritans, were supposed to technologize sex, to dilute its juices, to contain its wilder fires, to scrub it clean, to order it uniform, to render it safe . . . (substituting these risks for the less mysterious, tamer risks of infection, hemorrhage, cancer, and hormone imbalance)?

Tom Robbins[15]

BITES

Things that bite are vast and varied and occasionally need to be identified by professionals, as some things are downright deadly. For very general first aid, like soothing a wasp sting or a mosquito's bite, a drop of peppermint essential oil right away will soothe the first initial sting or itch. Peppermint is very nice and acts like a drop of ice to calm and cool the reaction. A simple mix of a teaspoon of clay moistened with peppermint (no water), covered by a cotton round and skin tape,[16] is also an effective remedy to speed up healing and draw out mild toxins.

Apothecary: peppermint and clay

BLACKHEADS AND WHITEHEADS

When tiny hair follicles get clogged, bumps called comedones are formed. If the skin over this congested follicle stays closed, it becomes a whitehead. If the skin over the comedone opens and is exposed and oxidized, it is called a blackhead. Typical treatments are only topical and are quite caustic, with chemical peels, over-the-counter chemicals of resorcinol, salicylic acid, and benzoyl peroxide, and prescriptions for retinol-A, tretinoin, tazarotene, adapalene, and antibiotics. Aside from mutating microbes, plugging pores with surfactants and residues, and the ablation of the stratum corneum, these options have some serious side effects and do not address underlying causes. The root of the issue is gut dysbiosis: clear up constipation, indigestion, and any **Leaky Gut Syndrome.** Cease toxic topical treatments and over-exfoliation that keep the skin in an endless loop, especially when there are effectively beautiful botanical options.

Balance with Botanicals: Oil cleanse with jojoba oil and a dash of baking soda, as it unplugs pores by dissolving sebum. Essential oils from the Brilliant Beauty Realm may be dabbed on the area morning and night. Support weekly with the **Pore Clarifying Mask.**

Super Supplements: pancreatic enzymes, probiotics and prebiotics, psyllium, aloe, triphala

BODY WEIGHT AND DIET

Optimal body weight is different for each person. Avoid comparing your body with that of friends and images in magazines and movies. Embrace your unique shape, form, and beauty.

> *A culture fixated on female thinness is not an obsession about female beauty, but an obsession about female obedience. Dieting is the most potent political sedative in women's history; a quietly mad population is a tractable one.*
>
> Naomi Wolf[17]

Calories Don't Count: Calories are not the villain the food industry has made them out to be, causing us to always try to cheat our way past them with foods that enable us to eat more in volume while consuming less in calories. The basic flaw in a calorie-counting diet, and most conventional diet programs that go along with it, is that they rarely take into account the nutritional value of the calorie. Not all calories are created equal. Calories from sugar will do different things in the body than calories from quality sources of fat (like ghee, coconut oil, nuts, seeds, olives, avocados, and clean animal sources). This means that calories from an apple, from an avocado, from a handful of gummy bears, or from a can of soda will all function differently. Our rate of calorie burning is affected by the foods we eat (we burn more calories digesting whole foods than processed foods), in combination with our age, whether we're male or female, our activity level, our stress level, and our metabolic type. If we focus on the nutrient concentration in every bite, then we can ditch that math equation from our plates. A calorie count becomes a weird way to measure whether a food is good for us or not. Somehow, the measure of calories in a food is what most of us have come to base our food choices on.[18]

Fats First: The foods we eat influence our body fat, our musculature, our microbiome, and our moods. And, contrary to cultural belief, dietary fat is not the problem. Fat is the solution—but not just any fat. . . .

Trans fats are found in vegetable oils that have been hydrogenated to increase the shelf life of the product, and they set off a cascade of negative reactions in the body: suppressed immunity, obesity, hardened arteries, inflammation, and elevated LDL or "bad" cholesterol. Monounsaturated fats help regulate insulin, blood sugar, and cholesterol levels. They also make your skin smooth and your hair shiny. Avocados, avocado oil, walnuts, flaxseeds and flaxseed oil, as well as olives and olive oil are great sources of monounsaturated fats.

Processed food is full of PUFA; however, not all PUFA are unhealthy. Omega-3 and omega-6 essential fatty acids are polyunsaturated fats that our bodies require. Omega-3 EFAs are needed for optimal cell growth, immune function, and good moods. They are anti-inflammatory, ease arthritis, and lower the risk of some cancers. Wild fatty fish (never farmed fish), walnuts, and meat and dairy from pasture-raised animals are great sources of omega-3s. Omega-6 fatty acids help reduce heart disease[19] and influence blood clotting. The standard Western diet is full of omega-6 fatty acids from processed food, oils from seeds and nuts, vegetable oils, and factory-farmed animals.

Saturated fat has unfairly been the victim of fad diets and much nutrition advice, due to a single study in the 1960s that declared a relationship between saturated fat and heart disease.[20] More recent research has discounted that correlation,[21] showing that it can improve immune function, improve bone density, and improve lung function (our lungs are coated with saturated fat). In fact, when we exercise or fast, our bodies use our own stores of body fat—which is saturated fat—for energy.

Our bodies require both carbohydrates and fat for fuel. Fat is converted to energy via an enzyme process, so carbs (glycogen) are used to fuel the body until fat is available. Fat provides a much longer energy source than glycogen, and improved physical fitness allows for faster access to fat stores for energy. For light physical activity, such as walking, and normal daily life, the natural carbs in fruit and vegetables can amply supply your muscles with glycogen for energy.

When it comes to how our bodies use the food we eat, including fats and carbs, there is a lot of individual variation. Play with your food! Experiment and see what feels right for you and makes your body feel good.

If you find it incredibly difficult to drop processed and sugary food from your diet, there is a good reason for it. Those foods may be addictive. Check out the book by Michael Moss called *Salt Sugar Fat: How the Food Giants Hooked Us*.

Food for Thought: There are lots of diet and food tips throughout this book. The foundation is a healthy, diverse gut microbiome.

Dive Deeper: Read: *Fat for Fuel: A Revolutionary Diet to Combat Cancer, Boost Brain Power, and Increase Your Energy* by Joseph Mercola; *The Skinny Gut Diet* by Brenda Watson and Leonard Smith; *The UnDiet Cookbook* by Meghan Telpner; *Clean Eats* by Alejandro Junger; *My New Roots* by Sarah Britton; *The Moon Juice Cookbook: Cosmic Alchemy for a Thriving Body, Beauty, and Consciousness* by Amanda Chantal Bacon; and *Women, Food and Desire* by Alexandra Jamieson.

BREAST MASSAGE

Breast massage is a simple step to keep our breasts healthy. Breasts contain an abundance of lymph vessels that support the circulatory system in moving nutrients and waste in and out of our bodies. The health of our lymphatic systems is intimately connected to our breast health (see Chapter Nine). Lymphatic flow can be obstructed by tight bras, poor posture, lack of exercise, shallow breathing, and tight neck, shoulder, chest, and back muscles. Massage encourages the tissues to release stored excesses of estrogen, move debris away from the spaces between cells, and return the fluid to the bloodstream to be eliminated. Over time, massaging the breasts may also enhance the elasticity of the ligaments in the chest, providing improved breast support.

Balance with Botanicals: Essential oils show promise in preventing or reversing imbalances that accumulate in adipose and lymph tissue. Grapefruit, frankincense, cypress, blood orange, laurel, and rose otto oils contain abundant amounts of monoterpenes, a class of botanical chemicals that are really great for the lymph, and some have demonstrated powerful anticancer properties. Working synergistically with massage, these botanicals may prevent or reverse cysts, rejuvenate cells, and increase immune-cell activity. See page 150 for the **Beautiful Breasts Therapeutic Massage Oil** recipe.

BREATHING

We all breathe. In and out, in and out, more than 20,000 times every day, and all without a single thought or a second of effort. But our breath is powerful; it can stimulate or relax us, inspire creativity, imbue with confidence and enlightenment. Controlled breathing has been studied as a successful treatment for PTSD, depression, inflammatory disease, pain, high blood pressure, and stress. It's free and easy and so worthwhile.

We are born obligate nose breathers, though over time, a variety of environmental conditions can influence us to breathe through our mouths instead. The Buteyko method is a simple breathing-therapy technique that can retrain you to nose-breathe naturally and to normalize breathing volume. It may help to ease asthma, sleep disorders, and chronic rhinitis. Practicing this method may quell panic attacks too. There are various books and websites that can guide you through this method. Here is a simplified version for you to relax with:

1. Breathe in and out of your nose one time quickly.

2. Immediately hold your breath, pinch your nose, and hold for five to ten seconds.

3. Release your breath and your nose, and breathe normally for ten seconds.

4. Repeat this series for a few minutes.

Breath Meditations: We have all heard that **Meditation** is good for us, and maybe your forward-thinking physician has recommended that you give it a try. Over the last twenty years, there have been nearly a thousand academic and scientific studies conducted on the benefits of daily meditation, and the conclusions are impressive. As little as twelve minutes of meditation every day can ease stress, anxiety, depression, pain, and panic.[22] It improves mood[23] and focus,[24] builds gray matter,[25] enhances decision making and memory,[26] builds resilience,[27] and fosters creativity.[28]

Breath meditations require very little technique and can be practiced just about anywhere. My favorite breath meditation is called Inner Fire Meditation, which opens the chakras and calls upon and channels inner vitality. A few minutes breathing Inner Fire helps me concentrate and come up with creative solutions.

Breathing Issues: Ease breathing issues from congested sinuses, sniffles, and allergies by reaching for essences that help you breathe easy. Inhale clarifying-camphorous-expectorant essences with the use of a **Salt Pipe Inhaler.** This positively purifying device cleanses the entire respiratory system by flushing out allergens and impurities. An **Aroma Diffuser** will help clear airborne bacteria too.

Balance with Botanicals: Essences distilled from leaves (eucalyptus, inula, rosemary, peppermint) have an affinity for the lungs and can clear congestion. Boost your body's fortification force with **Sinus Soother.**

BRUISES

Contusions form on skin when blood vessels burst from bumping into something. Peppermint and immortelle essential oils are effective antihematoma essences that help reduce localized swelling. Apply a drop of each neat to the area, or dilute 10:90 with an organic oil and massage into larger bruised areas.

Apothecary: peppermint and immortelle

CELLULITE

How did this common physical occurrence become the jinx of women? A "problem" as defined by the so-called beauty industry, statistics tell us that more than 80 percent of women have cellulite somewhere on the body.

Women are energy-storage experts. The female body is very efficient at fat storage to sustain us and our babies through motherhood. Cellulite is part of our expert fat-storage capacity. A myriad of components contributes to the formation of cellulite, including: circulation insufficiencies, a clogged vascular system, high cortisol levels, immobility or a sedentary lifestyle, nutritional deficits, increased body fat, estrogen dominance, genetics, and collagen and connective-tissue breakdown.

Overnight cellulite-banishing lotions are marketing tools developed to separate you from your body, and the results are less than promised. There are no quick fixes for cellulite's complex nature. Even so, there are things you can do to address the factors contributing to cellulite and thus curtail it and minimize its appearance. One of those steps is **Dry Brushing.** The best treatment for cellulite is to learn to love your body just as it is. Steer clear of critical thoughts and caustic comparisons. Appreciate the beauty of your unique form, and gaze in amazement at the stunningly intricate functions going on inside your body.

Move and Groove: Improved circulation from moving and grooving will keep the skin and connective tissue healthy by speeding up the elimination of waste and excess fluid. Also, movement helps to manage stress and lower cortisol levels. So play, swim, sweat, sauna, hike, dance, hula-hoop, rebound, or chase your children—go have fun!

Food for Thought: Simple changes to your diet will help balance hormones and clear out excess estrogen. Eliminate soy, as it stimulates estrogen production, which leads to a hormone surplus. Daily water retention can be relieved with a gentle dandelion root tincture or tea. Hormone-harmonizing herbs and foods are listed in the **Hormones** section. Iodine helps strengthen connective tissue and balances the three types of estrogen. Vitamin C and bioflavonoids are important nutrients for collagen and elastin, as well as for improving general circulation and lymphatic health.

Balance with Botanicals: Massage the area with circulation-stimulating, water-retention-releasing, and lymph-loving essential oils of cypress, rosemary, grapefruit, and laurel in jojoba oil. Massaging these oils into the skin will also benefit the connective and adipose tissue.

CHERRY ANGIOMAS

Cherry angiomas appear as small red or purplish spots on the skin. These crimson dots are papules on the skin comprising an atypical proliferation of blood vessels made of clusters of capillaries at the surface of the skin. They are usually flat, yet they can also emerge as slightly raised spots. Why these spots surface on the skin was a mystery until it was discovered that their appearance comes from the body detoxing bromide. This came to light when researchers found that ample cherry-colored dots appeared on their bodies after working with brominated compounds for prolonged periods of time.[29] As the body's intelligence works to move bromide poisoning away from vital organs, bromide gets pushed to the skin's surface. Bromide is a toxic halogen that gets stored in our fat tissues and blocks the assimilation of much-needed iodine. Plentiful in our factory food supply, bromide is an additive listed on labels as potassium bromate and brominated vegetable oil (BVO) that can be found in breads, sports drinks, and fruit-flavored drinks.

Bromide is also prolific as methyl bromide, a pesticide that is often used in growing strawberries,[30] and is used in asthma inhalers and anesthesia, in the production of plastic, mattresses, carpets, and flame-retardant fabrics, in the form of polybrominated diphenyl ethers (PBDEs), and in bromine-based swimming pool and hot tub cleaning agents.

Supplementing with iodine to reach sufficient levels will most likely make more cherry angiomas appear as the iodine begins to push out endocrine-disrupting bromides and other toxic halogens from the body. Thankfully, reaching iodine sufficiency shrinks these spots to tiny red pinprick-sized dots until they fade away. Removing bromide from the body will also boost breast and thyroid health.

Balance with Botanicals: Spot-treat the area with frankincense and sandalwood applied neat, or make a moisturizer with these essential oils and jojoba. Iodine may be applied topically with these oils too.

Dive Deeper: Read: *Iodine* by Dr. David Brownstein; and *The Iodine Crisis* by Lynne Farrow.

COUPEROSE

Couperose can manifest as tiny red areas on the cheeks, on the chin, and around the nose. These broken capillaries, called telangiectasia, appear as tiny red spider veins and are the result of dilated veins either from pressure or from a loss of tenacity in the vein wall. Broken blood vessels appear for some after menopause or from rosacea.

Balance with Botanicals: Apply a dab neat to the area with the essential oils (immortelle, cypress, rose otto, frankincense, cape chamomile, yarrow) from the Blithe or Benevolent Beauty Realms.

Super Supplements: vitamins C, B complex, K2, and D3. Tinctures or teas of horse chestnut, butcher's broom, bilberry, ginkgo, and pycnogenol.

CUTS

Nicks and cuts can range from annoying to serious, and essential oils act as excellent first-aid responders that can help to clean, heal, and seal the skin. Essential oils are all antibacterial, antifungal, and antiviral to varying degrees, and their astringent nature helps to cleanly "suture" the skin. Peppermint essential oil's ice-cube-in-a-drop effect is essential for soothing the first initial sting. Simply apply neat to the area. Frankincense, rose otto, and immortelle are also top choices, as they disinfect, remedy, and prevent scar formation. For non-life-threatening yet serious cuts, apply peppermint neat to the skin, cover with an organic cotton pad, and then apply skin tape or a Band-Aid to wrap up the cut and inhibit bleeding.

Apothecary: peppermint, immortelle, frankincense, lavender, and rose otto

CYSTS

There are almost fifty types of skin cysts, and they can be found anywhere on the body. They are sac-like lumps in the skin that are filled with fluid, pus, or a gas. Some cysts are caused by an infection, though the etiology of many types of cysts is unknown.

Balance with Botanicals: Apply a Blithe or Benevolent Beauty Spot Treatment or apply neat one or a combination of cape chamomile, cypress, lavender, or frankincense.

DARK CIRCLES UNDER THE EYES

For periorbital circles, the official scientific name for dark circles under the eyes, the first things to consider are stress and lack of sleep. Dark circles may also result from hormonal shifts, spiked insulin levels, toxic accumulation (especially chlorine in water), anemia, adrenal stress, and thinning collagen that causes the skin under the eyes to be more translucent. Lack of dietary iron can cause dark circles as well. Iron deficiency is the most common type of anemia, and this condition is a sign that not enough oxygen is getting to the body tissues.

Yet another reason to get a shower filter: chlorine is a cumulative burden on the skin and kidneys and could contribute to dandruff, skin irritation, fungal conditions, skin sensitivity, brittle hair, undereye puffiness, and dark circles. In Traditional Chinese Medicine (TCM), the undereye area has an affinity to the kidneys. Kidneys filter fluids for our bodies. Inflammation and adrenal stress (with increased cortisol) added to less-than-optimal kidney flow can cause retention of fluids, and this subtle form of edema can manifest as puffy bags and a darker undereye area. Be sure to stay hydrated, and consider looking for deeper issues with your integrative doctor, or explore acupuncture.

Food for Thought: To boost collagen production, be sure to include plenty of amino acids in the diet. There is also organic collagen that you can add to smoothies and such. It is also important to get plenty of fat-soluble vitamins—vitamin D3 (from supplements and sunshine) and vitamin K2—for carboxylation of osteocalcin. These substances usher key minerals into the bones from the blood, and this prevents calcification of the soft tissues and kidneys. Calcification creates reduced kidney filtration, which can be from an excess of inactive Matrix Gla-Protein (MGP). Dark circles under the eyes may also be an indication of a vitamin K2 deficiency.

Balance with Botanicals: Many women have reported a noticeable difference with oils from the Blithe Beauty Realm and the **Blithe Beauty Splendid Serum.**

DRY BRUSHING

Glow with good health by simply dry brushing. It involves coating a dry brush with a drop of a lymph-loving essential oil (laurel, cypress, eucalyptus, rosemary, or a blend of all four) and then very gently brushing every inch of skin, like butterflies on the skin—a very light touch. Always brush in the direction of the heart, and avoid brushing damaged or inflamed skin. Dry brushing 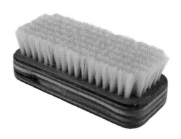 is so worth the two minutes it takes before a bath or shower. Simply pour 1-2 drops of an essential oil on the palm of your hand, and then glide a dry brush across your palm, coating the bristles. Then gently brush your body, starting with your toes, all the way up to your head. Of the many benefits, here are the top three reasons why I dry brush:

Love Your Lymph: Dry brush your skin for the love of your lymphatic system, because a flowing lymphatic system helps support healthy immune response and circulation. Lymph fluid bathes all of the cells of the body with oxygen and nutrients and carries away wastes and excess fluid.

Boost Blood Circulation: Just two minutes of whole-body dry brushing boosts blood supply (both in volume and in area) to the skin for an hour. Blood vessels weave through the skin in an elegant tapestry, delivering vitamins, minerals, proteins, fats, and fluids that build and sustain it. Blood also picks up the vitamin D made in skin cells and delivers it to the rest of the body. Stagnant blood supply to the skin leads to loss of vitality, paleness, and a cascade of complexion and immune issues. The light pressure on the skin from dry brushing promotes temporary blood-capillary dilation, which allows for a higher volume of blood flow and more efficient give-and-take with the cells. Dry brushing also recruits dormant capillaries back into action. This is why the skin has a rosy glow after a thorough brushing.

Curtail Cellulite: The thighs, especially the back of the thighs, are poorly vascularized compared to the rest of the body. So, blood and lymph circulation is low there from the start, which is one reason why **Cellulite** forms. The circulation-activating effects of dry brushing improve vascular efficiency in nutrient delivery and reduce the edema that exacerbates the bumpy appearance of cellulite.

Tools: a natural-bristle brush with medium-soft bristles (loofahs are too rough, and synthetic bristles are too listless). Upgrade your dry-brushing game with a copper natural-bristle brush that has fine bronze bristles made of copper and zinc. Due to the molecular structure of the bristles, they have a negative ion charge. When brushed on the skin, the negatively charged oxygen ions, key to our energetic well-being, are generated right on the skin.

DRYNESS

If your skin tends to be dry, be absolutely sure to use a gentle, nonstripping, nonsoap cleanser as well as a water filter to remove chlorine and fluoride (fluoride has been shown to disrupt collagen and enzymes and makes skin stiff).[31] Reduced levels of the hormone androgen may lead to inefficient skin oil (sebum) production. Dryness can also be an indication of iodine deficiency, dehydration, and thyroid imbalances. Hydrate with pure water.

Food for Thought: Increasing healthy fats in your diet will boost your skin (and hair) hydration. Try adding more omega-3 fatty acids, grass-fed butter and ghee, virgin coconut oil, olive oil, chia, and evening primrose to your diet.

Balance with Botanicals: from the Beloved Beauty Realm

EAR HEALTH

Healthy ears are usually self-cleaning. Earwax lubricates and protects the ear while trapping dirt. As the earwax migrates to the outer ear, it carries debris with it. Tissues and cotton swabs moistened with saltwater and a drop of frankincense can be used to clean the external, visible part of the ear, yet leave the ear canal alone.

Ear infections are common, especially among children. In 2004, the American Academy of Pediatrics advised doctors to hold off on prescribing antibiotics for ear infections. Most ear infections are caused by viruses, and antibiotics are ineffective against them. Most ear infections will clear up on their own after a few days.[32]

Preventing earaches is not always possible, yet always worth a try. Food allergy is one of the most common causes of recurring ear infections. If ear infections recur, then try a diet change with the **Elimination Diet.**

Breastfeeding babies for at least six months is linked to fewer ear infections. Also, boost the immune system with probiotics, vitamin C, and sunshine. If you or your child is predisposed to ear infections, massage **Dear Ear Oil** around the ear and neck area, and try holding a hair dryer set on the cool setting up to the ear for a few minutes every day, especially after bathing or swimming. The added air flow will keep the ear dry and the bacteria balanced.

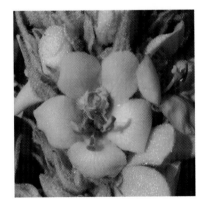

Balance with Botanicals: Herbal-infused mullein oil is an ear health classic, as mullein is revered for its ability to ease discomfort with plant constituents of coumarin and hesperidin, which studies have shown to be analgesic and anti-inflammatory. Or try the **Dear Ear Oil** formula, which is slightly analgesic and stimulates circulation and lymphatic flow.

ECZEMA

The etiology of eczema is unknown, yet it is categorized as "atopic," meaning it is an inherited allergic response. Eczema is an itchy rash that can occur on any part of the body in response to an inflammation-causing irritant. It is common among children (about 10 percent), who outgrow it as preteens.

Strictly avoid all synthetic skin products and synthetic laundry detergents; they will only exacerbate the issue.

There appears to be a strong correlation between healthy microbial diversity and the development of eczema. Infants with eczema tested at one month old and at twelve months old had reduced microbial diversity in the gut.[33] Ninety percent of people with eczema also have the common staph bacteria (*Staphylococcus aureus*) on their skin. The staph bacterium produces a substance called delta toxin that kills competing bacteria, thus reducing overall bacterial diversity. The delta toxin also stimulates the skin's immune system to react via an eczema rash. But not all staph bacteria produce the gene for making the toxin. Researchers are not quite ready to state definitively that this is the cause of eczema, yet it is good reason to foster a healthy microbial environment on the skin.[34]

Two studies have examined the influence of seabuckthorn on atopic dermatitis, a form of eczema. The bright-orange seabuckthorn berry is a rich source of fatty acids, including healthy alpha-linolenic acid, oleic acid, and palmitoleic acid. The participants consumed 5 grams of seabuckthorn per day. In just one month, the results noted an improvement in the fat content of the skin and improvement of symptoms.[35]

Be sure to heal any symptoms of a leaky gut and indigestion. Try an **Elimination Diet,** and boost with probiotics and prebiotics.

Balance with Botanicals: The Blithe Beauty Splendid Serum and Spot Treatment contain anti-inflammatory, anti-itch essential oils (peppermint, blue tansy) that will provide comfort to areas of the skin affected by eczema.

ELIMINATION DIET

If you have persistent diarrhea, gut pain, migraines, gastroesophageal reflux disease (GERD), bloating, constipation, eczema, or acne, or if there are issues with learning or concentration, an elimination diet may be helpful for you, as all of these issues may be caused by a food allergy. In an elimination diet, foods that may cause allergic reactions are eliminated and then reintroduced one at a time to see which foods are or are not well tolerated. The foods that account for most food allergies are: dairy/lactose, refined sugar, peanuts, soy, alcohol, gluten, all packaged, processed, or fast foods, and caffeine.[36]

For GERD and acid reflux, an acidic-food elimination diet may prove helpful. A great resource for this is a book by Dr. Jamie Koufman, Dr. Jordan Stern, and master chef Marc Bauer entitled *Dropping Acid: The Reflux Diet Cookbook & Cure.*

EXFOLIATION

Recommendations of exfoliation abound in beauty blogs and magazines, yet we cannot tackle our skin's imbalances by scrubbing away our stratum corneum. This perfectly protective top layer of skin is mostly composed of dead skin cells. The presence of dead cells has given rise to the practice of plastic-bead cleansers, synthetic scrubs, chemical peels, laser ablation, and excessive exfoliation. Yet this vital layer is like our topsoil and feeds our friendly flora. Exfoliating cells away too quickly tips the balance so that cell loss exceeds cell production. When we remove it prematurely, the young cells underneath are left stressed and vulnerable. With this juicy layer jeopardized, chemicals irritate the new skin, inducing a vicious cycle of inflammation. If this layer is disturbed regularly, *and it is,* an ongoing health deficit of missing microbes develops, as well as abnormal cells and easy entrance to toxins (especially when skincare involves chemicals). Balanced digestion and a flowing lymph system help to sustain the supple surface of the skin. Seal, heal, and keep the integrity of the top layer intact by oil cleansing with a cloth. The cloth and oil provide the perfect level of gentle daily exfoliation. Deeper spa-like exfoliation may be done weekly with the simple suggestions below.

Balance with Botanicals: Use one of the Renegade Beauty Realms All Over Oils for daily cleansing. Add a dash of baking soda to your oil and cloth for gently effective exfoliation; and for a more spa-like, yet still soft, exfoliation, use the Pore Clarifying or Pore Calming Mask for your face and the Grapefruit Glow Body Scrub to get your glow on. Stock your apothecary with jojoba, frankincense, sandalwood, sea salt, baking soda, clay, rosemary, and rosehips powder.

EYELASHES AND EYEBROWS

Coat lashes and brows with the botanicals suggested below to thicken and grow your lovely lashes. Switch to a more natural mascara and makeup that are gentler on the delicate eye area, and, pretty please, do not use harsh chemicals to remove eye makeup! Jojoba on a wet cotton round works wonders for cleaning off makeup. Brows that are thinning at the outer edge may be an indication of thyroid imbalance.

Balance with Botanicals: If you have a history of overplucking or if you just want to thicken those lashes, see our **Beautiful Brow + Lash Blend** that doubles as an eye-makeup remover.

EYES

The sky is the daily bread of the eyes.

Ralph Waldo Emerson[37]

In the wink of an eye, people can experience a decline in their vision; and when the underlying causes are addressed, there are more options than prescription glasses. Eyes need to see horizon lines and real light; lack of daylight replaced by lightbulbs and computer screens causes eyestrain, and this causes crow's-feet and deterioration of vision. Eyes are surrounded by muscles; and when these muscles tighten and contract due to eyestrain, tension in the neck, jaw, and occipital ridge can cause nearsightedness. Nearsightedness can be perceived as hereditary, yet what we often inherit is how we hold our bodies and relate to stress. Open your eyes to the wonder of the world, and relax those burrowed, furrowed brows.

When I was sixteen, I went to school one day and discovered the chalkboard was blurry from the back of the room. This led to getting glasses. Luckily, by my nineteenth year when I delved deeper into the world of health and healing, I practiced the Bates Method for a few months. I also read *Light: Medicine of the Future,* which led to sungazing; and with these methods and some liver cleansing, I never needed glasses again.

Lutein and zeaxanthin are potent plant compounds that are great for our eyes. Our bodies can't synthesize them, so we must get them from our diet. Dark-green leafy vegetables and peas are great sources. Orange, yellow, and red peppers are full of zeaxanthin. Lutein and zeaxanthin are also found in egg yolks, and pasture-raised hens produce bright-orange yolks from their own leafy diets. Astaxanthin is also particularly potent for eyes. It is a reddish-colored carotenoid that occurs in some algae and causes the red coloring in salmon.

Food for Thought: Eat a beautiful, colorful diet: green leafy plants, orange peppers, and peas, as well as egg yolks from pasture-raised hens, and wild-caught red/pink fish and seafood.

Balance with Botanicals: The Blithe Beauty Splendid Serum filled with anti-inflammatory oils from the Blithe Beauty Realm will ease tension in the temples and the back of the neck.

Super Supplements: blueberry, bilberry, lutein, zeaxanthin, astaxanthin, vitamins C and E, zinc, grapeseed extract, omega-3 fatty acids, CoQ10, green tea, alpha lipoic acid

Tools: Install f.lux on your computers to reduce blue light. Use your smartphone in night-shift mode twenty-four hours a day. Wear blue-blocking sunglasses.

Dive Deeper: Read: *Light: Medicine of the Future* and *Take Off Your Glasses and See* by Dr. Jacob Liberman; and *The Art of Seeing* by Aldous Huxley. Visit Jake Steiner's site: endmyopia.org.

FUNGAL FLARE-UPS, THRUSH, AND INFECTIONS

Tinea versicolor is a fungal infection of the skin caused by a fungus that normally lives on the skin but grows out of control. The yeast bleaches the skin in patches and causes a rash. People who have oily skin or sweat a lot or live in a hot climate are more likely to develop tinea versicolor.

Nail infections, jock itch, *Candida,* vaginal yeast infections, and ringworm are also common fungal infections.

Food for Thought: Real, organic yogurt, probiotics, and fermented food provide exposure to a wide variety of microbes that will help keep fungi in proper balance. Eliminating sugar from your diet will help to stem recurrent infections.

Balance with Botanicals: All essential oils are antifungal, though some are antifungal superpowers. Use essential oils from the Brilliant Beauty Realm for antifungal blends with coconut oil, as it is antifungal too.

GLYCATION

Glycation occurs both inside and outside of the body. When food is cooked at a high temperature and it browns, that is glycation. Inside the body, glycation occurs in the bloodstream to a small amount of blood sugar. The sugars found in the blood include fructose, galactose, and glucose, though there is ten times more glycation activity in fructose and galactose than with glucose.[38] The glycation process occurs when the sugar attaches to tissue proteins and rearranges their structures—these are called advanced glycation end products, or AGEs. Some AGEs are benign, but some are highly reactive and are especially damaging to long-lived tissues such as nerves, collagen and elastin, and brain cells. These AGEs are implicated in age-related disease such as heart disease, deafness, neuropathy, and even Alzheimer's disease. They may also damage DNA over time.

AGEs negatively impact the skin too. Collagen is a long-lived protein that is susceptible to glycation. It can degrade collagen and impair it from forming healthy structures, which leads to wrinkling, sagging, and creping skin.

Food for Thought: Avoid sugar and keep your blood sugar balanced. Eat plenty of anti-inflammatory foods that can halt the AGE-caused breakdown of collagen.

Balance with Botanicals: Apply skin serums from the Beloved Beauty Realm.

Super Supplements: glutathione, vitamins C, B complex, and E, alpha lipoic acid

HAIRCARE

We all want shiny, smooth, and manageable hair. Healthy hair feels good and wears well. If your hair has a mind of its own and you urgently need some hair repair, resist the urge to stock up with synthetic shampoo, conditioner, masks, and sprays touting miraculous hair-repair technology. The prescription for a good hair day, every day, is simple: undress your tresses from chemical duress, and bless them with bioactive botanicals and a healthy-hair diet. And wave bye-bye to waxy buildup. Drive out dandruff. Tame wild tresses. Love your locks. Ordain your mane. Consecrate your curls. Bounce your hair with bioactive botanical wisdom, and you will enjoy a good hair day, every day.

Many drugstore and salon products contain twenty or more synthetic ingredients. Some of these substances strip natural oils from the hair and scalp, leaving both seriously dry, while others leave behind a heavy waxy buildup, bolstering bad hair. The more damaged hair is, the higher its negative atomic charge; and softening, smoothing, and shining synthetics are drawn to that negative charge. If there is a lot of damage, you might see a lot of buildup on the hair.

Start with a Healthy Scalp: Our scalp has more than 200 blood vessels, 650 sweat glands, and 1,000 nerve endings. It, of course, is also the mother to our hair. Depending on our hair color, we have between 90,000 and 200,000 hair follicles nurtured by the scalp, and beautiful hair grows from healthy scalps. The core cause of many scalp issues arises from hormone imbalances, high blood sugar, dietary zinc deficiency, internal fungal infections, and even digestive and constipation issues. The following suggestions will help solve those root issues.

Dry, Itchy, and Flaky: The essential oils of rosemary, peppermint, eucalyptus, geranium, nettles, and pine are antibacterial and anti-inflammatory. Eucalyptus heals skin infections and stimulates blood flow. Sandalwood is a serene scalp soother. Peppermint is cooling and provides itch relief. Pine, geranium, nettles, and rosemary are antibacterial and antifungal as well as excellent astringents.

Hair Loss: Hormones play a major role in both male and female hair loss. DHT is an androgen hormone synthesized in the adrenal glands, hair follicles, testes, and prostate. Changes and imbalances in DHT may lead to hair loss by slowing the hair-growing cycle or shrinking and clogging hair follicles. The dermal papillae are the cells in the hair follicle responsible for hair growth. The papillae receive essential nutrients for follicle growth from the capillaries in the skin. Also, the papillae have a lot of DHT receptors. Too much DHT in the bloodstream undermines nutrient absorption, which slows, and sometimes stops, hair growth. DHT also shrinks the hair follicle by stimulating the deposit of a wax-like substance around the hair roots. If you are noticing hair loss, have your DHT levels tested, and increase your dietary zinc to recalibrate your androgen-to-DHT conversion. See the sections on **Hormones, Thyroid,** and **Adrenals** for bringing balance to the endocrine system.

General hair shedding, especially for women, is often the result of a thyroid imbalance, especially postpregnancy. Avoid gluten and soy, as they block nutrients from absorbing through the gut and into the bloodstream to nourish hair roots. First inside the gut and then in the scalp, gluten triggers inflammation in the hair follicles, which causes shedding. Removing wheat and gluten may cease this type of hair loss right away.

Seal Split Ends: Four years ago, I decided not to cut my hair anymore and see what happens. I am enjoying the natural layers and shape that flows as it grows, and it is nice to see hair tips remain healthy. I have been using seabuckthorn shampoo for years and years and find I need to wash my hair only once every two weeks, sometimes less often, sometimes more, depending on my schedule. (In the summertime, I plan hair washing on sunny days so I can let it sun dry.) I think decades of not using sodium lauryl sulfates and other harsh surfactants has been a boon. I also love conditioning my hair before and after shampooing. Before I shampoo, I like to massage oil onto my scalp. The amount of time I leave it on varies from a few minutes to overnight. Oiling the hair and scalp is a great way to stimulate cells and deliver nourishing essential oils to hair roots too. I like to keep my hair loose in the day and while sleeping. I use gentle elastics when needed. Natural-bristle brushes and wooden combs feel so good on the scalp, prevent static, and distribute oils evenly throughout my hair.

Styling Secrets: My favorite way to wash and dry my hair is in our lake after a morning swim, and then letting my hair dry in the fresh air and sunshine while I languidly apply sun-loving botanicals to build my skin's solar power. When my hair is close to being dry, I run a wooden comb through the strands to organize my mane. In the winter, I like to wash my hair at night, wrap it up in an organic Turkish towel[39] for a few minutes, and then go to sleep and wake up with dry hair; or I let it dry by the fire. This is all very different from the days when I would have a fainting spell when my mom blow-dried my hair, and in my teenage years when I indulged in devoted blow-drying sessions, slowly drying my hair in sections with big, round brushes. I would experiment with a curling iron, straighten with a flat iron, and preserve the moment with hair spray, or use the new fad at the time: foaming hair mousse. It all felt like a fun transition from styling sessions with my Barbie dolls' hair to playing with my own; yet now I know that overstyling with chemical-laden gels of goop, sprays, shampoos, and polymers with heated tools cooks those chemicals in, and that dries and damages hair swiftly. Then you find yourself, once again, in a loop of cutting hair to clear split ends, or on a never-ending search for the holy grail of hair conditioner to glue those split

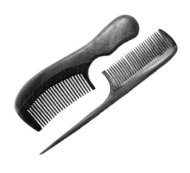

ends back together. Understandably, sometimes you just want to get your hair dry and get out the door. Luckily, there are now gentler hot curlers instead of an iron, and ceramic, ionic, tourmaline options for hair dryers and straighteners. And perhaps their use can be spread out. Now that you will be free of chemical haircare, these styling tools won't be baking in the butane. (Can you believe dry shampoos with butane as an ingredient exist?) For natural curls and waves, I like to twist up smaller sections of hair while damp and let it dry. Beauty blogs have tons of tips for no-heat hairstyles and beachy-bouncy tresses.

The loose hair strands of a woman don't have to be combed.

Food for Thought: Eat today for beautiful hair tomorrow. Your hair is a reflection of your internal health, and what you eat today will show up in your hair. Eat healthy fats. A diet rich in olive oil, flaxseeds, chia seeds, wild-caught cold-water fish, and walnuts will give your hair a super softness and a high-gloss sheen. Eat enough protein. Hair is made of protein; and if the diet is deficient in the full spectrum of amino acids that constitute complete proteins, then your hair will suffer for it. Ingest culinary creations rich in omega-3 fatty acids, iron, vitamin B12, and zinc, which are important for strong hair and a healthy scalp. Brittle hair is sometimes caused by a biotin deficiency. Organic, free-range eggs are rich in protein, happy-hair fats, and B vitamins. Dark-green leafy vegetables are good sources of vitamins A and C, which the body needs to produce natural hair oils that keep the hair soft and shiny.

Gluten is less than the best for healthy hair. It blocks nutrients from absorbing through the gut and into the bloodstream to nourish you. Reduced nutrition and inflammation of the gut and hair follicles from gluten sensitivity may cause shedding. Gluten and nonfermented soy (as well as radiation, bromide, mercury fillings, and other things) can put your thyroid in a tailspin. An underactive thyroid is often the cause of dryness, thinning, or loss of hair.

Balance with Botanicals: Switch to a chemical-free conditioner and shampoo. When switching, add a little baking soda to the shampoo for the first few washes to cleanse chemical residues and surfactants out of the scalp from previous shampoos. Chapter Sixteen has easy formulas for an anti-itch **Sandalwood Scalp Oil** for dandruff and scalp health, **Happy Hair Rinse, Happy Hair Dry Shampoo, Beach Breeze Hair Spray, Everything Balm,** and no-poo instructions. Pure petal perfumes and decadent essential oils like jasmine, sandalwood, rose, ylang, and neroli are a sensual adoration streaked through the hair. The aroma lasts until your next shampoo too!

Super Supplements: zinc, biotin, omega-3 fatty acids, B vitamins, *he shou wu*, pumpkin seed oil[40] to prevent hair loss, evening primrose and borage oils. Iron deficiency, especially in premenopausal women, can also play a role in hair loss, and an iron bisglycinate supplement is more absorbable.

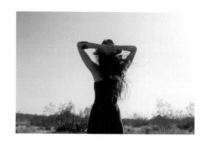

Tools: wooden combs, natural-bristle brush

Dive Deeper: There are tons of chemicals in hair dyes, yet if you are dismayed by gray, look for a gentler alternative at the health food store, henna, and a new revolutionary product called Hairprint. Read *Almond Eyes, Lotus Feet: Indian Traditions in Beauty and Health* by Sharada Dwivedi and Shalini Devi Holkar.

HEMORRHOIDS

When people refer to having hemorrhoids, their complaint is actually enlarged or irritated hemorrhoids, because we all have little pillows of tissue just inside the anus that are called hemorrhoids. When these little pillows are irritated, they get inflamed and itch and burn and make passing bowel movements very unpleasant. Because they are filled with tiny blood vessels, it isn't unusual for enlarged hemorrhoids to bleed a little. There are several causes, and the most frequent are: constipation or frequent diarrhea, straining to go, pregnancy and childbirth, genetics, and sitting on the toilet too long (this is not the place to check your email!). Most of the time, hemorrhoids are not a serious medical condition, though if they are a frequent or chronic problem or if there is more than a drop or two of blood when you go, you may want to seek professional guidance.

Stop the itch and burn! A sitz bath can relieve symptoms quickly. Simply fill up the tub with warm water twice a day and relax for about ten minutes. You can also add magnesium or epsom salts and a couple drops of peppermint essential oil to the bath.

Food for Thought: Eat more fiber and wholesome foods. Stay hydrated to encourage free elimination. Avoid alcohol and spicy food.

Balance with Botanicals: The quorum-sensing inhibitors of essential oils pacify pathogens while cooperating with our beneficial bacteria. Spot-treat with **Everything Balm.**

Super Supplements: probiotics and prebiotics, fermented food, psyllium, aloe, triphala

HERPES SIMPLEX

For herpes zoster, see **Shingles.**

Herpes simplex is a viral infection that demonstrates with fluid-filled blisters on the mouth, genitals, and mucous membranes.

Viral infection is yet to be completely cured; however, many people learn to hold outbreaks at bay. Here are a few tips:

- Keep your immune system optimized.
- L-lysine is an amino acid found in supplement form that may help avoid outbreaks.
- Carotenoids in red and orange vegetables raise immunity and speed healing.
- Zinc, both dietary and topical, can shorten and prevent outbreaks.
- B complex vitamins as well as vitamin C help the body deal with stress, which can drag down our immune system and make us vulnerable to illness.

Raw honey mixed with essential oils and applied topically has been shown to be an effective treatment of an outbreak. Honey diminishes pain, itching, and inflammation, and the moisturizing and natural antibacterial properties help the lesion heal.

Balance with Botanicals: The quorum-sensing inhibitors of essential oils pacify pathogens while cooperating with our beneficial bacteria. Target treat with **Brilliant Beauty Spot Treatment** and seal with **Calm Balm.** Stock the apothecary with honey, frankincense, rose otto, peppermint, blue tansy, and immortelle.

Super Supplements: L-lysine and immune-boosting nutrients of probiotics, vitamin C, B complex vitamins, zinc, iodine, vitamin D3, and sunshine

HORMONES

Also see **Menstruation, Thyroid,** and **Adrenals.**

Our hormones transcend our fertility—they are key players in our whole-body health. Some women are told that acne, cramps, irritability, breast tenderness, bloating, and back pain are the result of normal shifts in female hormones throughout the menstrual cycle. Au contraire, *ma soeur!* These symptoms are signs of hormone imbalance. A few simple steps bring perfect symmetry back to our bodies. Improve your nutrition and digestion with healthy fats, fiber, and fresh food filled with vitamins and minerals. Keep your blood sugar stable. Avoid soy. Find your internal space of centered calm to soften the effects of stress; try meditation or your favorite physical movement to get yourself in the flow. Well-selected herbs can also help, so find a trusted practitioner, or ask an integrative medical doctor for advice.

Balance with Botanicals: Herbs to boost healthy estrogen (estriol) and help with hot flashes: panax ginseng, black cohosh, kacip fatimah, and white kwao krua *(Pueraria mirifica).* Iodine, chamomile (acts as an aromatase inhibitor), and passionflower help to release excess estrogen. Vitex chaste tree and evening primrose oil stimulate progesterone, and maca helps as a general adaptogenic superfood to boost the body's DHEA. Pine pollen, tongkat ali, tribulus, and nettle root encourage the body's natural testosterone and magnesium levels. Boron supplementation raises serum estrogen and testosterone levels. For menopausal women, coconut-based DHEA suppositories are available from some compounding pharmacies; and the lubrication, increased orgasms, and finer hormone-balancing results have made many women happy.

Dive Deeper: Revolutionary hormone testing now exists with the DUTCH method. Read: *The Hormone Cure* by Dr. Sara Gottfried; *Ageless* and *I'm Too Young for This!* by Suzanne Somers; and *Natural Remedies for Low Testosterone* by Stephen Buhner.

HYPERPIGMENTATION[41]

Dotted, spotted, dappled, and discolored skin, referred to as hyperpigmentation, is a pervasive skin concern. There are a myriad of reasons why the skin develops these spots, referred to as melasma. *Melasma,* derived from the Greek word *melas,* which means "black," is irregular, uneven-skin-tone patches usually found on the face, especially across the upper lip and fore-head. There are a few medical causes for hyperpigmentation that require a doctor's diagnosis and care. Haemochromatosis, too much iron circulating in the bloodstream, can cause bronzy skin pigmentation; and congenital diseases such as Peutz–Jeghers syndrome, Cushing's disease, and Addison's disease, as well as other hormonal imbalances, can cause diffuse dappling pigmentation, cancerous lesions, and mercury poisoning. Also, some prescription medications and topicals make the skin more sensitive to ultraviolet rays and environmental exposures. If you are taking a medication and see changes in your skin, tell your doctor or pharmacist. Here are a few types of prescription drugs that may affect the skin: antibiotics, antiseizure medicines, diuretics, dyes, retinoids, aspirin, salicylic acid, nonsteroidal anti-inflammatories, heart medicines, antiemetics, antidepressants, contraceptive pills, hormone replacement pills, steroids, and cancer treatments.

Usually, though, flat, darkened skin spots are considered "benign" hyperpigmentation that can be faded and prevented without medical attention. Women tend to develop melasma more than men, who represent only 10 percent of the melasma cases seen by dermatologists. Elevated estrogen and hormone imbalance are major contributors to melasma. Excess hormones usually occur from overproduction, toxin stimulation, and inefficiency in the natural hormone-elimination process performed by the liver. The American Academy of Dermatology states that birth control pills and hormone replacement therapy can cause melasmas and sensitivity to the sun. Hormones stimulate the growth of cells that make brown pigment (melanocytes), and natural light stimulates the production of even more brown pigment (melanin). **Thyroid** dysfunction can also lead to hormone imbalances that affect the skin. Hyperpigmentation can also occur from facial chemical peels, microdermabrasion, and laser treatments.

To prevent melasma from occurring, worsening, or reoccurring, it is important to avoid endocrine-disrupting products, pass on the Pill and all artificial hormones, and if possible, keep hormones in balance. Pregnancy is the exception. When melasma occurs during pregnancy, it is commonly referred to as "pregnancy mask." Although this is a hormone issue, pregnancy mask is considered normal. Dietary changes and botanical skincare may prevent pregnancy pigmentation.

Post inflammatory hyperpigmentation, or PIH, is a darker or blotchy patch that remains after a skin trauma or disease—such as rashes, contact dermatitis, burns, allergic responses, injury, acne, and infections—has resolved. PIH is caused when the inflammation process alters the function of the immune cells and the melanocytes in the injured cells so that excess melanin is dispersed. African, Asian, and other skin with deep melanin is more prone to PIH. In time, with healthy cell turnover, PIH spots will fade on their own.

Age spots, or liver spots, are flat and brown or blackish, and generally they are larger than a freckle. These spots are most often on the face, arms, hands, chest, and back. Dermatologists largely consider age spots to be a cosmetic issue that occurs as part of the aging process, though medical researchers may now be establishing that these spots are a skin-surface indicator of a deeper issue called lipofuscin accumulation. Lipofuscin is a type of cellular waste that causes metabolic damage in the cell and slowly drains away cellular vitality. It is composed of brown pigment, oxidized proteins, lipids, and metals: iron, copper, zinc, aluminum, and manganese. Lipofuscin is also found in the liver, kidneys, heart, nerve cells, brain, and adrenal glands, where it fuels a cascade of age-related disease and health issues. If you have age or liver spots, it may mean that lipofuscin is also accumulating in other organs. Age spots are often confused with, or used synonymously for, solar lentigines (lentigo), which are accumulations of melanocytes (in lieu of melanin, as with freckles) in a small group of cells.

The sun is blamed for many skin issues, including melasma and age spots. While it is important to interact wisely with our ancient erudite accomplice, we do not want to be burned by the sun yet set aglow. Well-nourished skin has a healthy response to sunlight, and most "sun damage" is the result of modern malnutrition with its bereft banquet of rancid PUFA oils, copious corn syrup, and vacant carbohydrates. Processed omega-6 polyunsaturated fats and trans fats (soy, corn, and canola oils), found in every processed food on the shelf, impair intercellular communication, cause fungus to flourish, and suppress immune functions, which is associated with skin aging and hyperpigmentation. These oils are chemically unstable and oxidize readily to form free radicals that prevent flourishing health and are indicated for premature aging. Free radicals pillage DNA, organs, blood vessels, and immunity, and make the skin susceptible to UV damage as the sun ignites these internal chain reactions and bakes these chemicals in, along with transdermal toxins from lifeless liquids being applied to the body. The Research Foundation for Plastic Surgery in Los Angeles compiled data from 1,000 women on premature aging. Bottom line: those who ate polyunsaturated or trans fats showed 78 percent more signs of facial premature aging, some appearing more than twenty years older than their age.[42] Organic healthy fats and essential fatty acids on and in the skin, direly depleted in the standard North American diet, are desperately needed to amplify the benefits of the sun's rays and to drive that D vitamin in. Sipping on spring water and consuming colorful meals of garden greens, fantastic fats, paleo proteins, tree-ripened fruit, and vivacious vegetables are the first step toward properly functioning melanocytes, reducing low-level inflammation and reversing oxidative damage.

"Out, damned spot! out, I say!"[43] Lady Macbeth had little success in removing her spot with severe scrubbing, and neither will scrubbing fade a skin spot. Surfactants, chemical cleansers, dermal laser ablation, and vigorous exfoliation scour the skin's topmost protective layer. With this top coat jeopardized, toxins and exposures irritate the underlying, emergent skin and induce inflammatory issues. Irritated, inflamed, and unprotected skin is more prone to pigmenting than intact, balanced skin. When it comes to pigmentation, alcohol is one of the chief culprits. It dries and shrinks skin cells, furthering free-radical damage that contributes to skin spots and blotches. Avoid all topical products containing methanol, benzyl alcohol, isopropyl alcohol, SD-40 alcohol, ethyl alcohol (also called ethanol), and denatured alcohol.

Balance with Botanicals: Nature generously provides us a few skin-clearing solutions. Rich in antioxidants and cell-regenerative energy, essential oils are superheroes for hyperpigmented skin. Bright-orange seabuckthorn berry oil contains lipids of about 70 percent linoleic acid and alpha-linolenic acid, and research has demonstrated that linoleic acid and alpha-linolenic acid applied topically lighten hyperpigmentations. It can be applied undiluted to the skin, and, ideally, it is applied at night because the undiluted oil will temporarily turn your skin orange. Look to botanicals from the Benevolent and Beloved Beauty Realms. Apply a botanical zinc-based block to hyperpigmentation patches when going out in the sun. Skip the soap, cleanse with one of the Renegade Beauty Realms All Over Oils, treat with Benevolent or Beloved Beauty Spot Treatment (be diligent in your application), and follow with Benevolent or Beloved Beauty Splendid Serum. Stock the apothecary with immortelle, rose otto, frankincense, myrrh, seabuckthorn, sandalwood, cypress, and rockrose.

Food for Thought: Replace all processed PUFA oils of Mazola, canola, soy, corn, cottonseed, fake olive oil,[44] and peanut oil with wholesome fats of grass-fed butter, ghee, olive oil, coconut oil, and avocados.

Super Supplements: Mitochondrial medicine of magnesium, glutathione (a master antioxidant that boosts liver function), indole-3-carbinol, vitamin C. Vitamins B3 and B12 may lower inflammation and clear out the lipofuscin hyperpigmentation; and N-acetylcysteine (NAC), an amino-acid derivative, boosts glutathione, helping the cells to resist damage from reactive oxygen species (ROS).

HYPOPIGMENTATION

Hypopigmentation, or depigmentation, is the loss of skin color in a part of the skin that has been injured, a.k.a. white scars. When the skin is damaged, sometimes the cells that make melanin or the enzyme required to make melanin are depleted; so as the skin heals, the skin is white or light instead of the normal pigmented color.

Some people have found that fresh ginger or ginger juice applied topically to the area entices the melanocytes to produce more pigment and return the scar to a natural color. Vetiver essential oils may also be helpful.[45]

Balance with Botanicals: The quorum-sensing inhibitors of essential oils help to take care of pathogens while cooperating with our beneficial bacteria. Target treat with the **Blithe Beauty Spot Treatment,** and seal with one of the **Renegade Beauty Splendid Serums** or **Calm Balm.** Stock the apothecary with vetiver, frankincense, rose otto, peppermint, and ginger.

ITCHY SKIN

See **Eczema** and **Rashes.**

JADE OR CRYSTAL ROLLING

Massaging the face and neck with a cool jade roller gives a gentle lift to the lymphatic system, clears congested lymph nodes, stimulates skin tissue, and helps care for undereye issues. This beauty secret has been used in China since the seventh century. Store in the fridge for an extra chill factor, and apply a cooling

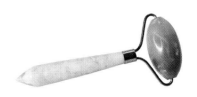

serum from the Blithe Beauty Realm or a soothing serum from the Benevolent Beauty Realm to the jade roller.

KERATOSIS PILARIS

Keratosis pilaris is rough, patchy bumps, a.k.a. "chicken skin," that occurs most frequently on the back of the arms, the thighs, and the buttocks. It is caused by an overproduction of keratin in the skin that blocks hair follicles and is considered an inflammatory condition that is sometimes coexistent with allergies and asthma. People with dry skin and those who live in dry environments are more likely to develop keratosis pilaris.

Balance with Botanicals: Apply oils from the Brilliant Beauty Realm, and use the Grapefruit Glow Body Scrub.

Food for Thought: Keratosis pilaris can be a sign of vitamin K2 or D3 deficiency. A diet rich in essential fatty acids, vitamin A, and the fat-soluble vitamins D3 and K2 helps lubricate the skin from the inside out, and many people find that this clears it up. Though no research studies have shown a dietary cause, because it is an inflammatory issue an Elimination Diet may help you to determine if a particular food is a source of inflammation.

LEAKY GUT SYNDROME, A.K.A. INTESTINAL HYPERPERMEABILITY

Leaky guts can result in rosacea, acne, eczema, fungal rashes, and psoriasis and are caused by a proliferation of *Candida* fungi. *Candida* is invasive pathogenic yeast that excretes a mycotoxin waste product. In advanced stages of overgrowth, *Candida* fungi grow root-like filaments that dig tiny holes in the intestines. This can cause leaky gut syndrome, when food, bacteria, and toxins escape the gut through tiny perforations and flow into the bloodstream. The mycotoxins it releases mimic estrogen and may deactivate our p53 gene, which is our anticancer superhero gene.[46] These mycotoxins are also prevalent in the factory food chain; it is in moldy corn, peanuts, and grains.

Many grains contain gliadin, which has been found to deregulate the gut protein zonulin. Zonulin modulates the tightness and laxness of spaces between the cells in the gut lining that regulate immunity.[47] In other words, gliadin damages the intestinal-barrier function by increasing its permeability. Gliadin is found in wheat and other grains in the *Triticeae* grass tribe, including kamut, spelt, barley, and rye. It is best to avoid these grains for optimal gut health.

A diverse, thriving microbiome protects the gastrointestinal tract from *Candida* and damage. Some species of microbes release anti-inflammation compounds to keep the gut working smoothly.[48] Daily doses of probiotics and fermented food will keep the flora flourishing. Avoid sugar; it upsets the balance of bacteria in the gut. Heal and seal the guts by eliminating these foods and recolonizing the guts with prebiotics and probiotics.

Super Supplements: Aloe vera, colloidal silver, and glutamine can help repair damaged guts.

Dive Deeper: Read: *The Body Ecology Diet* by Donna Gates; *Grain Brain* by Dr. David Perlmutter; and *Gut and Psychology Syndrome: Natural Treatment for Autism, Dyspraxia, A.D.D., Dyslexia, A.D.H.D., Depression, Schizophrenia* by Natasha Campbell-McBride.

LYMPHATIC SYSTEM

The lymph system is right under the surface of the skin, comprising a vast network of superficial capillaries that lead to larger collection vessels throughout the body. These capillaries consist of loosely overlapping cells so that they are permeable to fluids, larger molecules, pathogens, and other smaller cells. Fluid from interstitial spaces drains into the lymph capillaries, is transported through lymph nodes, and then flows into large ducts on either side of the spine. From there, the fluid along with the waste and unneeded cellular "stuff" is passed into the bloodstream to be processed and eliminated. Unlike the circulatory system, which has the heart for a pump, the circulation of lymph fluid relies on physical motion to get it moving. Muscle contractions massage the fluid along through the capillaries in the skin. Inactivity and loss of muscle tone are major obstacles for healthy lymph flow. The lymph fluid can also be roused by the dry and stiff bristles of a brush gently swept across the skin. The tiny muscles in your skin, the same muscles that make your hair stand up when you are cold, are stimulated by the motion of the brush and provide gentle contractions that get the lymph moving. Essential oils have such a lovely affinity to the lymph system that they can really help to stimulate flow with **Dry Brushing.**

Balance with Botanicals: Rosemary, eucalyptus, frankincense, and laurel are effective. Laurel *(Laurus nobilis)* is particularly known for moving the lymph and clearing the lymphatic system. In *Advanced Aromatherapy,* Dr. Kurt Schnaubelt states, "rubbing a few drops of bay laurel on swollen lymph nodes may have an immediate, noticeable effect. The positive and pleasant effect of this oil is so distinct and strong that one application will normally suffice to convince the most hardened skeptic to use it."[49]

MAKEUP

According to a survey conducted by the Environmental Working Group, 1 out of every 13 women and 1 out of every 23 men use every day a cosmetic that has an ingredient that is a known carcinogen.[50] Do you know all of the ingredients in your makeup?

Almost daily I receive emails from women who now feel so confident with their skin tone and texture that they feel free to leave their home without makeup! So the best foundation is to create a foundation of radiant skin. Get evenly toned and glowing skin so you feel ready to rock the world without makeup. There are many options with more natural mineral makeup for eye shadows, eyeliners, mascara, and blushes. I have yet to find a makeup line that is 100 percent pure, yet far cleaner options are found at the health food store than at the drugstore. You will find a **Cleopatra Charcoal Mascara** formula in Chapter Sixteen.

Hold on to your divine blush, your innate rosy magic . . .

Tom Robbins[51]

MEDITATION

Also see **Breathing.**

You know, your phone has a charger, right? It's like having a charger for your whole body and mind. That's what Transcendental Meditation is!

Jerry Seinfeld[52]

For the last few years, meditation has been a media buzzword. Articles inform us that it is good for us. Meditation, of course, is not new. Buddhist monks, Desert Fathers and Desert Mothers, and yogis discovered the life-centering power of meditation millennia ago.

There are so many ways to meditate, yet many people feel daunted, as they cannot control mental chatter. (This is true for most people, which is why meditation is called a practice, not an act. Keep practicing.) Meditation is about being *aware* of the stream of thoughts, observing the constant stream, and being aware of the momentum. There is a form of meditation that is a good fit for you: moving meditations, just taking a moment to breathe meditations, kundalini *kriyas*, group meditations, audio guided meditations, and binaural beats. There are even headbands that help and of course, nowadays, there is an app for that too.[53] I have recorded a meditation for beauty too: *Being Beauty: A Guided Meditation to Feeling Beautiful.*[54]

Balance with Botanicals: Simply anoint frankincense or your favorite essential oils to your pineal gland. (Since ancient times, this gland has been referred to as the mind's eye, the third eye, or the inner eye. This area, the center of the brow, is perceived to be the seat of the soul and an extension of our mind's intuitive perception.) A drop applied under your nose will elevate your focus. Using the salt pipe for fifteen minutes of aromatherapeutic breathing is meditative too.

MELASMA

See **Hyperpigmentation.**

MENSTRUATION

Also see **Hormones.**

It is truly time to be fine with our menstrual moon cycles. I promise, if you suffer from PMS symptoms and cramps, there are so many ways to solve these symptoms, and many women feel the results by their next cycle.

PMS is caused by a combination of factors: **Adrenal** stress, unstable blood sugar, thyroid issues, toxins, and nutrient deficiencies. A few changes in diet and lifestyle can help you make friends with your luteal phase and menstruation:

Avoid nonfermented soy as well as plastic water bottles, canned foods, and synthetic skincare. They contain chemicals known to disrupt hormones. Create calming **Sleep** habits and **Meditation** for optimal rest, and find stress-busting (and fun) activities that get you moving and grooving.

Food for Thought: Be sure that you are getting enough vitamins D, B6, E, and A as well as magnesium and iodine. Ingest evening primrose oil and healthy fats, and avoid sugar, wheat, and processed food to maintain level blood sugar.

Catch the Flow: How do you catch the flow? Personally, I wouldn't plug this pinnacle with any synthetic objects or materials. Some women sleep on an old flannel sheet to let their flow freely flow while they sleep. Nonorganic pads and tampons can be filled with pesticide residues, bleach, and manufacturing chemicals. They may also be moldy! Organic pad and panty liner options are easily available. Thinx brand underwear is a good option too. Their lightweight, leak-proof, and reusable panties absorb up to two tampons' worth of blood, and they come in several styles . . . now if they could just make an option with organic cotton.

Balance with Botanicals: Massage the **Marjoram Moontime Blend** to your belly, or even better, apply it with the Arvigo Techniques of Maya Abdominal Therapy. This type of massage guides internal abdominal organs into their proper position for optimal well-being, resulting in improved organ function, release of congestion, and improved flow of the circulatory, lymphatic, and nervous systems. See **Yoni Steam Baths.**

Super Supplements: Vitex, black cohosh, and peony help regulate hormones. Passionflower, panax ginseng, and schizandra support good energy and mental function. Smooth digestion is also optimal for easing cramps, so be sure to tweak any gut and liver imbalances. Tone up the liver with DIM, milk thistle, and dandelion, so that it has the ability to filter the flux of hormones every month. Probiotics and enzymes also help move things through the body so that all of your energy is not getting cramped.

MENTAL HEALTH AND MOODS

The gut–brain axis is a superhighway for our microbiome, and the highway goes both ways. The brain interacts with the gastrointestinal system, and immune functions in the gut and the gut microbes make neurochemicals and neurotransmitters that act on the brain. For decades, the theory held that depression and other mental health issues were caused by chemical imbalances in the brain, but breakthroughs in microbiology seem to be dismantling that theory.

The science is still nascent, yet future research may help ease the burden of mental illness without the side effects of pharmaceutical drugs.

Food for Thought: Dr. Kelly Brogan, a brilliant holistic psychiatrist, urges people to make some dietary changes before considering an antidepressant: stop eating GMO food, gluten, and sugar.[55] Build your bacterial reserve with probiotics, balance hormones, and be sure to test your **Thyroid** if you are experiencing anxiety and/or depression.

Mood Lifter: Elevate with the elegance of euphoric essential oils: ylang, jasmine, bergamot, rose, fragonia, neroli, blood orange, and grapefruit. These essences alight with levity. Inhale, anoint, or blend with honey and eat. They are perfect to share for communions and sacred unions.

Mental Clarity: Essential oils are stellar at assisting with mental clarity, especially when the wheels of the mind are spinning. Tame monkey-mind mode with essential oils of rosemary, inula, eucalyptus, lemon, frankincense, laurel, and peppermint to pull up the socks of mental focus and unleash whirlwinds of creativity too. Let the essential oils take your thoughts into ease and flow. They require no effort, and upon inhalation their miraculous molecules immediately shift states of being, your mind, and your emotions. You can get into a new headspace without effort. All of a sudden you are in a place of lucid thought and meditation.

Anxiety and Panic Attacks: This is the time when any essential oil you have on hand is going to help, as inhaling aroma molecules will immediately reach your limbic system and start working on releasing neurotransmitters. Without any effort, your breathing is going to change. Your whole physiology is going to change. Even your central nervous system is going to change. I recommend lavender, bergamot, spikenard, chamomile, marjoram, and frankincense for these moments.

Tools: salt pipe, aroma diffuser

Dive Deeper: Read: *A Mind of Your Own: The Truth about Depression and How Women Can Heal Their Bodies to Reclaim Their Lives* by Dr. Kelly Brogan, and do view her blog and online conversations with luminaries such as Marianne Williamson and Marie Forleo; *Brain Maker* by Dr. David Perlmutter; *White Hot Truth: Clarity for Keeping It Real on Your Spiritual Path from One Seeker to Another* by Danielle LaPorte; *How to Be a Bawse* by Lilly Singh; *A Return to Love* by Marianne Williamson; and *Why Isn't My Brain Working? A Revolutionary Understanding of Brain Decline and Effective Strategies to Recover Your Brain's Health* by Dr. Datis Kharrazian.

MILIA

Milia are very small, white bumps commonly found on the nose, cheeks, and eyelids. They often occur on infant skin, though no one knows why, and are inaccurately called acne. They form when a little bit of keratin gets stuck under the surface of the skin. Adults also develop milia occasionally; usually milia form on skin that has been injured somehow. Essential oils can help to resolve milia.

Balance with Botanicals: Use the Spot Treatments from the Blithe and Brilliant Beauty Realms.

MOLES

Moles are growths that are usually brown, black, or flesh colored. Moles occur when skin cells grow in a cluster. It isn't unusual for them to darken a little with sun exposure and during hormone shifts—puberty, pregnancy, and menopause. They may also change slowly with age by gaining size or disappearing.

Melanoma and Moles: Fewer than 1 in 33,000 moles become malignant, even in men over sixty years old, which is the highest risk group.[56] However, melanoma is an aggressive cancer; so if you see a new skin lesion, a black spot, or rapid changes in a mole, then it is pertinent to seek advice from a medical practitioner. It is a good idea to keep an eye on any moles larger than a pencil eraser, too. Look for a specialized clinic with high-tech equipment that offers a higher degree of accuracy in pre-excision diagnosis. General practitioners and nonspecialized dermatologists tend to overexcise moles and lesions for pathology. A ten-year study that included both specialized and nonspecialized clinics found that of 300,215 excised moles and suspicious spots, only 17,172 were malignant.[57] That means that 283,043 surgeries occurred to remove nonmalignant lesions—that is a lot of unnecessary surgery. To find a specialized clinic near you, visit the website for the Melanoma International Foundation. See page 276 for details about applying iodine to moles.

NAILS

Healthy fingernails are pink with white half-moons near the base. Strong nails are usually a reflection of a healthy diet full of protein, iron, B vitamins, silicon, vitamin D, zinc, and omega-3 fatty acids. Imbalances in nail texture and color reflect injury to the nail and nail bed or a dietary deficiency. For example, vertical ridges in the nails may reflect inadequate dietary magnesium. Also, white spots on the nails, called leukonychia, are usually caused by injury to the nail or nail bed.

Green, blue, or yellow nails as well as nails with red streaks or dark spots may reflect bigger underlying health issues and may require the intervention of a trusted medical practitioner.

Thickened nails may be the result of a fungal infection of the nail.[58] Fungal infections of the nail result when microbes of the nail are out of balance, allowing the fungal infection called onychomycosis to take over. The most common symptoms of infection are pain around the nail bed and white or yellow patches or discoloration on the nail. Athlete's foot, nail damage, dirty and tight shoes and socks, and compromised immune function all make the nails more susceptible to onychomycosis. Replenishing healthy gut bacteria with probiotics and healing leaky guts are a good place to start to resolve fungal nail infections. Oregano essential oil (5 percent) diluted in tea tree essential oil (95 percent) may be applied directly to the nail neat a few times every day to fight infection and encourage bacteria rebalance.

Nail polish is full of undesirable toxins that are absorbed dermally. A 2015 study found triphenyl phosphate in 100 percent of test subjects with painted nails, and it may disrupt hormone regulation, healthy development, metabolism, and reproduction.[59] Other toxic ingredients commonly found in nail polish include formaldehyde, toluene, and dibutyl phthalate. Although there are many formaldehyde-free nail polishes available these days, your nails need to breathe! The use of any type of nail polish will result in less-than-healthy nails in the buff. Then you may find yourself in a cyclical situation where you feel you need to wear nail polish to cover up.

Balance with Botanicals: Simply keep nails clean with a daily, natural-bristle brushing and an anointment with one of the **Renegade Beauty Realms All Over Oils** as cuticle oil. To make nail tips extra white, use the **Lemon + Baking Soda Nail Brightening Soak** and apply a drop of tea tree under each nail. And by making some of the dietary changes suggested in this book, your nails will gain strength with better nutrition.

Tools: Perfectly manicured nails can be achieved with a crystal nail file, and any of the **Renegade Beauty Realms All Over Oils** as a cuticle blend.

NOSE HEALTH

The nose and sinus cavity are lined with tiny hairs, millions of bacteria, and soft, slick mucous membranes that warm and moisten incoming air and trap foreign intruders. The nose is the first line of defense against inhaled infectious agents, so keeping it in good working order is important. "Contracting and overcoming a cold is connected to the immune functions of the respiratory tract . . . remaining in overheated or extremely dry rooms for long periods of time in the winter is a common prelude to upper respiratory infections."[60]

Anointing the inside of the nose with a soothing and hydrating oil will protect the nasal mucosa, especially during dry winter months and air travel. Coconut oil is a great carrier, or use **Everything Balm.**

Nose Microbiome: The microbiome of the nose and sinuses mostly remains a mystery. The sinuses themselves—what they do and why they are there—are yet to be understood by doctors and researchers. What we do know is that diverse populations of bacteria live in the warm caverns of the nose and sinuses at all times and that people with smaller "nose gardens" are more likely to suffer from sinonasal disease. (Interestingly, men tend to have about twice as many total bacteria in their noses as women.[61])

In a recent study of people with chronic sinusitis, persistently inflamed sinuses, researchers discovered that their noses were heavily populated with one bacterium called *Corynebacterium tuberculostearicum*. The researchers think that perhaps viral infections may be causing inflammation in the person's nose and that the inflammation may be killing off some of the other protective diverse bacteria.[62] Oral probiotics may help keep the nose and sinuses healthy. A study conducted in 2009 found that children who were fed a probiotic containing either *Lactobacillus* or *Bifidobacterium* or a combination of the two for six months saw improvements in fevers, coughs, runny, congested noses, and upper-airway infection.[63]

Nasal Polyps: These are small, benign growths in the mucous membrane of the nose and sinuses. They occur from chronic inflammation in the nose and sinuses. Most polyps are small and are no problem. Larger polyps can make the nose feel stuffy, obstruct air movement and mucus drainage, and influence the sense of smell and taste. They may also cause headaches, snoring, chronic colds, or runny noses. Apply the **Luxor Nose Balm** or frankincense and jojoba to your olfactory inner sanctum.

OIL CLEANSING THE BODY AND FACE

We can feed our skin from the outside in with a transdermal botanical bouquet that purifies, calms, and clears the skin. Consider adopting the ancient method of washing the skin with oil. Washing with botanicals gently and effectively cleanses and exfoliates the skin while maintaining moisture and the integrity of the precious top layer.

Plants evolved alongside us, and their oils harmonize with our skin. The antimicrobial properties of essential oils combined with the gentle dirt-dissolving fatty oils lift away the daily accumulation of dirt, toxins, and makeup while healing, not harming, the skin's surface. Seabuckthorn berry supercritical extract is highly concentrated and heals the root causes of skin imbalances by regenerating the skin from the inside out; combined with jojoba oil, it is a beautiful way to wash the skin.

It may seem strange, washing with oils. People think that oil will leave their skin feeling oily and less than clean, yet the exact opposite is experienced when washing with the right oils. Beauty glows with a balanced biome.

How to Wash with Oils: Three Easy Steps: Washing with oils is an easy and super effective way to keep the skin clean and healthy. Use jojoba or any of the Renegade Beauty Realms All Over Oils for an excellent experience. These same steps can be followed to oil cleanse the body.

1. Dampen a small area of an organic cotton cleansing cloth with water. Squeeze it out.

2. Apply a squirt of jojoba or your favorite combination of oils to the damp cloth.

3. Gently massage the face with the cloth. Massage gently to cleanse, or vigorously to exfoliate the skin. Rinsing your skin is optional. If you would like added moisture, squirt a few drops of jojoba or a skin serum onto your fingertips and massage into face.

ORAL OIL PULLING

Although most of us have been brushing diligently for decades, receding and bleeding gums are still the norm; unexpected cavities form, and millions of root canals are performed. The definition of insanity, doing the same thing and expecting different results, applies to our current state of oral care.

Enter ancient techniques and botanical extracts for oral swishing. When we swish our saliva with soothing serums of botanical extracts rich in phytonutrients known for their anti-inflammatory, lipid-soluble, lymph-stimulating nature that nurtures, the very thin skin of the oral epithelium can heal and seal, and teeth can gleam white and bright.

Oil swishing, otherwise known as oil pulling, is an ancient Ayurvedic medicinal practice used to detoxify the mouth, teeth, gums, and the entire oral cavity. Although this practice has been used throughout the ages, it has only recently begun to gain traction in the Western world. Scientists, holistic practitioners, and dentists are singing the praises of oil swishing and its ability to draw toxins from the mouth and flush them from the body.

A Quick Swish through Time: From ancient Egypt to ancient India, archaeologists have found the remains of human beings with beautiful, strong, perfectly intact teeth . . . long before fluoridated toothpastes and bristled toothbrushes were invented. Ancient peoples did not use synthetic commercial toothpastes and alcohol-based mouthwashes. They used natural means to keep teeth and gums healthy, including teeth picking and oil pulling. The oil-pulling process involves swishing in the mouth about a tablespoon of oil for fifteen minutes. Oil swishing draws toxins and tartar from the oral cavity and from between the teeth. It facilitates the flow of tooth- and tongue-bathing saliva, and balances the pH in the mouth. The warm, liquefied oil dissolves and traps food and tartar on the teeth and "brushes" your teeth as you swish.

Strategic Swishing: A small number of studies have been conducted on oil swishing and its impact on halitosis and oral health. Researchers concluded that oil swishing may eliminate the bacteria that cause oral issues.[64] Ideally, you want to swish with pure coconut oil or coconut MCT oil (read about these oils in the "Cosmoetic Materia Medica" in Chapter Fifteen).

Balance with Botanicals: Coconut or MCT oil is a great swisher alone; and if you want to pump up the potential (and the pleasure), consider mixing in a few optimizers to your morning swish. Essential oils are the mouth's best friend. They are gently antimicrobial and antiplaque, both of which cause tooth decay, bad breath, and gum disease. A drop of oregano, frankincense, peppermint, and tea tree essential oils is great for swishing. When added to swishing oil, probiotic powder can replenish the diversity of healthy bacteria in the mouth so that the oral ecology stays balanced and healthy. Simply pop open a capsule and add to the oil. Activated charcoal can help remove stains (like coffee and tea stains) from tooth enamel. Adding these nutrients to swishing oil takes tissue-healing nutrients right where they are needed most—gum pockets and between the teeth.

Oil-Swishing How-to: It is best to oil swish first thing in the morning before you eat or drink. Measure about 20 drops of oil and 2 drops of an essential oil or Minty Mouthwash and swish in your mouth. Swish without swallowing for up to fifteen minutes, and then spit. If you swish with coconut oil, it may solidify in cold water and clog your pipes, so spit it into a trash can. Then, follow your regular routine including the **Successful Self-Dentistry** steps.

POISON IVY

Leaves of three, let them be! But if you have already walked through the poison ivy (or poison oak) patch, there are a few things you can try to ease the itch and ditch the urushiol oil from your skin and clothes.

Get to know jewelweed (*Impatiens capensis*). It is a three-foot-tall herb that grows in wet areas with decent sun exposure. It has a small yellow-orange flower in the summer that develops into a long seedpod that will pop like magic between your fingers and spray seeds everywhere. It is easy to grow from seed. To use jewelweed for poison ivy, crush the plant in your hand and rub it over where you were exposed to the poison ivy leaves. You can also make a jewelweed "tea" by steeping it in hot water (freeze some in ice-cube trays) and then apply to the skin.

Baking soda and apple cider vinegar combined are effective at temporarily easing the ivy itch. (Don't forget your science-class volcano-eruption experiment with vinegar and baking soda. . . . Make sure that your mixing jar has room for foam!) And good old-fashioned soap helps to removes urushiol from the dermal layers to speed up healing.

Balance with Botanicals: Use peppermint essential oil to ease itch and redness.

PSORIASIS

Psoriasis occurs when the skin grows an excess of cells in the deepest basal layers of skin. These cells push cells to the top layer of the skin that are not aged enough to die and slough off as they normally would. So patches of cells build up that are often itchy and silvery looking. Psoriasis is an inflammatory response, so it is important to identify and avoid irritants that trigger inflammation. Some common triggers include soap, cleaning chemicals, laundry detergent, skin injuries and burns, animal dander, perfume, alcohol, cold and dry weather, jewelry, food sensitivities or allergies, and some medications.

Sunshine has proved to be an effective treatment for the most common kinds of psoriasis. Vitamin D improves immune function, and that shift may improve the interplay between skin and the immune system. Also, vitamin D changes how skin cells grow and may slow down the overgrowth associated with psoriasis.[65]

Some people have found that a honey and turmeric dressing can improve symptoms and aid in healing lesions. Mix turmeric with aloe or coconut oil, and apply to the skin. Turmeric will stain just about everything, so be sure to cover it with a cloth. Exposing turmeric stains to sunlight is the best treatment. Apple cider vinegar applied at a 50 percent dilution may also reduce inflammation and decrease the rate of infection.

Balance with Botanicals: Apply fresh aloe vera, coconut oil, or honey and turmeric. Also try the anti-itch essential oils and soothing serums from the Blithe Beauty Realm.

RASHES

A skin rash is any inflammation or discoloration of the skin. The most common causes of rashes are contact (poison ivy, laundry detergent), photosensitivity (a topical agent reacts in the sun), bacterial, viral, fungal, and hives (a response to an allergen or stress). Regardless of the cause, a rash needs exposure to fresh air and mild sunshine. Bacterial and fungal rashes respond really well to essential oils, and viral rashes can be eased with oils.

Balance with Botanicals: It is simple to soothe skin with the anti-inflammatory, anti-itch oils (frankincense, peppermint, blue tansy, chamomile, and yarrow) in the Blithe Beauty Realm and with **Calm Balm.**

ROSACEA

Rosacea typically begins to appear midlife. It is more frequently an issue with fair-skinned women who are prone to flushing. The first sign of rosacea is flushed, red skin, and from there it may progress to visible blood vessels, bumps, dry and scaly patches, pimples, and swelling. The cause of this conglomeration of symptoms is yet unknown, though scientists are getting close to determining a bacterial cause. The *Journal of Medical Microbiology* reports that some recent research raises the possibility that rosacea is caused by an increase of *Demodex* mites and their bacterial associates that thrive in damaged skin.[66]

Members of the American Academy of Dermatology are exploring the topical use of probiotics to rebalance a dysbiotic skin microbiome that contributes to rosacea and acne. Probiotics applied to the skin run "bacterial interference" by interfering with the bad bacteria. The live probiotics also calm the cells that react to the bad flora with inflammation, to reduce flares.[67]

Recent research indicates that pathogenic small intestine bacterial overgrowth (SIBO) may contribute to the development of rosacea. Eliminating those pathogens corresponded to a significant improvement in skin lesions.[68]

Probiotic supplements may improve the function of the "gut–brain–skin axis" and reverse the effects of stress, poor diet, and slow digestion that encourage unfriendly bacteria. When these bacteria are prevalent, the gut becomes leaky, and toxins spread through the body via the bloodstream, causing inflammatory conditions, including rosacea. In a dermatologic study in Italy, half of the participants were given the standard medical treatment and the other half were given an oral probiotic supplement in addition to their standard treatment. The people who took the probiotics saw the rosacea clear up faster.[69]

According to the National Rosacea Society, 41 percent of their members state that certain skincare products and 27 percent state that certain cosmetics trigger an outbreak.[70] These synthetic ingredients were listed as irritants: alcohol (66 percent), witch hazel (as it is mainly alcohol) (30 percent), fragrance (30 percent), and menthol (21 percent).[71]

Here is a good protocol for healing the skin:

1. Seal and heal the skin with the systems in this book to rebuild and maintain the integrity of the skin's outer barrier to protect the inner layers from irritants. Be gentle: Cleanse with oil using your fingertips and lukewarm water.

2. Start simple: Introduce one ingredient at a time, and start with jojoba.

3. Avoid triggers. Heat, humidity, hot foods, hot emotions, and hot baths are common triggers. Keeping cool is key.

4. Experiment with an **Elimination Diet,** as many foods are triggers. Eat an anti-inflammation, antihistamine diet that includes plenty of B vitamins. Consider keeping a food journal to map out what foods are triggers.

5. Heal and seal **Leaky Gut Syndrome** by clearing up symptoms of gut dysbiosis. Boost body with bountiful prebiotics and probiotics.

Balance with Botanicals: All of the oils in the Beloved Beauty Realm will help clear up rosacea.

SAGGING SKIN

Hormones out of whack can be the culprits responsible for sagging skin. As estrogen levels fall below normal, the skin can thin and sag from less collagen and elastin. **Glycation** and **Thyroid** imbalances can also make skin prone to sagginess. Testosterone stimulates the skin's oil glands, so if testosterone is low, the skin may be dry and dehydrate—another cause of sagging skin. Weight-bearing exercise also boosts testosterone.

Balance with Botanicals: The Beloved Beauty Realm is full of beautiful oils to prevent and reduce the appearance of sagging skin.

Super Supplements: Herbs to boost healthy estrogen (estriol): panax ginseng, hops, shatavari, black cohosh, and white kwao krua *(Pueraria mirifica)*. Pine pollen, tongkat ali, tribulus, and nettle root encourage the body's natural testosterone. Omega-3 fatty acids, maca, and minerals of magnesium, iodine, and boron raise serum estrogen and testosterone levels. Flaxseeds as well as broccoli sprouts can gently boost and balance estrogen.

SALT PIPE INHALER

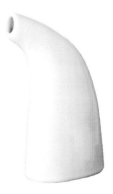

These positively purifying devices cleanse the entire respiratory system by piping in essential oil molecules and flushing out allergens and impurities. The pipe contains salt to which essential oils are added. It works by inhaling the beneficial micron-particles of salt along with molecules of essential oils that are absorbed by and penetrate the entire respiratory system. This cleanses the sinuses, nasal cavities, throat, and lungs of smoke particulates, allergens, asthma triggers, and respiratory irritants. This simple tool strengthens lungs and respiration. The salt pipe inhaler is also terrific for treating sinus issues and colds (try **Sinus Soother**), and it is great for purifying the inhaled air during flight travel. It is easy to use: inhale deeply through the mouth and exhale through the nose for ten to twenty minutes. Inhalation by alternate nostril breathing is also effective: hold the inhaler to each nostril, inhale deeply, and then exhale through the other nostril.

Apothecary: frankincense, black spruce, eucalyptus, peppermint, lavender, chamomile, grapefruit, laurel, marjoram, inula

SAUNAS, FAR-INFRARED

Infrared saunas use infrared light to radiate heat into the body instead of warming the air. Heat from infrared light penetrates the body, creating ample sweat and greater detoxification at lower, more comfortable temperatures.

Balance with Botanicals: Dry brush before saunas with laurel, eucalyptus, frankincense, inula, and rosemary and use these oils in the sauna too.

SCARS AND KELOIDS

Scars are marks on the skin or in the tissue where fibrous connective tissue forms as the injury heals. Keloids are firm, shiny elevated scars from an overgrowth of tissue after a skin injury. We usually think of scars and keloids as cosmetic issues, though there may be more to them than that. Life energy, or qi, flows along meridians in our body like superhighways. These meridians penetrate every cell in our bodies. Deep scars can act like blockades in our qi superhighways by preventing vitality from flowing through and beyond the scar. Restoring the area with acupuncture and essential oils is beneficial.

Balance with Botanicals: Both old and new scars can fade fantastically with essential oils. Use a **Spot Treatment** from the Beloved and Benevolent Beauty Realms. Apply twice a day, especially on fresh scars; once sealed, apply **Spot Treatments** with one of the **Renegade Beauty Splendid Serums.** Stock your apothecary with rose otto, myrrh, frankincense, lavender, sandalwood, and immortelle.

SEBORRHEIC DERMATITIS

Researchers are still studying the etiology of this skin issue. The key contributors to developing seborrheic dermatitis in adults are stress, genetic predisposition, immune health, and living in a cold and dry climate. *Malassezia* and *Candida,* common yeasts that normally live on the skin, could be cofactors. The symptoms are dry, flaky skin and itchiness that can turn into a weeping, oily rash. It is often found on the face, scalp, and neck. Cradle cap and diaper rash are instances of seborrheic dermatitis affecting babies. Babies usually grow out of it in the first year, though seborrheic dermatitis is often a recurrent issue with adults.

Balance with Botanicals: Use botanicals from the Brilliant Beauty Realm, and for itchy spots use the **Blithe Beauty Spot Treatment.**

Food for Thought: See **Leaky Gut Syndrome** and **Elimination Diet.**

SHAVING

The pubic hair that covers our lady lair is not just a biological mishap that propels women to wax. It serves the paramount purpose of protection: it protects the delicate skin from friction and it protects the native friendly flora colonies. Waxing and shaving irritate and inflame hair follicles, leaving microscopic open wounds. Combined with a moist environment, perhaps exacerbated by unbreathable polyester underwear, this creates a breeding ground for pathogens and STDs. Shaving our armpits also disrupts the skin's surface, which makes it more susceptible to absorbing harmful metals and synthetics found in cosmetics-aisle deodorants and antiperspirants.

When left unprotected from friction, the vulvar skin tends to thicken and get dry and wrinkly. After years of no pubic-hair protection, the labia may begin to look almost scrotal.[72] Moreover, the hair down there (and in our armpits) is a pheromone blanket, ensorcelling the scents that attract lovers.

Balance with Botanicals: For nicks and ingrown hairs, use the calming and cooling **Blithe Beauty Spot Treatment.**

SHINGLES

Shingles, a.k.a. herpes zoster, is an uncomfortable condition resulting from a reactivation of the chicken pox virus, called the varicella zoster virus. Shingles is characterized by very sore blisters that form along paths of nerves around the body. They most often form on the torso. Even after the blisters heal, some people experience lasting nerve pain, or neuralgia. The best prevention is to optimize your immune system. Medical reviews of antiviral medications are mixed on the results. Anecdotal evidence supports the use of supplemental L-lysine (an amino acid) as a low-dose preventive and as a treatment at higher doses. Tamanu oil and essential oils are excellent at alleviating symptoms.

Balance with Botanicals: Use the Blithe Beauty Spot Treatment or use these essential oils: tea tree, peppermint, lavender, frankincense, myrrh, and immortelle with tamanu, jojoba, and/or MCT oils; and very gently apply to blisters several times a day for healing, soothing, and pain relief. It may also be helpful to break open a fresh aloe leaf and apply the juice to tender areas.

SKIN TAGS

Skin tags, or acrochordons, are tiny flaps of skin that are normally flesh colored. Why they occur is not perfectly understood yet; they tend to appear more in skin folds, areas where skin rubs skin or where clothes rub skin. Some theories suggest they are a symptom of an internal fungus or *Candida*.

Balance with Botanicals: A dab of Blithe Beauty Spot Treatment or a drop of frankincense, peppermint, sandalwood, or blue tansy twice a day for a few weeks often is sufficient to remove them.

SLEEP

Be still as the lake is for the moon, emotions and mind in buoyant, still water guided by the evening star. Deep insight and peace are the order of the eve. Mind flows into an expanded chest. Quiet darkness restores, gathering strength to meet the light of day. Lay and play in an open sacred bed. Let tension unravel; relax the jaw and tongue. Open the gateway; there is no more explaining to do. Die to the day. Enter into absorption. Disintegrating. Integrating. Dream a voyage into the lion, the witch, and the wardrobe corridors of your being. Emptiness calls without invitation, to whisper and renew, a visit to the infinite nighttime parts of ourselves. From room to room, this emptiness is existence too. A simple, quiet mind emits a most sublime fragrance, dreams deep insights to rejuvenate the body, and emanates innumerable light beams vaster than a starry night field. Soar to sites within sights. Yet some nights be awake till dawn, be the moon meeting the sun.

Sweet sleep is an essential beauty protocol. The body repairs and reenergizes and the mind reorganizes at night as your body relaxes and your mind dreams. Shortchanging yourself of all the zzz's you need will cause grumpy attitudes and spike your cortisol level (which in turn boosts carb cravings, because your body feels the need for a power surge since it did not get recharged at night). Too little sleep also increases the chance of a foggy brain, dark circles under the eyes, and puffy eyes. Before falling asleep, think of all the best parts of the day and what you are grateful for. Upon rising, think about all the things in your life that you appreciate and then, if you can, create space for a fifteen-minute meditation.

As researchers learn the importance of deep, sweet sleep, their studies have resulted in some easy-to-implement tips for good zzz's:

- Keep your bedroom cool, quiet, and dark. If you don't have window coverings, use a silk cloth or an eye mask to shield your eyes from all light.
- In the morning, step outside into the sun to synchronize your circadian rhythm.
- Remove electronics from your bedroom: blue light and electromagnetic frequencies suppress melatonin production.
- Avoid caffeine and alcohol for eight hours before bed.
- Maintain a consistent sleep schedule.

Nature's Nightcaps: Nestle your nerves with these calming herbs that may be enjoyed in a tea or ingested in a night capsule: lemon balm, lavender, skullcap, catnip, and chamomile.

Balance with Botanicals: If you toss and turn with restlessness or insomnia, essential oils of calming chamomile, languid lavender, serene sandalwood, mollifying marjoram, or soporific spikenard will take you to lullaby land. These sedating aromas may be enjoyed by the drop in a bedtime bath, dispersed by a diffuser, dropped onto your pillow, dabbed under the nose, or combined in a pillow spray.

Super Supplements: GABA, Relora (a blend of Chinese cork bark and magnolia that reduces cortisol and boosts DHEA), and magnesium

STRETCH MARKS

Stretch marks (also called striae distensae) are a type of scar caused when the elastic fibers in the skin tear, leaving pinkish lines in the skin that eventually fade to a more natural skin color. Stretch marks often occur during pregnancy, during puberty, and whenever there is significant weight gain. For more information on pregnancy, see Chapter Eleven.

Due to the frequency of stretch marks in women and during pregnancy, scientists think that they are possibly hormone related. Researchers have found two times as many hormone receptors in skin with stretch marks compared to the unscarred skin next to it. They think that the stretching of the skin causes the increase in hormone-receptor activity, which then damages the skin's extracellular matrix, those structures that provide skin with its tensile strength and elasticity.[73]

Other factors that contribute to forming stretch marks include genetics, suppressed immune function, and chronic liver disease. Contributing to stretch-mark formation are high blood levels of steroid hormones that break down fibroblasts and decrease collagen in the skin.

Laser therapy that stimulates collagen production may slightly decrease the visibility of stretch marks if used when the stretch marks are fresh, yet neither hot nor cold laser is particularly effective or a "cure." Laser treatments can also cause hyperpigmentation in skin.[74] Additionally, each abrasion treatment must abrade to the point of bleeding, and it requires many treatments, up to twenty, in a short period of time.[75]

Essential oils are the only thing I have seen that provides results with stretch marks. As with cellulite, the very best remedy of stretch marks is to love your body as it is and to appreciate the intricacies of your moist envelope.

Balance with Botanicals: Soothe with Spot Treatments and Serums from the Beloved and Benevolent Beauty Realms. Some of the most effective essential oils are palmarosa, neroli, patchouli, spikenard, rose otto, grapefruit, cypress, immortelle, petitgrain, geranium, and frankincense.

SUN CARE

We can revel in the sun without being burned. See "Sun Wise: Gracefully Interface with Sunlight" in Chapter Seven.

THYROID

Dry skin, hair loss, loss of libido, low energy, mental fog, anxiety, depression, menstrual cycle askew, weight gain that won't budge . . . it could be your thyroid. With radiation in the air, bromide in the food supply, and iodine vanished from the food supply, thyroid imbalances are thought to be experienced by twelve million Americans.[76] The thyroid, sometimes called the third ovary, as it governs hormonal secretions of the ovaries, seems to create more imbalances for women post-partum and can affect the harmony of all other hormones.

Endocrine disrupters can create or mask issues with thyroid hormones too. Alas, these substances are pretty widely found: fluoride in water and oral-care products, bromine in leavening agents in baked goods, and heavy metals. There are also medicines that can disrupt thyroid function: beta-blockers, cholesterol-lowering drugs, and steroids. Then there are the endocrine-disrupting chemicals found in common cosmetics and household products: BPA, phthalates, and lead.

Regular screening and blood tests for thyroid hormones are not accurate, so be sure to consult a thyroid-literate naturopath or integrative medical doctor.

Dive Deeper: Read: *Hypothyroidism Type 2: The Epidemic* by Dr. Mark Starr; *Why Do I Still Have Thyroid Symptoms? When My Lab Tests Are Normal: A revolutionary breakthrough in understanding Hashimoto's disease and hypothyroidism* by Dr. Datis Kharrazian; *Your Healthy Pregnancy with Thyroid Disease* by Dana Trentini and Mary Shomon; *The Iodine Crisis* by Lynne Farrow; *Thyroid Healthy* by Suzy Cohen; and *The Paleo Thyroid Solution: Stop Feeling Fat, Foggy, and Fatigued at the Hands of Uninformed Doctors—Reclaim Your Health!* by Elle Russ.

VARICOSE VEINS

For facial spider veins, see **Couperose.**

Varicose veins are enlarged blood vessels that look like red and blue ribbons on the surface of the legs and feet. Usually, varicose veins are a cosmetic issue, though they can be a medical problem if they cause swelling and aching. At this point, if they are untreated there could be complications such as phlebitis, ulcers, and blood clots. There are a variety of causes; the most likely are genetics, age, weight, and hormones. Hormonal shifts, as well as birth control pills and estrogen drugs, can increase the risk of varicosity. It is common for pregnant women to notice enlarged veins in their legs; luckily, those varicose veins tend to vanish after delivery. Activity keeps muscles and veins strong and elastic. And, believe it or not, constipation can cause varicose veins. Straining can close off blood flow through the big leg veins and force the blood to flow through small superficial veins, and this enlarges them.[77]

Balance with Botanicals: Apply a dab neat to the area of Spot Treatments from the Blithe or Brilliant Beauty Realms.

Super Supplements: vitamins C, B complex, K2, and D3; tinctures or teas of horse chestnut, butcher's broom, bilberry, ginkgo, and pycnogenol

WARTS

A wart is a hard, benign growth on the skin caused by a virus. Warts usually occur on the knees, fingers, and elbows.

Balance with Botanicals: Warts can be stubborn, yet topical applications of antifungal oils of oregano (diluted), white cedar, and peppermint can be helpful. Another tip is to apply a strong dilution of hydrogen peroxide with a cotton swab.

WATER

Water is the spring of life. Pure water is imbued with eight qualities. "The ideal water of pure lands is cool, clear, sweet, soft, lustrous, settled, nourishing, able to ally hunger and thirst."[78] Pure spring water (to find a spring near you, go to the FindASpring website) is great just as it is, yet you can add a few things to water to make it just a little bit better. If you add a squeeze of lemon to a glass of water, you are getting a quick boost of vitamin C, as well as a little potassium and magnesium. Lemon water also buffers indigestion. A pinch of salt in a glass of water is a good boost too. It will replenish essential trace minerals found in unrefined salt, and a pinch of salt in water is slightly more hydrating than plain water. Also, salt is antibacterial and alkalinizing, so a little swish in your mouth before swallowing will ease oral acidity. (If you have hypertension, talk to a medical professional before increasing your salt intake.)

According to Dr. Chris Exley, silicon is also a good addition to drinking water. Exley is a professor of bioinorganic chemistry and specializes in aluminum. He found that silicon binds with aluminum, so if we drink silicon-enriched water, it will leach aluminum out of the body.[79]

When it comes to buying bottled water, buyer beware. Some water is bottled from pristine sources, and some is bottled right from the tap. Moreover, there are no federal standards regulating pharmaceutical-residue levels in bottled water (or in tap water!). Reverse osmosis is handy for removing contaminants from water, yet with it essential minerals are removed too. Removing the minerals makes the water more acidic and "hungry" for seeking minerals. Thus, when this type of water is consumed, it seeks to leach buffering, more alkaline minerals from the body. Avoid buying it, or any water, in plastic bottles. BPA and other synthetics can seep from the plastic and spoil the purity of the water. What makes water in plastic bottles more hazardous than drinking out of a plastic cup is that most plastic bottles are made on-site at the bottling factory. This means warm, freshly formed plastic is what the water is injected into, and chemical leaching from the plastics is high. Glass bottles are best.

> Pollution is nothing but the resources we are not harvesting. We allow them to disperse because we've been ignorant of their value.
>
> Buckminster Fuller[80]

You may also want to whisper a blessing over your drinking water. Dr. Masaru Emoto has used expert photography to capture glimmering water crystals. In his experiment, beautiful and symmetrical crystals formed when exposed to kind words or beautiful music; however, deformed crystals formed when exposed to unkind words and heavy-metal music.[81] Our bodies are mostly water, so if Dr. Emoto is on to something about water's consciousness and memory, this is another reason to only say kind words to your body.

Balance with Botanicals: The addition of a drop of lemon, peppermint, or frankincense is lovely to imbibe.

> The water in your jug
> is brackish and low.
> Smash the jug
> and come to the river!
>
> Rumi

YONI

Keep your vulva (the exterior part of the yoni) vivacious by caring for it gently. The lovely labia protects its tissues by generously secreting oils that defend it from clothing friction and natural discharges. Steer clear of underwear made with irritating chemicals, as well as laundry detergents and dryer sheets with harsh chemicals, dyes, and perfumes that irritate vulvar skin. Scrubbing and harsh cleansers wash away these natural oils and the friendly flora that keeps the vulva vital. For the most part, warm water and a salt bath is all that is needed to refresh. There is also an Ayurvedic method of oil washing the vulva called Yoni Prakshalanam. Oil washing with jojoba infused with essential oils is used to reduce inflammation, irritation, and dryness, to strengthen weak tissue, and to prevent fungal and yeast infections. Ylang oil is lovely for yoni health. For day-to-day dryness, massage a little dab of jojoba on the inner labia and the outside opening of the vagina to keep the tissue hydrated.

Yoni Eggs for Strength Training: A crystal egg stone is an ancient Taoist tool for yoni and pelvic-floor strength training, and crystal eggs are perfect because the shape makes it comfortable and it is organic and easy to clean. Yoni eggs have a hole running through the middle so that organic yarn can be strung through it, to allow you to remove it more easily and also to introduce weight on the outside of the yoni as your yoni muscles strengthen over time. The ancient Taoists believed that as the yoni grew in strength, the woman grew in intuition, power, and wisdom.

Dive Deeper: Read: *Healing Love through the Tao: Cultivating Female Sexual Energy* by Mantak Chia; and watch *Vaginal Kung Fu* videos with Kim Anami.

Yoni Steam Baths: Yoni steam baths are an age-old Mayan practice to reduce bloating, cramps, backaches, and imbalances associated with menstruation. Steaming may also ease uterine fibroids, ovarian cysts, and uterine weakness. People who experience hemorrhoids may find some relief with the steam bath too.

Yoni tissues of the vagina are lined with mucous membranes that are soft and absorbent. Herbs and essential oils steeped in hot water release their therapeutic properties in the steam and are carried to the surface of the skin, where they are absorbed. Simply steep herbs in a basin of hot water, or add a few drops of essential oils. Be sure that the water is warm enough to produce steam yet not too hot. Squat with the steam below your yoni for twenty minutes. You can also put the basin inside the toilet bowl and sit on the seat for more comfort.

Balance with Botanicals: Fresh herbs of black cohosh, rose, and yarrow are great for steaming, along with rose otto, ylang, and frankincense. Finish by applying the soothing Yoni Serum found in Chapter Ten.

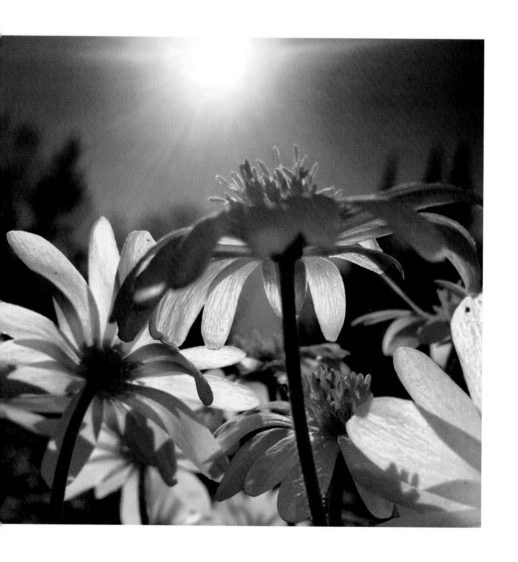

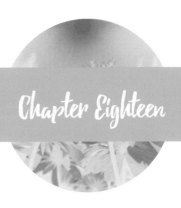

Chapter Eighteen

BEING BEAUTY

The moon smiles bright knowing it is holy night. The flower blooms knowing it is ethereal perfume. The embryo grows knowing it is the delight of infinite light.

Do you want to be perfectly pretty when you peer into the magnifying mirror? Is the purpose to free our faces of fine lines? Is the goal perfectly pore-less skin? Or do you want to *feel* beautiful from within?

Beyond the what-was and what-will-be comparison world of commercial beauty is a reality that communes with the cosmos. Beauty is not a skincare regimen of incessant becoming. Beauty is not another adrenal-driven ambition of self-improvement clashing against the rocks of time. Be free of the dangling carrot that endlessly entices with the chimera of idealized and never fully realized beauty. Let the unseen alchemist of ether whisper in your ear about being in beauty's revered reception, and move away from the hazy gaze of the convoluted fears of comparison. The desire to be beautiful is beauty. The yearning is desire's reply. This is the benediction of beauty—it is all right here.

Your beautiful nature verifies that you are already everything, divine. Look no further. Your own beauty is here: that near, that clear. The wonder and mysterious depths of the starlit sky are the wonder and mysterious depth of your being. Wild roses and wooded hills are not your opposite. The source that unfurls leaves on a tree is the same source that unfurls the beauty of your being. You are nature; and naturally, nature is you. You are an elegant elixir of life, a vessel of vibrant vitality, a chalice of creation, a living libation pouring forth your unique beingness integral to the universe. Open to this vast cosmos of your being with wide-eyed wonder, and be the ever-blossoming beauty you are.

Every living thing is immersed in an atmosphere of elements. Everything is in relation. There is no separation from creation. In the moment of this sentence, you may nod yes, yes! Yet is it possible in all of one's waking moments for this to be the shape of your lips, the song pulsing in your heart, and the utterance of your thoughts?

This is life's adventure: to understand that there is no separation from creation, and to grow branches of ecstasy to all living things. Embracing the elements' presence is the pure medicine you desire, receiving sunbeams to be a serum, welcoming water's refreshing ways, allowing air to tousle your hair, and accepting the earth to rebirth your self-worth.

MEDITATION FOR BEAUTY

Loving the Skin You Are In

Let's create a fresh moment of feeling good, a new to-do list, a renewed set of goals that speaks to your soul. This remedy of revivification is to bathe your body in the light of creation and turn your thoughts to the elixir of appreciation.

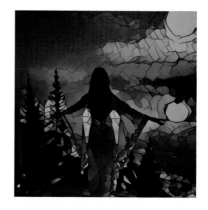

May this be an invitation to the billions of bacteria and cells in the body that contain billions of points of consciousness. This cellular and bacterial beingness desires balance and continually seeks improved conditions from the contrasts of life. So, let us take a moment to allow the consciousness of our skin to come into alignment by appreciating all the good that our bodies, bacteria, cells, and DNA do without us even thinking about it. Let's dive into our divine skin, into the brilliance of our beings, and nourish the billions of pores that are parched for a real-to-the-feel reunion with the gorgeous garden of the cosmos.

Let us begin by deepening our breathing.

Inhaling.
Exhaling.

This time is a gift to your being and aligns you to the natural rhythm of
your beauty.
Each breath tunes your Self to the beauty of who you really are.
Focus softly on these words and allow this fine-tuning on a cellular level.
Feel your breath, feel life breathing you.
Feel that your body is naturally guided by the light of all creation.

Feel the sun. Imagine warm, golden beams of sunlight pouring upon your
hair, pouring upon your head, pouring upon your face.
As this light pours into your body, feel it restoring and revitalizing every cell.
Pouring upon your back, flowing down your torso, and flowing down your legs.
Feel this light on your skin.

Submerge into your skin and nourish your body with this light of creation.
Receive this light into every pore of your skin and every cell within.
Invite this light elixir to travel throughout your body.
Feel this bright light in your bloodstream.
Feel this light loving your lymph, liver, and lungs.
Feel this light guiding your glands and your body's internal rhythms.

Wherever your skin and health are at, decide to feel good about it.
Honor how your body and skin serve you so well.

Appreciate how your skin and senses consistently decipher life for you.
Feel life's innate wisdom, its infinite reliability, its beauty.

It is natural for you to feel well-being and to feel beautiful.
Relax into this renewed radiance and for the next few moments let your
breath guide you.

Inhaling.
Exhaling.

Feel life's luminous effervescence shining through the skin you are in!
Feel radiance glowing from your skin.
Feel brightness beaming from your cheeks and shining from your eyes.
Feel the stream of well-being pouring into you.
Feel the cells in your skin tuning in to your appreciation, and feel the life
*   within lighting up the beneficial bacteria and cells that make you a*
*   beautiful you.*

There is vast light-filled beauty in the universe and within you.
Feel this Light of Creation circulating throughout your body.
Gather the light into your heart. Inhale.

And, as you slowly exhale, let your being beam this illuminating beauty
*   from your chest, allowing the Light of Life to do the rest.*

Tune in to the concert of reciprocating cosmic rhythms, feel the vital cadence of confluencing elements, the eternal streams of well-being, the source that makes the sunrise—give up to the grace of that goodness. Give your beauty the benefit of the doubt, and ripen with the morning glory of that knowledge. Receive your beauty.

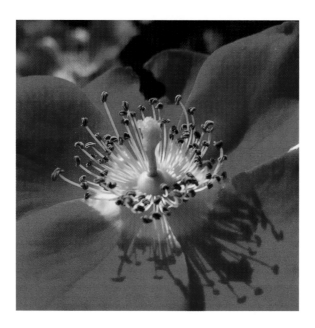

Acknowledgments

This distillation of my mind's outpouring is decanted into the basin of this book. May it be a repository of beauty to revive your being.

To swirl and twirl plant essences, to delve into living libraries, to gather the highlighted prose from treasured books and open the apothecary of the elements' infinite intelligence, to combine this with the countless questions from clients about their beauty concerns and desires and bundle it all in a book: I am in deep appreciation to all the billions of countless components that brought you and me together and placed this book in your realm.

It takes a village to birth a book and I am thankful to these dream teams:

The dream team of all the wisdom that has gone on before me: it imprints the ethers of eternity and inspires me to connect continually to the universe within. It is delightful to bring forth ancestral advice . . . antidotes of Avicenna with ruminations of Rumi mixed with alchemy and the muse of modernity keeps the continual conversation of the cosmoetic cocktail party aglow.

To the dream team of the intelligent joy-juice of flora, the muse for all my creations: my hands serve at the pleasure of plants and flowers, the original owners of essences and oils. They teach through total immersion. The cosmic chemists of plants and their beautiful botanical essences and their reviving verdant vespers teach so much about health, beauty, and illuminable immunity. Much praise to the diligence of the distillers who capture delicious drops of plant quintessence.

To the dream team of Living Libations ladies and gentlemen: each of you shines in the work you do, and you all contribute greatly to creating our engaged enterprise, which continually contributes to the flowering of Living Libations. In turn, we get to pour more into the universe.

And this book could not have been birthed into being without Lacey Bloom, who midwifed the manuscript with great care. Special thanks to Tim McKee and the team at North Atlantic Books that bring this book to you.

To my pantheon of soul sisters who illuminate the beauty of our world through their innovative, artistic, and entrepreneurial work: Anne, Carrie-Anne, Kristin, Camille, Christine, Kelly, Kim, Bonnie Rose, Lilly, Laurie, Bunni, Brooke, Barbara, Amanda Chantal, Shiva, Sima, Julia, Mea, Maya, Rebecca, Angela, Alanis, Sarah, Shailene, Sass, Nicole, and Meghan. Thank you for daring to be all that you are.

Mahalo to the day-making Wagner family for our beautiful times in Hawaii with so much aloha abundance and beauty inspirations that were nurtured in numerous ways.

Endless thanks to the essential oil wisdom and curiosity of my aroma colleagues in our verdant world: Christa Obuchowski, Jack Chaitman, John Steele, Kurt Schnaubelt, Monica Haas, Michael Scholes, and Robert Tisserand. Where would the scent trail be without you?

To Ron, my love, I am a garden of gratitude that blooms in the shower of your infinite love and spirited song. To Leif, I look forward to the life and legacy you will bequeath. You are my eternal son shine.

And the land, to all the land of this earth and specifically the land I live on. It has held, melded, and allowed me to engage with the elements in endless ways of play that have brought to fruition the early whisperings and the blending of these beauty endeavors closer to the elements. To live on the outside of the land I live inside is an earthly embrace I drink in daily.

Endnotes

FRONTMATTER

1 Rumi, "How Does God Keep from Fainting?" *Love Poems from God*, trans. Daniel Ladinsky (New York: Penguin Compass, 2002), 77.

2 J. Krishnamurti, *Talks in Europe 1968*, Conversation 3, March 17, 1968, www.jkrishnamurti.com/krishnamurti-teachings/view-text.php?tid =3&chid=3&w=&s=Text.

3 Tom Robbins, *Skinny Legs and All* (New York: Bantam Books, 1990), 380.

4 Alicia Keys, interview on *Jimmy Kimmel Live!*, February 2017.

5 J. Krishnamurti, Chapter 19, *This Matter of Culture* (London: Victor Gollancz, 1964), 158.

6 Kahlil Gibran, *The Prophet* (New York: Alfred A. Knopf, 1923), 76.

CHAPTER ONE

1 Statista, "Revenue of the Cosmetics Industry Worldwide from 2007 to 2012 (in Billion U.S. Dollars)," www.statista.com/statistics/307411/ revenue-of-the-global-cosmetics-industry/.

2 Wendy Steiner, *Venus in Exile: The Rejection of Beauty in Twentieth-Century Art* (Chicago: University of Chicago Press, 2002), xx.

3 Kahlil Gibran, "On Beauty," *The Prophet* (Mumbai: Jaico Publishing House, 1988), 74.

CHAPTER TWO

1 Hafiz, *I Heard God Laughing: Poems of Hope and Joy* (New York: Penguin Books, 2006), 18.

2 J. Krishnamurti, Chapter 7, *Freedom from the Known* (San Francisco: Harper SanFrancisco, 2009).

3 J. Krishnamurti, *This Light in Oneself* (Boston: Shambhala, 1999), 121.

4 Martin Luther King Jr. spoke of cosmic companionship: *"I am convinced that the universe is under the control of a loving purpose and that in the struggle for righteousness man has cosmic companionship."* Martin Luther King Jr., "Pilgrimage to Nonviolence," Chicago, April 13, 1960, http://kingencyclopedia.stanford.edu/encyclopedia/documentsentry /pilgrimage_to_nonviolence/.

5 Gustav Fechner, *Nanna, or on the Soul Life of Plants* (Leipzig: Voss, 1848).

6 Esther Hicks and Jerry Hicks, "Are You Worthy?" *You Can Heal Your Life,* www.healyourlife.com/are-you-worthy.

7 Danielle LaPorte, quoted in Cindy Heath, *Real Beautiful: The Secret Energy of the Mind, Body, and Spirit* (Bloomington, IN: Balboa Press, 2014), 279.

8 J. Krishnamurti, *The Benediction Is Where You Are: The Last Bombay Talks 1985* (Chennai, India: KFI Publications, 1985).

9 Coleman Barks and John Moyne, trans., *The Drowned Book: Ecstatic and Earthly Reflections of Bahauddin, the Father of Rumi* (San Francisco: HarperOne, 2005), 88.

CHAPTER THREE

1 *The Empire Club of Canada Addresses,* February 16, 1989, Toronto, Canada, 234–249, http://speeches.empireclub.org/61201/data.

2 George William Askinson, *Perfumes and Their Preparation* (New York: Henley & Co., 1892).

3 R. S. Cristiani, *A Comprehensive Treatise on Perfumery* (Philadelphia: Baird & Co., 1877).

4 Oscar Wilde, *De Profundis* (Project Gutenberg, 2007), www.gutenberg .org/files/921/921-h/921-h.htm.

CHAPTER FOUR

1 John Muir, Chapter 1, "Puget Sound and British Columbia," *Travels in Alaska*, 1915, http://vault.sierraclub.org/john_muir_exhibit/writings/travels_in _alaska/chapter_1.aspx.

2 Nikhat Parveen, "Fibonacci in Nature," University of Georgia, http://jwilson .coe.uga.edu/emat6680/parveen/fib_nature.htm.

3 Emily Dickinson, *The Complete Poems of Emily Dickinson*, ed. Thomas H. Johnson (New York: Back Bay Books, 1960), 516.

4 Elaine Scarry, *On Beauty and Being Just*, reprint ed. (Princeton, NJ: Princeton University Press, 2001).

5 Carl Jung, *Man and His Symbols* (New York: Doubleday, 1964), 95.

6 Richard Louv, *Last Child in the Woods* (Chapel Hill, NC: Algonquin Books of Chapel Hill, 2005), 3.

7 Richard Louv, *The Nature Principle* (Chapel Hill, NC: Algonquin Books of Chapel Hill, 2011), 3.

8 John Ruskin, *Modern Painters*, vol. II (London: George Allen, 1906). Read it in its entirety at http://archive.org/stream/modernpaintersvo030029mbp#page /n15/mode/2up.

9 John Ruskin, *The Works of John Ruskin*, XI (New York: John B. Alden, 1885), 345.

10 George P. Landow, "Chapter Two, Section III: Ruskin's Theories Beauty—Vital Beauty," *The Aesthetic and Critical Theories of John Ruskin*, www .victorianweb.org/authors/ruskin/atheories/2.3.html.

11 Joke Brouwer, Arjen Mulder, and Lars Spuybroek, eds., *Vital Beauty: Reclaiming Aesthetics in the Tangle of Technology and Nature* (Rotterdam: V2_publishing, 2012), 133.

12 John Ruskin, *The Works of John Ruskin*, XVI (London: George Allen, 1905), 378.

13 Brouwer, Mulder, and Spuybroek, *Vital Beauty*, 7.

14 Vigen Guroian, *Inheriting Paradise: Meditations on Gardening* (Grand Rapids, MI: William B. Eerdmans, 1999), 7.

15 George P. Landow, *The Aesthetic and Critical Theories of John Ruskin* (Princeton, NJ: Princeton University Press, 2015), 63.

16 Ruskin, *The Works of John Ruskin,* XVI, 384.

17 John Ruskin, "The Work of Iron," *The Two Paths: Being Lectures on Art and Its Application to Decoration and Manufacture* (Kent, England: George Allen, 1878), 112.

18 Mark Frost, "'Entering the Circles of Vitality': Beauty, Sympathy, and Fellowship," in Brouwer, Mulder, and Spuybroek, *Vital Beauty,* 144.

19 Edward Abbey, *Down the River* (New York: Plume, 1991), 148.

20 Johann Wolfgang von Goethe, *Maxims and Reflections* (Project Gutenberg, 2010), #481, www.gutenberg.org/files/33670/33670-h/33670-h.htm.

21 Parveen, "Fibonacci in Nature."

22 Makini Brice, "Golden Ratio of a Woman's Uterus Is Linked with Her Fertility," *Medical Daily,* August 14, 2012, www.medicaldaily.com/golden-ratio-womans-uterus-linked-her-fertility-241942.

23 "The Torus—Dynamic Flow Process," *Cosmometry,* www.cosmometry.net/the-torus---dynamic-flow-process.

24 Ralph Waldo Emerson, *The Collected Works of Ralph Waldo Emerson* (Cambridge, MA: Belknap Press of Harvard University Press, 1971), 27.

CHAPTER FIVE

1 Gibran, "Clothes," *The Prophet,* 36.

2 Hafiz, "Faithful Lover," *The Gift* (New York: Penguin Compass, 1999), 159.

3 Charles Eisenstein, Chapter 10, "The Law of Return" (Pt. 11), *Sacred Economics,* http://realitysandwich.com/116895/sacred_economics_chapter_10/.

4 Hafiz, "The Sun Never Says," *The Gift,* 34.

5 Herbert M. Shelton, *The Hygienic System, Vol III. Fasting and Sun Bathing* (Pomeroy, WA: Health Research Books, 2005), 208.

6 "Medicine: Heliotherapy," *Time* magazine, August 6, 1923.

7 Hafiz, "A Lot to Digest," *A Year with Hafiz* (New York: Penguin Books, 2011), 327.

8 Tatanka Iyotake, quoted in Neil Philip, ed., *In a Sacred Manner I Live: Native American Wisdom* (New York: Clarion Books, 1997), 20.

9 Kahlil Gibran, *The Essential Kahlil Gibran: Aphorisms and Maxims* (New York: Citadel Press, 1966), 69.

10 Jalaloddin Rumi, quoted in Annemarie Schimmel, *The Triumphal Sun: A Study of the Works of Jalaloddin Rumi* (Albany, NY: State University of New York Press, 1993), 21.

11 Callum Coats, *Living Energies: Viktor Schauberger's Brilliant Work with Natural Energy Explained* (Bath, UK: Gateway Books, 1996).

12 "An AP Investigation: Pharmaceuticals Found in Drinking Water," http://hosted.ap.org/specials/interactives/pharmawater_site/index.html.

13 www.findaspring.com.

14 Viktor Schauberger, quoted in Olof Alexandersson, *Living Water: Viktor Schauberger and the Secrets of Natural Energy* (Dublin: Gill & MacMillan, 2002), 52.

15 Guroian, *Inheriting Paradise*, 9–10.

16 Viktor Schauberger, *The Water Wizard: The Extraordinary Properties of Natural Water*, trans. Callum Coats (Bath, UK: Gateway Books, 1998), 3.

17 Heart, "Dreamboat Annie," *Dreamboat Annie* (Vancouver, BC: Mushroom Records, 1975), http://genius.com/Heart-dreamboat-annie-lyrics.

18 J. H. Schulz, *Le training autogene* (Paris: Presses Universitaires de France, 1958), 37.

19 J. W. Goethe, quoted in G. Bachelard, *The Poetics of Reverie: Childhood, Language, and the Cosmos*, trans. Daniel Russell (Boston: Beacon Press, 1971), 180.

20 Neil deGrasse Tyson, *Astrophysics for People in a Hurry* (New York: W. W. Norton, 2017), 202.

21 Guy Murchie, *The Seven Mysteries of Life: An Exploration of Science and Philosophy* (New York: Mariner Books, 1999), 320.

22 Henry David Thoreau, *Walden* (Boston: Ticknor and Fields, 1854), 150.

23 Hafiz, *The Subject Tonight Is Love: 60 Wild and Sweet Poems of Hafiz*, trans. Daniel Ladinsky (New York: Penguin Compass, 2003), 40.

24 "Are We Really All Made of Stardust?" www.physics.org/article-questions.asp?id=52.

25 Paracelsus, *Hermetic Medicine and Hermetic Philosophy*, trans. L. W. de Laurence (Chicago: de Laurence, Scott & Co., 1910), 289.

26 "How Much of the Human Body Is Made Up of Stardust?" Physics Central, www.physicscentral.com/explore/poster-stardust.cfm.

27 Zora Neale Hurston, *Their Eyes Were Watching God* (Chicago: University of Illinois Press, 1937), 120.

28 Van Morrison, "Moondance," *Moondance* (Warner Bros. Records, 1970).

29 Jim Nollman, *Why We Garden: Cultivating a Sense of Place* (New York: Henry Holt, 1994), 216–17.

30 Josie Glausiusz, "Is Dirt the New Prozac?" June 14, 2007, *Discover* magazine, http://discovermagazine.com/2007/jul/raw-data-is-dirt-the-new-prozac.

31 A. C. Bittner et al., "Prescript-Assist Probiotic-Prebiotic Treatment for Irritable Bowel Syndrome: A Methodologically Oriented, 2-Week, Randomized, Placebo-Controlled, Double-Blind Clinical Study," *Clinical Therapeutics* 27, no. 6 (June 2005): 755–61.

32 Mike Amaranthus and Bruce Allyn, "Healthy Soil Microbes, Healthy People," *The Atlantic,* June 11, 2013, www.theatlantic.com/health/archive/2013/06/healthy-soil-microbes-healthy-people/276710/.

33 Hafiz, *I Heard God Laughing,* 25.

34 Franklin D. Roosevelt, "Letter to All State Governors on a Uniform Soil Conservation Law," February 26, 1937; available online: Gerhard Peters and John T. Woolley, The American Presidency Project, www.presidency.ucsb.edu/ws/?pid+15373.

35 Rumi, *The Illuminated Rumi,* trans. Coleman Barks (New York: Broadway Books, 1997), 31.

36 Eisenstein, *Sacred Economics.*

37 John Muir, *Our National Parks* (Boston: Houghton Mifflin, 1901), 56.

38 Mary Oliver, "When I Am Among the Trees," *Thirst* (Boston: Beacon Press, 2006), 4.

39 C. S. Lewis, *Prince Caspian* (New York: Harper Entertainment, 2008), 227.

40 Gustav Fechner, "Nanna: On the Soul of Plants," in Brouwer, Mulder, and Spuybroek, *Vital Beauty,* 188.

41 Florence Williams, "Take Two Hours of Pine Forest and Call Me in the Morning," *Outside Magazine,* November 28, 2012, www.outsideonline.com/fitness/wellness/Take-Two-Hours-of-Pine-Forest-and-CMe-in-the-Morning.html.

42 Muir, *Our National Parks,* 1.

43 B. J. Park, Y. Tsunetsugu, T. Kasetani, T. Kagawa, and Y. Miyazaki, "The Physiological Effects of *Shinrin-yoku* (Taking in the Forest Atmosphere or Forest Bathing): Evidence from Field Experiments in 24 Forests across Japan," *Environmental Health and Preventive Medicine* 15, no. 1 (2010): 18–26, http://doi.org/10.1007/s12199-009-0086-9.

44 Q. Li, "Effect of Forest Bathing Trips on Human Immune Function," *Environmental Health and Preventive Medicine* 15, no. 1 (January 2010), 9–17, www.ncbi.nlm.nih.gov/pubmed/19568839.

45 Rick J. Willis, *The History of Allelopathy* (Berlin: Springer Science+Business Media, 2007), 287.

46 Q. Li et al., "Effect of Phytoncide from Trees on Human Natural Killer Cell Function," *International Journal of Immunopathology and Pharmacology* 22, no. 4 (Oct.–Dec. 2009), 951–59, www.ncbi.nlm.nih.gov/pubmed/20074458.

47 Li, "Effect of Forest Bathing Trips on Human Immune Function."

48 "Report by National Chung Hsing University Reveals the Secrets of Phytoncides," *Campus News,* Ministry of Education, Republic of China (Taiwan), February 7, 2013, http://english.moe.gov.tw/ct.asp?xItem=10743&ct-Node=11020
&mp=1. This experiment gave rats extremely high doses of essential oil without a toxic reaction, demonstrating that these oils are safe.

49 Dalė Pečiulytė, Irena Nedveckytė, Vaidilutė Dirginčiūtė-Volodkienė, and Vincas Būda, "Pine Defoliator Bupalus piniaria L. (Lepidoptera: Geometridae) and Its Entomopathogenic Fungi," *Ekologija* 56, nos. 1–2 (2010): 34.

50 Kahlil Gibran, *Sand and Foam* (North Charleston, SC: CreateSpace Independent Publishing Platform, 2014), 9.

51 Li et al., "Effect of Phytoncide from Trees on Human Natural Killer Cell Function."

52 Saint Hildegard of Bingen, "O Ignis Spiritus Paracliti," *Symphonia: A Critical Edition of the Symphonia armonie celestium revelationum,* trans. Barbara Newman (Ithaca, NY: Cornell University Press, 1998), 150.

53 Charles Darwin, *The Variation of Animals and Plants under Domestication,* vol. 2 (London: William Clowes and Sons, 1868).

54 Ronnie N. Glud, Frank Wenzhöfer, et al., "High Rates of Microbial Carbon Turnover in Sediments in the Deepest Oceanic Trench on Earth," *Nature Geoscience* 6 (March 17, 2013): 284–88.

55 Rob Knight, "How Our Microbes Make Us Who We Are," TED Talk transcript, February 2015, www.ted.com/talks/rob_knight_how_our_microbes_make_us_who_we_are/transcript?language=en.

56 "NIH Human Microbiome Project Defines Normal Bacterial Makeup of the Body," National Institutes of Health, June 13, 2012, www.nih.gov/news/health/jun2012/nhgri-13.htm.

57 Ibid.

58 Kelly Brogan MD blog, "Microbiome—Let's Get Into It," September 11, 2014, http://kellybroganmd.com.

59 Richard Matthews, *The Symbiont Factor: How the Gut Microbiome Redefines Health, Disease and Humanity*, 67.

60 Explore all of Dr. Ben-Jacob's images at the Bacteria Art Gallery: http://tamar.tau.ac.il/~eshel/html/Bacteria_art_gallery.html.

61 Matthews, *The Symbiont Factor*, 41.

62 Christine M. Dejea, "Microbiota Organization Is a Distinct Feature of Proximal Colorectal Cancers," *Proceedings of the National Academy of Sciences of the United States of America* 111, no. 51.

63 "NIH Human Microbiome Project Defines Normal Bacterial Makeup of the Body."

64 Matthews, *The Symbiont Factor*, 75.

65 Terry L. Powley and Robert J. Phillips, "Morphology and Topography of Vagal Afferents Innervating the GI Tract," *American Journal of Physiology* 283, no. 6 (December 1, 2002): G1217–25, http://ajpgi.physiology.org/content/283/6/G1217.full.

66 Matthews, *The Symbiont Factor*, 74.

67 Ibid., 69–75.

68 Ibid., 75.

69 Ibid., 73.

70 Ibid., 80.

71 Andrew Weil, "Love Me, Love My Microbiome," 2011, www.drweil.com/drw/u/ART03452/Love-Me-Love-My-Microbiome.html.

72 Matthews, *The Symbiont Factor*, 332.

73 Ibid., 182.

74 Ibid., 328.

75 "Why Are Allergies Increasing?" UCLA Food and Drug Allergy Care Center, 2010, http://fooddrugallergy.ucla.edu/body.cfm?id=40.

76 Martin Blaser, *Missing Microbes* (New York: Henry Holt, 2014).

77 Andrew Martin, "Antibacterial Chemical Raises Safety Issues," *New York Times*, August 19, 2011, www.nytimes.com/2011/08/20/business/triclosan-an-antibacterial-chemical-in-consumer-products-raises-safety-issues.html?pagewanted=all&_r=0.

78 "Strategic and Technical Advisory Group (STAG) on Antimicrobial Resistance," World Health Organization, www.who.int/antimicrobial-resistance/events/stag/en/.

79 Cloflucarban, fluorosalan, hexachlorophene, hexylresorcinol, iodine complex (ammonium ether sulfate and polyoxyethylene sorbitan monolaurate), iodine complex (phosphate ester of alkylaryloxy polyethylene glycol),

nonylphenoxypoly (ethyleneoxy) ethanoliodine, poloxamer–iodine complex, povidone-iodine 5 to 10 percent, undecoylium chloride iodine complex, methylbenzethonium chloride, phenol (greater than 1.5 percent), phenol (less than 1.5 percent), secondary amyltricresols, sodium oxychlorosene, tribromsalan, triclocarban, triclosan, triple dye.

80 Food and Drug Administration, "FDA Issues Final Rule on Safety and Effectiveness of Antibacterial Soaps," September 2, 2016, www.fda.gov/NewsEvents/Newsroom/PressAnnouncements/ucm517478.htm.

81 G. Avendaño-Pérez and C. Pin, "Loss of Culturability of Salmonella enterica subsp. enterica Serovar Typhimurium upon Cell-Cell Contact with Human Fecal Bacteria," *Applied and Environmental Microbiology* 79, no. 10 (2013): 3257–63.

82 Matthews, *The Symbiont Factor*, 167.

83 Ibid., 80.

84 Mike Amaranthus and Bruce Allyn, "Healthy Soil Microbes, Healthy People," *The Atlantic*, June 11, 2013, www.theatlantic.com/health/archive/2013/06/healthy-soil-microbes-healthy-people/276710/.

85 Matthews, *The Symbiont Factor*, 87.

86 Rob Dunn, *The Wild Life of Our Bodies: Predators, Parasites, and Partners That Shape Who We Are Today* (New York: Harper, 2011), 57.

87 Read about some of these stories at jasper-lawrence.com.

88 Agatha Christie, *Murder in Mesopotamia* (New York: HarperCollins, 2011), 262.

89 Tom Robbins, *Jitterbug Perfume* (New York: Bantam, 1990), 319.

90 Weil, "Love Me, Love My Microbiome."

91 Ibid.

92 Brouwer, Mulder, and Spuybroek, *Vital Beauty*, 176.

93 Neil Diamond, "Done Too Soon," *Tap Root Manuscript*, 1970.

94 Brouwer, Mulder, and Spuybroek, *Vital Beauty*, 177.

CHAPTER SIX

1 Jane Fonda, *Jane Fonda's Workout Book* (New York: Simon and Schuster, 1981).

2 Bruce Agnew, "The Skin Microbiome: More Than Skin Deep," National Human Genome Research Institute of the NIH, November 21, 2014, www.genome.gov/27559614.

3 Matthews, *The Symbiont Factor*, 328.

4 Agnew, "The Skin Microbiome."

5 Ibid.

6 Russel M. Walters, Guangru Mao, Euen T. Gunn, and Sidney Hornby, "Cleansing Formulations That Respect Skin Barrier Integrity," *Dermatology Research and Practice*, 2012: 495917, www.ncbi.nlm.nih.gov/pmc/articles/PMC3425021/.

7 "An AP Investigation: Pharmaceuticals in Drinking Water."

8 Matthews, *The Symbiont Factor*, 94.

9 Under the Fair Packaging and Labeling Act, the U.S. Food and Drug Administration requires all retail cosmetic products to list ingredients. However, this requirement can't force manufacturers to reveal trade secrets, and "fragrance" is often a complex mixture of ingredients, which falls under the scope of "trade secret." This is why fragrance ingredients can be labeled as just "fragrance."

10 "A New Approach in Topical Hyaluronic Acid: Going Beyond Instant Benefits to Restore Epidermal HA Homeostasis," *Journal of Drugs in Dermatology* 15, no. 1 (January 2016).

11 Matthews, *The Symbiont Factor*, 79.

12 Ibid.

13 S. Macfarlane, G. T. Macfarlane, and J. H. Cummings, "Prebiotics in the Gastrointestinal Tract," *Alimentary Pharmacology and Therapeutics* 24, no. 5 (September 1, 2006): 701–14.

14 S. Hylla, A. Gostner, G. Dusel, H. Anger, et al., "Effects of Resistant Starch on the Colon in Healthy Volunteers: Possible Implications for Cancer Prevention," *American Journal of Clinical Nutrition* 67, no. 1 (January 1998): 136–42.

15 K. L. Johnston, E. L. Thomas, J. D. Bell, G. S. Frost, and M. D. Robertson, "Resistant Starch Improves Insulin Sensitivity in Metabolic Syndrome," *Diabetic Medicine* 27 (2010): 391–97.

16 Danielle Alexander, "Postprandial Effects of Resistant Starch Corn Porridges on Blood Glucose and Satiety Responses in Non-overweight and Overweight Adults," Iowa State University Digital Repository, 2012.

17 M. B. Purba, A. Kouris-Blazos, N. Wattanapenpaiboon, et al., "Skin Wrinkling: Can Food Make a Difference?" *Journal of American College of Nutrition* 20 (2001): 71–80.

18 Kahlil Gibran, *The Collected Works* (New York: Random House, 2007), 112.

19 www.Soaphistory.net.

20 Dig deeper into the antimicrobial properties of fatty acids in Halldor Thormar, ed., *Lipids and Essential Oils as Antimicrobial Agents* (West Sussex, UK: John Wiley & Sons, 2011).

21 "'Super' Bacteria Live on Sheets, Fingernails: Study," June 6, 2005, *ABC News*, www.abc.net.au/news/2005-06-07/super-bacteria-live-on-sheets-fingernails-study/1587380.

22 C. M. Lin et al., "A Comparison of Hand Washing Techniques to Remove Escherichia coli and Caliciviruses under Natural or Artificial Fingernails," *Journal of Food Protection* 6, no. 12 (December 2003): 2296–301.

23 Tom Robbins, *Still Life with Woodpecker* (New York: Bantam, 1980), 20.

CHAPTER SEVEN

1 Barks and Moyne, *The Drowned Book*, 59.

2 Simon N. Young, "How to Increase Serotonin in the Human Brain without Drugs," *Journal of Psychiatry and Neuroscience* 32, no. 6 (2007): 394–99, www.ncbi.nlm.nih.gov/pmc/articles/PMC2077351/.

3 Bernard Ackerman, *The Sun and the "Epidemic" of Melanoma: Myth on Myth!* (New York: Harmony, September 1998), 126.

4 Richard Hobday, "Sunbathing: The Benefits Are More Than Skin Deep," *Creations Magazine*, www.creationsmagazine.com/articles/C114/Hobday.html.

5 Pliny the Elder, quoted in Shelton, *The Hygienic System*, 206.

6 Richard Hobday, *The Healing Sun: Sunlight and Health in the 21st Century* (Forres, Scotland: Findhorn Press, 1999), 58–59.

7 Elana Conis, "The Rise and Fall of Sunlight Therapy," *Los Angeles Times*, May 28, 2007, http://articles.latimes.com/2007/may/28/health/he-esoterica28.

8 From *Nobel Lectures, Physiology or Medicine 1901–1921* (Amsterdam: Elsevier, 1967), www.nobelprize.org/nobel_prizes/medicine/laureates/1903/finsen-bio.html.

9 Follow this link to see some of the before and after photos of children at the Lysine Clinic: http://digital.library.mcgill.ca/sun/browse.php?p=005.

10 *The Spectator* Archive, October 17, 1925, http://archive.spectator.co.uk/article/17th-october-1925/8/o-n-the-simplon-line-easy-to-reach-a-few-miles.

11 Jacob Hoban, "Sunlight for Your Health," Dr. Hoban Natural Healing Center, July 16, 2015, www.drhoban.com/sunlight-for-your-health/.

12 J. J. Cannell et al., "Epidemic Influenza and Vitamin D," *Epidemiology and Infection* 134, no. 6 (December 2006): 1129–40.

13 Edgar Mayer, *The Curative Value of Light: Sunlight and Sun Lamp in Health and Disease* (Whitefish, MT: Literary Licensing LLC, 2013).

14 Thank-you to Sayer Ji of GreenMedInfo.com for bringing this study to my attention: Chen Xu et al., "Light-Harvesting Chlorophyll Pigments Enable Mammalian Mitochondria to Capture Photonic Energy and Produce ATP," *Journal of Cell Science* 127 (2014): 388–99.

15 Sayer Ji, "Amazing Discovery: Plant Blood Enables Your Cells to Capture Sunlight Energy," GreenMedInfo, May 12, 2015, www.greenmedinfo.com/blog/chlorophyll-enables-your-cells-captureuse-sunlight-energy-copernican-revolution.

16 Caroline Myss, *Why People Don't Heal and How They Can.*

17 Xu, "Light-Harvesting Chlorophyll Pigments Enable Mammalian Mitochondria to Capture Photonic Energy and Produce ATP."

18 Ji, "Amazing Discovery."

19 Dianne Godar, Madhan Subramanian, and Stephen Merrill, "Cutaneous Malignant Melanoma Incidences Analyzed Worldwide by Sex, Age, and Skin Type over Personal Ultraviolet-B Dose Shows No Role for Sunburn but Implies One for Vitamin D_3," *Dermato-Endocrinology* 9, no. 1 (2017), www.tandfonline.com/doi/full/10.1080/19381980.2016.1267077.

20 Valerie Beral, Helen Shaw, Susan Evans, and Gerald Milton, "Malignant Melanoma and Exposure to Fluorescent Lighting at Work," *The Lancet* 320, no. 8293 (August 1982): 290–93.

21 J. Mark Elwood and Janet Jopson, "Melanoma and Sun Exposure: An Overview of Published Studies," *International Journal of Cancer* 73 (1997): 198–203.

22 Ackerman, *The Sun and the "Epidemic" of Melanoma,* 134.

23 Beral, Shaw, Evans, and Milton, "Malignant Melanoma and Exposure to Fluorescent Lighting at Work."

24 Environmental Working Group, "Imperfect Protection: EWG's Analysis of UV Protection Offered by U.S. Sunscreens," https://www.ewg.org/sunscreen/report/imperfect-protection/.

25 Ackerman, *The Sun and the "Epidemic" of Melanoma,* 134.

26 "Sunscreen Can Damage Skin, Researchers Find," August 29, 2006, University of California, Riverside, http://newsroom.ucr.edu/1399.

27 Joseph Mercola, "The Bottom Line on Sunscreens," June 6, 2011, *Mercola*, http://articles.mercola.com/sites/articles/archive/2011/06/06/do-you-know -which-sunscreen-products-to-avoid.aspx.

28 Hafiz, *I Heard God Laughing*, 8.

29 D Minder, http://dminder.ontometrics.com/.

30 Stephanie Seneff, "Sulfur Deficiency," July 2, 2011, Weston A. Price Founda-tion, www.westonaprice.org/vitamins-and-minerals/sulfur-deficiency.

31 Charles A. Strott and Yuko Higashi, "Cholesterol Sulfate in Human Physiol-ogy: What's It All About?" *Journal of Lipid Research* 44 (2003): 1268–78.

32 Richard Cohen, *Chasing the Sun: The Epic Story of the Star That Gives Us Life* (New York: Simon and Schuster, 2011).

33 Jordan Lite, "Vitamin D Deficiency Soars in the US, Study Says," *Scientific American*, March 2009.

34 From *Nobel Lectures, Physiology or Medicine 1901–1921*.

35 Sif Hansdottir et al., "Respiratory Epithelial Cells Convert Inactive Vitamin D to Its Active Form: Potential Effects on Host Defense," *Journal of Immu-nology* 181, no. 10 (November 15, 2008): 7090–99, www.jimmunol.org /content/181/10/7090.short; M. Mangin, R. Sinha, and K. Fincher, "Inflamma-tion and Vitamin D: The Infection Connection," *Inflammation Research* 63, no. 10 (2014): 803–819, www.ncbi.nlm.nih.gov/pmc/articles/PMC4160567/.

36 Philip T. Liu, Steffen Stenger, Huiying Li, Linda Wenzel, Belinda H. Tan, Stephan R. Krutzik, Maria Teresa Ochoa, et al., "Toll-Like Receptor Trigger-ing of a Vitamin D-Mediated Human Antimicrobial Response," *Science* 311, no. 5768 (March 24, 2006): 1770–73, http://science.sciencemag.org /content/311/5768/1770.

37 Herbert M. Shelton, *Fasting and Sun Bathing*, 3rd rev. ed. (San Antonio, TX: Dr. Shelton's Health School, 1950), http://soilandhealth.org/wp-content /uploads/02/0201hyglibcat/020127shelton.III/020127.toc.htm.

38 G. Goodman and D. Bercovich, "Melanin Directly Converts Light for Verte-brate Metabolic Use: Heuristic Thoughts on Birds, Icarus and Dark Human Skin," *Medical Hypotheses* 71, no. 2 (August 2008): 190–202, www.ncbi.nlm .nih.gov/pubmed/18479839.

39 "Ultrafast Photodynamics of Nucleic Acids," Kohler Research Group, Ohio State University, http://cbc-wb01x.chemistry.ohio-state.edu/~kohler/dna.html.

40 E. D. Gorham, S. B. Mohr, C. F. Garland, G. Chaplin, and F. C. Garland, "Do Sunscreens Increase Risk of Melanoma in Populations Residing at Higher Latitudes?" *Annals of Epidemiology* 17, no. 12 (December 2007): 956–63.

41 Beth A. Glenn, Tiffany Lin, L. Cindy Chang, Ashley Okada, Weng Kee Wong, Karen Glanz, and Roshan Bastani, "Sun Protection Practices and Sun Exposure among Children with a Parental History of Melanoma," *Cancer Epidemiology, Biomarkers & Prevention: A Publication of the American Association for Cancer Research, Cosponsored by the American Society of Preventive Oncology* 24, no. 1 (2015): 169–77.

42 C. W. Saleeby, *Sunlight and Health* (London: Nisbet & Company, 1923).

43 "Tomato Paste Helps Fight Sunburn and Wrinkles," News-Medical, April 2008, www.news-medical.net/news/2008/04/29/37863.aspx.

44 Cleveland Clinic, "Protecting Yourself from Sun Damage," http://my.clevelandclinic.org/health/articles/protecting-yourself-from-sun-damage.

45 Beinsa Douno, *The Sacred Power of the Sun*, ed. C. J. Todd (High Place Publishing, 2013), 247.

46 Susan Brown, "Sunscreen Wipes Out Corals," *Nature*, January 29, 2008, www.nature.com/news/2008/080129/full/news.2008.537.html.

47 Daniel Cressey, "Coral Crisis: Great Barrier Reef Bleaching Is 'The Worst We've Ever Seen,'" *Nature*, April 13, 2016, www.scientificamerican.com/article/coral-crisis-great-barrier-reef-bleaching-is-the-worst-we-ve-ever-seen/.

48 Inga Vesper, "Hawaii Seeks to Ban 'Reef-Unfriendly' Sunscreen," *Nature*, February 3, 2017, www.scientificamerican.com/article/hawaii-seeks-to-ban-reef-unfriendly-sunscreen1/.

49 Douno, *The Sacred Power of the Sun*, 194.

50 Fechner, "Nanna."

51 M. Kaur et al., "Skin Cancer Chemopreventive Agent, {Alpha}-Santalol, Induces Apoptotic Death of Human Epidermoid Carcinoma A431 Cells via Caspase Activation Together with Dissipation of Mitochondrial Membrane Potential and Cytochrome c Release," *Carcinogenesis* 26, no. 2 (February 2005): 369–80, www.ncbi.nlm.nih.gov/pubmed/?term=sandalwood+kaur.

52 T. Akihisa, K. Tabata, N. Banno, H. Tokuda, R. Nishimura, Y. Nakamura, Y. Kimura, K. Yasukawa, and T. Suzuki, "Cancer Chemopreventive Effects and Cytotoxic Activities of the Triterpene Acids from the Resin of Boswellia carteri," *Biological and Pharmaceutical Bulletin* 29, no. 9 (September 2006): 1976–1979; Parduman R. Sharma, Dilip M. Mondhe, Shanmugavel Muthiah, Harish C. Pal, Ashok K. Shahi, Ajit K. Saxena, and Ghulam N. Qazi, "Anticancer Activity of an Essential Oil from Cymbopogon flexuosus," *Chemo-Biological Interactions* 179, nos. 2–3 (May 15, 2009): 160–68.

53 Douno, *The Sacred Power of the Sun*, 275.

54 Mary Oliver, "Why I Wake Early," *Why I Wake Early: New Poems* (Boston: Beacon Press, 2004), 3.

CHAPTER EIGHT

1 "Dentists Vary Widely on Diagnosis and Cost," CBC News Canada, October 18, 2012, www.cbc.ca/news/canada/dentists-vary-widely-on-diagnosis-and-cost-cbc-marketplace-finds-1.1279371.

2 William Ecenbarger, "How Dentists Rip Us Off," *Reader's Digest,* www.dentistat.com/ReaderDigestArticle.pdf.

3 James Wynbrandt, *The Excruciating History of Dentistry: Toothsome Tales & Oral Oddities from Babylon to Braces,* 1st ed. (New York: St. Martin's Griffin, 2000), 181.

4 "Amalgam/Mercury—Dental Filling Toxicity," Huggins Applied Healing, www.hugginsappliedhealing.com/amalgam-mercury.php.

5 U.S. Environmental Protection Agency, "Mercury Releases and Spills," www.epa.gov/mercury/spills/.

6 Parin Shah, January 22, 2004, www.fda.gov/ohrms/dockets/dockets/06n0352/06N-0352-EC22-Attach-6.pdf.

7 G. Sällsten, J. Thorén, L. Barregård, A. Schütz, and G. Skarping, "Long-Term Use of Nicotine Chewing Gum and Mercury Exposure from Dental Amalgam Fillings," *Journal of Dental Research* 75, no. 1 (January 1996): 594–98.

8 Jay W. Friedman, "The Prophylactic Extraction of Third Molars: A Public Health Hazard," *American Journal of Public Health* 97, no. 9 (September 2007): 1554–59.

9 Ibid.

10 Corinne Vizcarra, "Incidence Levels and Chronic Health Effects Related to Cavitations," www.biodentistrydrvizcarra.com/?s=8&sub=8.

11 *The Tooth Truth: Cavity-Free Conversations with Dentists, Doctors and Health Heroes* (White Lake, ON: The Raw Divas, Inc., December 1, 2012), www.wishsummit.com/book.

12 Erwin P. Vernon, DDS, "Ozone and Root Canals," The Holistic Dentist, April 20, 2012, http://theholisticdentist.wordpress.com/2012/04/20/ozone-root-canals/.

13 Stuart M. Nunnally, "In Vitro Enzymatic Inhibition Associated with Asymptomatic Root Canal Treated Teeth: Results from a Sample of 25 Extracted Root Fragments," *Journal of Minerals, Metals, and Materials Society* 27,

no. 3 (2012): 112–16, https://iaomt.org/wp-content/uploads/Nunnally-RC
-Enzyme-Inhibition.pdf.

14 See Nadine Artemis, *Holistic Dental Care: The Complete Guide to Healthy Teeth and Gums* (Berkeley, CA: North Atlantic Books, 2013) for questions to ask your dentists before making an appointment.

15 R. F. Gerlach, A. P. de Souza, J. A. Cury, and S. R. Line, "Fluoride Effect on the Activity of Enamel Matrix Proteinases in Vitro," *European Journal of Oral Sciences* 108, no. 1 (2000): 48–53.

16 Marilyn Chase, "Rat Studies Link Brain Cell Damage with Aluminum and Fluoride in Water," *Wall Street Journal,* October 28, 1992.

17 Michael Connett, "Mechanisms by Which Fluoride May Reduce Bone Strength," April 2012, http://fluoridealert.org/studies/bone06/.

18 Milton A. Saunders Jr., "Fluoride Toothpaste: A Cause of Acne-like Eruptions," *Archives of Dermatology* 111 (1975): 793.

19 H. A. Cook, "Fluoride Studies in a Patient with Arthritis," *The Lancet,* October 9, 1971.

20 National Research Council, "Fluoride in Drinking Water: A Scientific Review of EPA's Standards," *NRC (2006): Fluoride's Impact on the Thyroid Gland,* 2006, 224–236, http://fluoridealert.org/studies/nrc_thyroid/.

21 Michael Connett, "Fluoride's Effect on the Male Reproductive System," April 2012, http://fluoridealert.org/studies/fertility01/.

22 Ahmad Al-Hiyasat, "Reproductive Toxic Effects of Ingestion of Sodium Fluoride in Female Rats," *Fluoride* 33, no. 2 (2000): 79–84, http://fluoridealert.org/wp-content/uploads/al-hiyasat-200011.pdf.

23 M. Bely, "Changes in Collagen Structure of Bone Tissue in Experimental Fluorosis," http://fluoridealert.org/wp-content/uploads/bely-1988.pdf.

24 Joel Griffiths, "Fluoride Linked to Bone Cancer in Fed Study," December 28, 1989, http://fluoridealert.org/articles/ntp01/.

25 "Impact of Fluoride on Neurological Development of Children," Harvard School of Public Health, July 25, 2012, www.hsph.harvard.edu/news/features/fluoride-childrens-health-grandjean-choi/.

26 S. J. Padilla et al., "Building a Database of Developmental Neurotoxitants: Evidence from Human and Animal Studies," Neurotoxicology Division, Environmental Protection Agency, 2009, https://cfpub.epa.gov/si/si_public_record_report.cfm?dirEntryId=200234; Artemis, *Holistic Dental Care,* 20

27 For further scientific research, explore the book about Dr. Ralph R. Steinman's pioneering work: Clyde Roggenkamp, *Dentinal Fluid Transport* (Loma Linda, CA: Loma Linda University Press, 2005).

28 Ralph R. Steinman and John Leonora, "Effect of Selected Dietary Additives on the Incidence of Dental Caries in the Rat," *Journal of Dental Research* 54 (May 1975): 570–77.

29 Melvin Page, *Your Body Is Your Best Doctor*, rev. ed. (New Canaan, CT: Keats, 1991).

30 Blaser, *Missing Microbes*.

31 Shodhganga, "Summary," http://shodhganga.inflibnet.ac.in/bitstream/10603 /63580/18/18_summary.pdf.

32 Joy L. Moelle, "Orofacial Myofunctional Therapy: The Critical Missing Element to Complete Patient Care," DentalTown.com, August 2010.

33 Dig deeper into oral ecology, self-dentistry, and botanical oils for the mouth in my book *Holistic Dental Care: The Complete Guide to Healthy Teeth and Gums*.

34 For a list of harmful ingredients in oral-care products, read "May Be Harmful if Swallowed" at www.livinglibations.com/default/may_be_harmful _if_swallowed.

35 Titik Nuryastuti et al., "Effect of Cinnamon Oil on icaA Expression and Biofilm Formation by Staphylococcus epidermidis," *Applied Environmental Microbiology* 75, no. 21 (November 2009): 6850–55.

36 R. M. Karuppaiah, S. Shankar, S. K. Raj, K. Ramesh, R. Prakash, and M. Kruthika, "Evaluation of the Efficacy of Probiotics in Plaque Reduction and Gingival Health Maintenance among School Children—A Randomized Control Trial," *Journal of International Oral Health* 5, no. 5 (2013): 33–37.

37 Matthews, *The Symbiont Factor*, 205.

38 W. Teughels et al., "Guiding Periodontal Pocket Recolonization: A Proof of Concept," *Journal of Dental Research* 86, no. 11 (November 2007): 1078–82.

39 Erin LaBlanc, "Hip Fracture and Increased Short-Term but Not Long-Term Mortality in Healthy Older Women," *Archives of Internal Medicine* 171, no. 20 (2011): 1831–37.

40 Frank Lloyd Wright, quoted in John Rattenbury, *A Living Architecture: Frank Lloyd Wright and Taliesin Architects* (San Francisco: Pomegranate Communications, 2000), 67.

41 Amanda Leigh Mascarelli, "Osteopenia Doesn't Mean Osteoporosis—So Should You Treat It?" *Los Angeles Times*, April 30, 2011.

42 Spiegel, "How a Bone Disease Grew to Fit the Prescription."

43 Zoltan P. Rona, "Bone Density Drugs and the Best Alternatives," *Vitality Magazine,* http://vitalitymagazine.com/article/bone-density-drugs-and-the-best-natural-alternatives/.

44 Laura Y. Park-Wyllie et al., "Bisphosphonate Use and the Risk of Subtrochanteric or Femoral Shaft Fractures in Older Women," *Journal of the American Medical Association* 305, no. 8 (February 23, 2011): 783.

45 Aaron P. Sarathy et al., "Bisphosphonate-Associated Osteonecrosis of the Jaws and Endodontic Treatment: Two Case Reports," *Journal of Endodontics* 31, no. 10: 759–63.

46 Frederick W. Fraunfelder and Frederick T. Fraunfelder, "Bisphosphonates and Ocular Inflammation," *New England Journal of Medicine* 348, no. 12 (March 20, 2003): 1187–88.

47 A. Sharma, S. Chatterjee, A. Arbab-Zadeh, et al., "Risk of Serious Atrial Fibrillation and Stroke with Use of Bisphosphonates," *CHEST* 144, no. 4 (2013): 1311–22.

48 Rona, "Bone Density Drugs and the Best Alternatives."

49 Fracture Risk Assessment Tool, www.shef.ac.uk/FRAX/index.aspx.

50 Anthony Samsel and Stephanie Seneff, "Glyphosate's Suppression of Cytochrome P450 Enzymes and Amino Acid Biosynthesis by the Gut Microbiome: Pathways to Modern Diseases," *Entropy* 15, no. 4 (2013): 1416–63.

51 C. M. Weaver, "Diet, Gut Microbiome, and Bone Health," *Current Osteoporosis Reports* 13, no. 2 (2015): 125–30, doi:10.1007/s11914-015-0257-0.

CHAPTER NINE

1 "Global Cancer Fact Sheet," Susan G. Komen, Greater New York City, www.komennyc.org/site/DocServer/Global_Breast_and_Cancer_Facts-_6-30-10.pdf?docID=3881.

2 CDC, "DES History," www.cdc.gov/des/consumers/about/history.html.

3 M. Bibbo, W. Haenszel, et al., "A Twenty-Five-Year Follow-up Study of Women Exposed to Diethylstilbestrol during Pregnancy," *New England Journal of Medicine* (1978): 763–67.

4 A. L. Herbst, H. Ulfelder, and D. C. Poskanzer, "Adenocarcinoma of the Vagina: Association of Maternal Stilbestrol Therapy with Tumor Appearance in Young Women," *New England Journal of Medicine* 284, no. 15 (1971): 878–81.

5 Janet Raloff, "Hormones: Here's the Beef," *Science News: Online*, 2002, www.phschool.com/science/science_news/articles/hormones_beef.html.

6 Margaret Hartmann, "Maxipads Get Cute and Sparkly for Young Menstruaters," April 15, 2011, *Jezebel*, http://jezebel.com/5792366/maxipads-get-cute -and-sparkly-for-increasingly-young-menstruaters.

7 Lindsey Konkel, "DDT Linked to Fourfold Increase in Breast Cancer Risk," *National Geographic*, June 16, 2015, http://news.nationalgeographic .com/2015/06/15616-breast-cancer-ddt-pesticide-environment/.

8 "Genetics," BreastCancer.org, www.breastcancer.org/risk/factors/genetics.

9 Susan Silberstein, "3-D Mammograms: Do They Save Lives?" June 28, 2014, http://beatcancer.org/2014/06/3-d-mammograms-do-they-save-lives/.

10 P. Hoekstra, "Quantitive Digital Thermology: 21st Century Imaging Systems," paper presented at OAND Conference, Hamilton, Ontario, 2001.

11 Arizona Center for Advanced Medicine, 2009, http:// arizonaadvancedmedicine.com/mammography-guidelines-revised- november-2009/.

12 U.S. Preventive Services Task Force, "Final Recommendation Statement: Breast Cancer: Screening, November 2009," 2009, www .uspreventiveservicestaskforce.org/Page/Document /RecommendationStatementFinal/breast-cancer-screening.

13 P. C. Gøtzsche et al., "Screening for Breast Cancer with Mammography," *Cochrane Database of Systematic Reviews* 4 (October 7, 2009): CD001877, www.ncbi.nlm.nih.gov/pubmed/19821284.

14 Mette Kalager et al., "Effect of Screening Mammography on Breast Cancer: Mortality in Norway," *New England Journal of Medicine* 363, no. 13 (September 2010), www.nejm.org/doi/pdf/10.1056/NEJMoa1000727.

15 Anthony Miller et al., "Twenty Five Year Follow-up for Breast Cancer Incidence and Mortality of the Canadian National Breast Screening Study: Randomised Screening Trial," *BMJ* 348 (February 11, 2014): g366 www.bmj.com /content/348/bmj.g366.

16 Gina Kolata, "Vast Study Casts Doubts on Value of Mammograms," *New York Times*, February 11, 2014, www.nytimes.com/2014/02/12/health/study -adds-new-doubts-about-value-of-mammograms.html?hpw&rref=health&_r=1.

17 National Breast Cancer Coalition, "Breast Cancer Facts and Figures," http://BreastCancerDeadline2020.org/BCFactsFigures.

18 Lori Jardines, Sharad Goyal, et al., "Stages 0 and 1 Breast Cancer," *Breast Cancer Network*, www.cancernetwork.com/cancer-management/stages-0 -and-i-breast-cancer.

19 Stephanie Saul, "Prone to Error: Earlier Steps to Find Cancer," *New York Times*, July 19, 2010, www.nytimes.com/2010/07/20/health/20cancer.html?_r=2&th&emc=th.

20 R. A. Hubbard, K. Kerlikowske, C. I. Flowers, B. C. Yankaskas, W. Zhu, and D. L. Miglioretti, "Cumulative Probability of False-Positive Recall or Biopsy Recommendation after 10 Years of Screening Mammography: A Cohort Study," *Annals of Internal Medicine* 155, no. 8 (2011): 481–92.

21 Elizabeth Fernandez, "High Rate of False-Positives with Annual Mammogram," *UCSF News Center*, October 17, 2011, www.ucsf.edu/news/2011/10/10778/high-rate-false-positives-annual-mammogram.

22 Breast Cancer Choices, "Biopsy FAQ," http://breastcancerchoices.org/faqbiopsies.html.

23 L. E. Esserman, M. A. Cura, and D. DaCosta, "Recognizing Pitfalls in Early and Late Migration of Clip Markers after Imaging-Guided Directional Vacuum-Assisted Biopsy," *Radiographics* 24, no. 1 (January–February 2004): 147–56, www.ncbi.nlm.nih.gov/pubmed/14730043.

24 Springer Science+Business Media, "Heavy Metal: Titanium Implant Safety under Scrutiny," July 26, 2011, www.sciencedaily.com/releases/2011/07/110725101257.htm.

25 Vidudala V. T. S. Prasad and Ramprasad O. G. Gopalan, "Continued Use of MDA-MB-435, a Melanoma Cell Line, as a Model for Human Breast Cancer, Even in Year, 2014," *Nature Partner Journals: Breast Cancer,* article 15002 (2015).

26 M. S. O'Reilly, L. Holmgren, Y. Shing, C. Chen, R. A. Rosenthal, Y. Cao, M. Moses, W. S. Lane, E. H. Sage, and J. Folkman, "Angiostatin: A Circulating Endothelial Cell Inhibitor That Suppresses Angiogenesis and Tumor Growth," *Cold Spring Harbor Symposia on Quantitative Biology* 59 (1994): 471–82.

27 Ibid.

28 P. D. Darbre and P. W. Harvey, "Parabens Can Enable Hallmarks and Characteristics of Cancer in Human Breast Epithelial Cells: A Review of the Literature with Reference to New Exposure Data and Regulatory Status," *Journal of Applied Toxicology* 34, no. 9 (September 2014): 925–38.

29 M. W. White, "Metabolism of the Malignant Cell, the Role of Bacterial Spores, and a Pictorial Presentation to Substantiate the Latter's Presence as an Etiological Factor in Carcinogenesis," *Medical Hypotheses* 39, no. 1 (September 1992): 95–109.

30 Ibid.

31 Katherine Harmon, "Saving Face: How Safe Are Cosmetics and Body Care Products?" *Scientific American,* May 5, 2009, www.scientificamerican.com /article/how-safe-are-cosmetics/.

32 E. C. Dodds and W. Lawson, "Synthetic Oestrogenic Agents without the Phenanthrene Nucleus," *Nature* 137, no. 3476 (1936): 996.

33 Y. Omura, Y. Shimotsuura, A. Fukuoka, H. Fukuoka, and T. Nomoto, "Significant Mercury Deposits in Internal Organs Following the Removal of Dental Amalgam, & Development of Pre-cancer on the Gingiva and the Sides of the Tongue and Their Represented Organs as a Result of Inadvertent Exposure to Strong Curing Light (Used to Solidify Synthetic Dental Filling Material) & Effective Treatment: A Clinical Case Report, along with Organ Representation Areas for Each Tooth," *Acupuncture and Electrotherapeutics Research* 21, no. 2 (April–June 1996): 133–60, www.ncbi.nlm.nih .gov/pubmed/8914687.

34 Tyrone Hayes, Vicky Khoury, et al., "Atrazine Induces Complete Feminization and Chemical Castration in Male African Clawed Frogs (Xenopus laevis)," *Proceedings of the National Academy of Sciences* 107, no. 10 (March 9, 2010): 4612–17.

35 Wallace Ravven, "Common Herbicide Disrupts Human Hormone Activity in Cell Studies," *Science Daily,* May 2008, www.sciencedaily.com/releases /2008/05/080507084013.htm.

36 Lynne Farrow, *The Iodine Crisis* (New York: Devon Press, 2013).

37 Kerry Scott Lane, "Aflatoxin, Tobacco, Ammonia and the p53 Tumor-Suppressor Gene: Cancer's Missing Link?" *Medscape General Medicine* 1, no. 2 (1999), www.medscape.com/viewarticle/717362.

38 E. V. Bandera, U. Chandran, B. Buckley, et al., "Urinary Mycoestrogens, Body Size and Breast Development in New Jersey Girls," *Science of the Total Environment* 409, no. 24 (2011): 5221–27.

39 Silent Spring Institute, "Testing Exposure Reduction Strategies," www .silentspring.org/research-area/testing-exposure-reduction-strategies.

40 "Fortifying Salt Pipe," International Council for Control of Iodine Deficiency Disorders, www.iccidd.org/pages/protecting-children/fortifying-salt.php.

41 J. E. Gunton, G. Hams, M. Fiegert, and A. McElduff, "Iodine Deficiency in Ambulatory Participants at a Sydney Teaching Hospital: Is Australia Truly Iodine Replete?" *Medical Journal of Australia* 171, no. 9 (November 1, 1999): 467–70.

42 S. A. Hoption Cann, "Hypothesis: Dietary Iodine Intake in the Etiology of Cardiovascular Disease," *Journal of the American College of Nutrition* 25, no. 1 (February 2006): 1–11.

43 Guy Abraham, "Serum Inorganic Iodide Levels Following Ingestion of a Tablet Form of Lugol Solution: Evidence for an Enterohepatic Circulation of Iodine," *Original Internist,* September 2004.

44 L. Patrick, "Iodine: Deficiency and Therapeutic Considerations," *Alternative Medicine Review* 13, no. 2 (June 2008): 116–27.

45 C. Spitzweg, K. J. Harrington, L. A. Pinke, J. G. Vile, and J. C. Morris, "Clinical Review 132: The Sodium Iodide Symporter and Its Potential Role in Cancer Therapy," *Journal of Clinical Endocrinology and Metabolism* 86, no. 7 (July 2001): 3327–35.

46 "Fibrocystic Breast Changes," Atlanta Women's Specialists, www.awsphysicians.com/health-topics/article/6/Fibrocystic-Breast-Changes.php.

47 W. Ghent et al., "Iodine Replacement in Fibrocystic Disease of the Breast," *Canadian Journal of Surgery* 35, no. 5 (October 1993): 453–60. C. Aceves, B. Anguiano, and G. Delgado, "Is Iodine a Gatekeeper of the Integrity of the Mammary Gland?" *Journal of Mammary Gland Biology and Neoplasia* 10, no. 2 (April 2005): 189–96.

48 J. H. Kessler, "The Effect of Supraphysiologic Levels of Iodine on Patients with Cyclic Mastalgia," *Breast Journal* 10, no. 4 (2004): 328–36; W. R. Ghent et al., "Iodine Replacement in Fibrocystic Disease of the Breast," *Canadian Journal of Surgery* 35, no. 5 (October 1993): 453–60; B. A. Eskin et al., "Mammary Gland Dysplasia in Iodine Deficiency," *Journal of the American Medical Association* 200 (1967): 115–19.

49 Guy E. Abraham, "The Historical Background of the Iodine Project," Iodine Study #8, Optimox, www.optimox.com/iodine-study-8.

50 David Perlmutter, *Brain Maker: The Power of Gut Microbes to Heal and Protect Your Brain—for Life* (Boston: Little, Brown, 2015), 11.

51 Sameer Kalghatgi, "Bactericidal Antibiotics Induce Mitochondrial Dysfunction and Oxidative Damage in Mammalian Cells," *Translational Medicine,* July 23, 2016.

52 Brijesh Kumar Singh et al., "Natural Terpenes Prevent Mitochondrial Dysfunction, Oxidative Stress and Release of Apoptotic Proteins during Nimesulide-Hepatotoxicity in Rats," *PLoS One,* April 3, 2012.

53 American Institute for Cancer Research, "Plant-Derived Monoterpenes May Help Fight Leukemia," *AICR Science Now* 13 (Summer 2005), http://

preventcancer.aicr.org/site/News2?page=NewsArticle&id=8708&news
_iv_ctrl=0&abbr=res_.

54 E. L. Cavalieri et al., "Molecular Origin of Cancer: Catechol Estrogen-3,4-Quinones as Endogenous Tumor Initiators," *Proceedings of the National Academy of Sciences of the United States of America* 94, 10937–42.

55 Douglas Hall, "Nutritional Influences on Estrogen Metabolism," *Applied Nutritional Science Reports,* 2001, www.afmcp-sa.com/ansr/MET451%20 Endocrine%20ANSR.pdf.

56 M. N. Gould, "Prevention and Therapy of Mammary Cancer by Monoterpenes," *Journal of Cellular Biochemistry* 59, Supplement S22 (1995): 139–44.

57 H. Yang and Q. P. Dou, "Targeting Apoptosis Pathway with Natural Terpenoids: Implications for Treatment of Breast and Prostate Cancer," *Current Drug Targets* 11, no. 6 (2010): 733–44.

58 M. Y. Chang and Y. L. Shen, "Linalool Exhibits Cytotoxic Effects by Activating Antitumor Immunity," *Molecules* 19, no. 5 (May 22, 2014): 6694–706.

59 Marianna Vieira Sobral, Aline Lira Xavier, et al., "Antitumor Activity of Monoterpenes Found in Essential Oils," *Scientific World Journal* (2014).

60 J. A. Miller, J. E. Lang, M. Ley, R. B. Nagle, C. H. Hsu, P. A. Thompson, C. Cordova, A. Waer, and H. H. Chow, "Human Breast Tissue Disposition and Bioactivity of Limonene in Women with Early Stage Breast Cancer," *Cancer Prevention Research* 6 (2013): 577–84.

61 J. A. Miller, P. A. Thompson, I. A. Hakim, A. M. Lopez, C. A. Thomson, W. M. Chew, C. H. Hsu, and H. H. Chow, "Safety and Feasibility of Topical Application of Limonene as a Massage Oil to the Breast," *Journal of Cancer Therapy* 3 (2012): 749–54.

62 J. A. Miller, P. A. Thompson, I. A. Hakim, H. H. Chow, and C. A. Thomson, "*d*-Limonene: A Bioactive Food Component from Citrus and Evidence for a Potential Role in Breast Cancer Prevention and Treatment," *Oncology Reviews* 66, no. 5 (2011): 31–42.

63 Rita de Cássia da Silveira e Sá, Luciana Nalone Andrade, and Damião Pergentino de Sousa, "A Review on Anti-Inflammatory Activity of Monoterpenes," *Molecules* 18 (2013): 1227–54.

64 Kurt Schnaubelt, *Advanced Aromatherapy: The Science of Essential Oil in Therapy* (New York: Healing Arts Press, 1995), 75.

65 Endocrine-disrupting parabens and metalloestrogen aluminum, common ingredients in deodorants and antiperspirants, are linked to increased breast-cancer risk. A study conducted by Pennsylvania State University on

dermal absorption of aluminum concluded that 0.12 percent of aluminum applied to the armpit is absorbed into the body. Dr. Chris Exley of Keele University in the United Kingdom has charted a correlation between the occurrence and location of breast-cancer tumors and the rise of aluminum-based antiperspirants. R. Flarend, T. Bin, D. Elmore, and S. L. Hem, "A Preliminary Study of the Dermal Absorption of Aluminum from Antiperspirants Using Aluminium-26," *Food Chemistry Toxicology* 39, no. 2 (February 2001): 163–68 and www.keele.ac.uk/lifesci/people/cexley/.

66 Joan M. Lappe, Dianne Travers-Gustafson, K. Michael Davies, Robert R. Recker, and Robert P. Heaney, "Vitamin D and Calcium Supplementation Reduces Cancer Risk: Results of a Randomized Trial," *American Journal of Clinical Nutrition* 85, no. 6 (June 2007): 1586–91; Sharif Mohr, Edward Gorham, John Alcara, Christopher Kane, Caroline Macera, J. Kellogg Parsons, Deborah Wingard, and Cedric Garland, "Serum 25-Hydroxyvitamin D and Prevention of Breast Cancer: Pooled Analysis," *Anticancer Research* 31, no. 9 (2011): 2939–48.

67 Maya Angelou, "Phenomenal Woman," *Phenomenal Woman: Four Poems Celebrating Women* (New York: Random House, 1994), 5.

CHAPTER TEN

1 Birth control pills are now manufactured with the "benefit" of not menstruating. An article featured on the Dr. Oz blog states, "The obvious benefit is that no period means no cramps, no menstrual headaches, no making a midnight run to buy tampons." The article avoids any mention of how cramps and headaches could be the body signaling that hormones could come further into balance. Lauren Streicher, "When No Period Is No Problem," *The Oz Blog*, January 22, 2014.

2 Recalled: 1,400 cases of Kotex tampons contaminated with a life-threatening bacterium that may cause vaginal infections, urinary-tract infections, and pelvic inflammatory disease. Sora Song, "Kotex Tampons Recalled over Bacterial Contamination," November 15, 2011, http://healthland.time .com/2011/11/15/kotex-tampons-recalled-over-bacterial-contamination/.

3 Robbins, *Still Life with Woodpecker*, 14.

4 D. A. Grimes, "Intrauterine Devices (IUDs)," in R. A. Hatcher et al., eds., *Contraceptive Technology*, 19th ed. (New York: Ardent Media, 2007), 117–43.

5   Andra James, "Women's Health," National Blood Clot Alliance, www
    .stoptheclot.org/learn_more/womens_health_faq.htm.

6   A Tantric word to describe the nectars that flow from the womb.

7   George C. Denniston, Frederick Mansfield Hodges, and Marilyn Fayre
    Milos, eds., *Circumcision and Human Rights* (Berlin: Springer Science
    +Business Media, 2008), 7.

8   "Circumcision for Women: The Kindest Cut of All," *Playgirl* magazine, Octo-
    ber 1973.

9   ACOG Committee on Gynecologic Practice, "Vaginal 'Rejuvenation' and
    Cosmetic Vaginal Procedures," ACOG Committee Opinion Number 378,
    September 2007 and Reaffirmed 2014, American Congress of Obstetri-
    cians and Gynecologists, www.acog.org/Resources-And-Publications
    /Committee-Opinions/Committee-on-Gynecologic-Practice/Vaginal
    -Rejuvenation-and-Cosmetic-Vaginal-Procedures.

10 Naomi Wolf, *Vagina: A Cultural History* (New York: Ecco, 2012), 208.

11 Fang Fu Ruan, *Sex in China: Studies in Sexology in Chinese Culture* (Berlin:
    Springer Science+Business Media, 2013), 59.

12 S. Freud, *The Question of Lay Analysis,* standard ed. (New York: W. W.
    Norton, 1990).

13 Produced by Lehn & Fink, New York. View the ad at http://thesocietypages
    .org/socimages/2008/08/21/vintage-zonite-douche-ads/.

14 Andrea Tone, *Devices and Desires: A History of Contraception in America,*
    1st ed. (New York: Hill and Wang, 2002).

15 Produced by the Lambert Pharmacal Company, 1920s.

16 M. McCullough and C. Farah, "The Role of Alcohol in Oral Carcinogenesis
    with Particular Reference to Alcohol-Containing Mouthwashes," *Australian
    Dental Journal* 53 (2008): 302–5.

17 Stephanie Ann Loesch, "Does Mouth Wash Cause Oral Cancer?" *SiOWfa15:
    Science in Our World: Certainty and Controversy,* October 22, 2015, https://
    sites.psu.edu/siowfa15/2015/10/22/does-mouth-wash-cause-oral-cancer/.

18 Andy Wright, "The 6 Weirdest Things Women Do to Their Vaginas," *Mother
    Jones,* February 2, 2012, www.motherjones.com/blogs/2010?page=560.

19 Youngs Drug Products Corporation, New York. View the ad at http://
    myria.com/22-vintage-ads-explain-how-smelling-bad-will-ruin-your-life
    /bidette-towelettes-1969.

20 Warner-Lambert Pharmaceutical Company, New Jersey. View the ad at
    http://myria.com/22-vintage-ads-explain-how-smelling-bad-will-ruin-your
    -life/pristeen-spray-deodorant-vintage-ad.

21 View the ad at www.newspapers.com/newspage/7926089/.

22 Nora Ephron, *Crazy Salad and Scribble Scribble: Some Things about Women and Notes on Media* (New York: Random House), 119.

23 Ibid., 120.

24 Norwich Pharmaceutical Company, New York, 1962. View the ad on page 16 of the August 1962 issue of *Ebony* magazine at https://books.google.com /books?id=59YDAAAAMBAJ.

25 View the ad at www.andrewburnett.com/tale-fannies/.

26 Amy Schumer, *The Girl with the Lower Back Tattoo* (New York: Gallery Books, 2016).

27 View at www.pinterest.com/livinglibations.

28 "Bacterial Vaginosis Fact Sheet," Office on Women's Health, U.S. Department of Health, www.womenshealth.gov/a-z-topics/bacterial-vaginosis.

29 Moises Velasquez-Manoff, "What's in Your Vagina?" *Slate*, January 11, 2013, www.slate.com/articles/health_and_science/medical_examiner/2013/01 /microbial_balance_in_vagina_miscarriage_infertility_pre_term_birth_linked.html.

30 Carey Hamilton, "Bacterial Vaginosis Often Goes Untreated," *Salt Lake Tribune*, March 2017, http://archive.sltrib.com/story.php?ref=/healthscience /ci_4820799.

31 E. H. Koumans, M. Sternberg, C. Bruce, G. McQuillan, J. Kendrick, M. Sutton, et al., "The Prevalence of Bacterial Vaginosis in the United States, 2001–2004: Associations with Symptoms, Sexual Behaviors, and Reproductive Health," *Sexually Transmitted Diseases* 34, no. 11 (2007): 864–69.

32 Andrea Donsky, "Is There Pesticide Residue on Your Tampons? Our Independent Testing Gets Specific," *Naturally Savvy*, August 15, 2013, http:// naturallysavvy.com/care/is-there-pesticide-residue-on-your-tampons-our -independent-testing-gets-specific.

33 "Persistent, Bioaccumulative and Toxic (PBT) Chemical Program: Dioxins and Furans," U.S. Environmental Protection Agency, www.epa.gov/pbt /pubs/dioxins.htm.

34 Cameron Diaz, *The Body Book* (New York: HarperWave, 2013).

35 D. E. Tourgeman et al., "Serum and Tissue Hormone Levels of Vaginally and Orally Administered Estradiol," *American Journal of Obstetrics and Gynecology* 180, no. 6 (1999): 1480–83, http://dx.doi.org/10.1016/S0002-9378(99) 70042-6.

36 Wolf, *Vagina*, 19.

37 B. Ottesen, B. Pedersen, J. Nielsen, D. Dalgaard, G. Wagner, and J. Fahren-krug, "Vasoactive Intestinal Polypeptide (VIP) Provokes Vaginal Lubrication in Normal Women," *Peptides* 8, no. 5 (September–October 1987): 797–800.

38 Lauren K. Wolf, "Studies Raise Questions about Safety of Personal Lubricants," *Chemical and Engineering News* 90, no. 50: 46–47.

39 Thomas R. Moench, "Microbicide Excipients Can Greatly Increase Susceptibility to Genital Herpes Transmission in the Mouse," *BMC Infectious Diseases* 10 (2010): 331.

40 Ibid.

41 L. Anderson, S. E. Lewis, and N. McClure, "The Effects of Coital Lubricants on Sperm Motility in Vitro," *Human Reproduction* 13, no. 12 (December 1998): 3351–56.

42 R. S. Sandhu, T. H. Wong, C. A. Kling, and K. R. Chohan, "In Vitro Effects of Coital Lubricants and Synthetic and Natural Oils on Sperm Motility," *Fertility and Sterility* 101, no. 4 (April 2014): 941–44.

43 "Shailene Woodley," *Into the Gloss*, March 2014, https://intothegloss.com/2014/03/shailene-woodley-hair/.

44 Joni Mitchell, "Woodstock," *Ladies of the Canyon*, A&M Studios, Los Angeles, March 1970.

CHAPTER ELEVEN

1 Beyoncé, 2017 Grammy performance, reciting poetry from Somalian-born poet Warsan Shire.

2 Robert Tisserand and Tony Balacs, *Essential Oil Safety: A Guide for Health Care Professionals* (London: Churchill Livingstone, 1995), 111.

3 Ibid., 3.

4 Ibid., 3, 105.

5 Ibid., 111.

6 Hafiz, "Circles," *I Heard God Laughing,* 26.

7 Mildred Seelig, *Magnesium Deficiency in the Pathogenesis of Disease: Early Roots of Cardiovascular, Skeletal and Renal Abnormalities* (New York: Goldwater Memorial Hospital, New York University Medical Center, 1980), www.mgwater.com/Seelig/Magnesium-Deficiency-in-the-Pathogenesis-of-Disease/chapter3.shtml.

8 Elise S. Pelzer et al., "Microorganisms within Human Follicular Fluid: Effects on IVF," *PLoS ONE* 8, no. 3 (2013).

9 Marie Ellis, "Stress in Pregnancy Linked to Offspring's Asthma Risk," *Medical News Today,* August 1, 2014, www.medicalnewstoday.com /articles/280514.php.

10 B. Xu, J. Pekkanen, M. R. Järvelin, P. Olsen, and A. L. Hartikainen, "Maternal Infections in Pregnancy and the Development of Asthma among Offspring," *International Journal of Epidemiology* 28, no. 4 (1999): 723–27.

11 "Premature Babies," U.S. National Library of Medicine, National Institutes of Health, www.nlm.nih.gov/medlineplus/prematurebabies.html.

12 Rajiv Saini, Santosh Saini, and Sugandha R. Saini, "Periodontitis: A Risk for Delivery of Premature Labor and Low-Birth-Weight Infants," *Journal of Natural Science, Biology and Medicine* 1, no. 1 (July–December 2010): 40–42.

13 Maria G. Dominguez-Bello et al., "Partial Restoration of the Microbiota of Cesarean-Born Infants via Vaginal Microbial Transfer," *Nature Medicine* 22, no. 3 (March 2016): 250–53.

14 Ewen Callaway, "Scientists Swab C-Section Babies with Mothers' Microbes," *Nature,* February 2016, www.nature.com/news/scientists-swab-c-section -babies-with-mothers-microbes-1.19275.

15 Anaïs Nin, quoted in Dan Millman, *Living on Purpose: Straight Answers to Life's Tough Questions* (Novato, CA: New World Library, 2000), 4.

16 Gibran, "On Children," *The Prophet,* 18.

17 O. R. C. Smales and R. Kime, "Thermoregulation in Babies Immediately after Birth," *Archives of Disease in Childhood* 53 (1978): 58–61.

18 H. T. Akinbi et al., "Host Defense Proteins in Vernix Caseosa and Amniotic Fluid," *American Journal of Obstetrics and Gynecology* 191, no. 6 (December 2004): 2090–96.

19 S. J. McDonald, "Effect of Timing of Umbilical Cord Clamping of Term Infants on Maternal and Neonatal Outcomes," *Cochrane Database of Systematic Reviews* 7 (July 11, 2013): CD004074.

20 T. N. K. Raju and N. Singhal, "Optimal Timing for Clamping the Umbilical Cord after Birth," *Clinics in Perinatology* 39, no. 4 (2012): 889–900, http:// doi.org/10.1016/j.clp.2012.09.006.

21 Hafiz, *I Heard God Laughing,* 3.

22 For further reading: Lisa Reagan, "Big Bad Cavities: Breastfeeding Is Not the Cause," *Mothering* 113 (July–August 2002), http://mothering.com /health/big-bad-cavities-breastfeeding-is-not-the-cause.

23 P. S. Pannaraj, F. Li, C. Cerini, J. M. Bender, S. Yang, A. Rollie, H. Adisetiyo, S. Zabih, P. J. Lincez, K. Bittinger, A. Bailey, F. D. Bushman, J. W. Sleasman,

and G. M. Aldrovandi, "Association between Breast Milk Bacterial Communities and Establishment and Development of the Infant Gut Microbiome," *Journal of the American Medical Association of Pediatrics*, May 8, 2017, doi:10.1001/jamapediatrics.2017.0378.

24 National Center for Environmental Health, "Perchlorate in Baby Formula Fact Sheet," CDC, April 2009, www.cdc.gov/nceh/features/perchlorate _factsheet.htm.

25 Laura McClure, "Which Infant Formulas Contain Secret Toxic Chemicals?" *Mother Earth News,* July 12, 2010, www.motherjones.com/blue-marble/2010 /07/infant-formula-similac-enfamil-melamine-bpa.

26 Sayer Ji, "Chemicals as 'Nutrients' in 'USDA Organic' Infant Formula," GreenMedInfo, www.greenmedinfo.com/blog/chemicals-nutrients-usda-organic -infant-formula.

27 Kenneth Setchell, "Exposure of Infants to Phyto-oestrogens from Soy-Based Infant Formula," *The Lancet* 350, no. 9070 (July 5, 1997): 23–27.

28 Joseph Mercola, "Soy Formula: The Popular Food You Should Never, Ever Feed Your Baby," April 2, 2011, *Mercola,* http://articles.mercola.com/sites /articles/archive/2011/04/02/soy-formula-linked-to-fibroid-tumors.aspx.

29 For more information, visit WestonAPrice.org or contact them at info@ westonaprice.org.

30 Additionally, tons of fabric baby wipes are available on Etsy.

31 Rumi, "Birdwings," *Rumi: Selected Poems* (London: Penguin Books, 1995), 174.

CHAPTER TWELVE

1 Heinrich Heine, *Wit, Wisdom, and Pathos: From the Prose of Heinrich Heine,* trans. John Snodgrass (Boston: Couples and Herd, 1888), 3.

2 Robbins, *Jitterbug Perfume,* 399.

3 Richard Le Gallienne, *The Romance of Perfume* (New York: Richard Hudnut, 1928), 19.

4 Ibid., 14.

5 Julia Lawless, *Aromatherapy and the Mind* (San Francisco: Thorsons, 1995), 15.

6 The Bastide du Parfumeur in Grasse, a conservatory of aromatic plants, preserves the history and local heritage of perfume plants.

7 Le Gallienne, *The Romance of Perfume,* 36.

8 Read more about the fascinating history of perfume: Eugene Rimmel, *The Book of Perfumes* (London: Chapman and Hall, 1867). Read it in full.

9 Patrick Süskind, *Perfume: The Story of a Murderer* (New York: Vintage, 2001).

10 Tisserand and Balacs, *Essential Oil Safety*, 28.

11 Le Gallienne, *The Romance of Perfume*, 9.

12 Exodus 30:22–31 (NIV).

13 Barks and Moyne, *The Drowned Book*, xxiii.

14 Ibid., 3.

15 "Citral," BASF, www.basf.com/group/corporate/en/news-and-media-relations /science-around-us/citral/story.

16 Lawrence Bergman, "Two-Hybrid Systems: Methods and Protocols," *Methods in Molecular Biology* 177: 9.

17 Iody Bomgardner, "The Sweet Scent of Microbes," *Chemical and Engineering News* 90, no. 29 (July 16, 2012): 25–29.

18 "Isobionics Introduces Natural Valencene Pure(TM)," 2010, www .thefreelibrary.com/Isobionics+Introduces+Natural+Valencene+Pure(TM) .-a0228250607.

19 Tanya Lewis, "Your Perfume May Soon Be Produced by Bacteria," *Wired*, July 19, 2012, www.wired.com/wiredscience/2012/07/bacteria -producing-aromas/.

20 Wiley-Blackwell, "Bacteria Manage Perfume Oil from Grass," November 7, 2008, www.sciencedaily.com/releases/2008/10/081031102053.htm.

21 Josep Peñuelas, Gerard Farré-Armengol, et al., "Removal of Floral Microbiota Reduces Floral Terpene Emissions," *Scientific Reports* 4 (October 22, 2014), www.nature.com/srep/2014/141022/srep06727/full/srep06727.html.

22 Juvenal, "Satires XIV," *Juvenal and Persius, vol. II* (Oxford, England: J. Vincent, 1839), 161.

23 Isonaline 70® is manufactured by DSM.

24 Becky M. Hess et al., "Coregulation of Terpenoid Pathway Genes and Prediction of Isoprene Production in *Bacillus subtilis* Using Transcriptomics," ed. Michael Otto, *PLoS ONE* 8, no. 6 (2013): e66104, www.ncbi.nlm.nih.gov /pmc/articles/PMC3686787/.

25 Kurt Schnaubelt, *Medical Aromatherapy: Healing with Essential Oils* (Berkeley, CA: Frog Books, 1999), 181.

26 Robbins, *Jitterbug Perfume*, 280.

27 Hsuan Hua, *The Flower Adornment Sutra*, http://cttbusa.org/fas1/fas _contents.asp.

28 Hada Bejar, quoted in Mary Mackenzie, *Peaceful Living* (Encinitas, CA: PuddleDancer Press, 2005), 236.

29 Robbins, *Jitterbug Perfume,* 76.

30 Rumi, quoted in William Chittick, *The Sufi Path of Love: The Spiritual Teachings of Rumi* (Albany, NY: State University of New York Press, 1983), 149.

31 Walt Whitman, *Leaves of Grass* (New York: Dover, 1982), 51.

32 Brian Handwerk, "Armpits Are 'Rain Forests' for Bacteria, Skin Map Shows," *National Geographic News,* May 28, 2009, http://news.nationalgeographic .com/news/2009/05/090528-armpits-bacteria-rainforests.html.

33 Diane Ackerman, *A Natural History of the Senses* (New York: Random House, 1990), 24.

34 Ibid.

35 Helen Keller, "Sense and Sensibility," *The Century Illustrated Monthly Magazine, vol. 75* (New York: Century Company, 1908), 574.

36 P. D. Darbre, "Underarm Cosmetics and Breast Cancer," *Journal of Applied Toxicology* 23, no. 2 (March–April 2003): 89–95.

37 John Emsley, "What's Inside Dove Original Deodorant," *Wired,* June 2010, www.wired.co.uk/magazine/archive/2010/07/start/whats-inside-dove -original-deodorant.

38 Melinda Wenner, "Birth Control Pills Affect Women's Taste in Men," *Scientific American,* December 1, 2008.

39 Sandalwood oil (at 5 percent dilution) was used topically for twenty weeks and decreased the incidence of skin papilloma and inhibited TPA and ODC activity, which are prominent in skin cancer. C. Dwivedi and Y. Zhang, "Sandalwood Oil Prevents Skin Tumor Development in Mice," *European Journal of Cancer Prevention* 8, no. 5 (October 1999): 449–55, www.ncbi.nlm.nih.gov /pubmed/10548401.

40 Oscar Wilde, *The Picture of Dorian Gray* (New York: Dover, 1993).

CHAPTER THIRTEEN

1 Plutarch, quoted in Martin Watt and Wanda Seller, *Frankincense & Myrrh* (Essex, England: C. W. Daniel Company, 1996), 71.

2 Martha Graham, "I Am a Dancer," *The Routledge Dance Studies Reader,* ed. Alexandra Carter (New York: Routledge, 1998), 68.

3 Avicenna, *Congelatione et conglutinatione lapidium* (1021–1023), trans. E. J. Hohnyard and D. C. Mandeville (Paris: Librarie Orientaiste, 1927), 20.

4 Hafiz, "It Felt Love," *The Gift,* 121.

5 Lawless, *Aromatherapy and the Mind,* 20.

6 Annick Le Guerer, *Scent: The Mysterious and Essential Powers of Smell,* trans. Philip Turner (New York: Kodansha International, 1994), 218.

7 Michel de Montaigne, "Of Smells," *Quotidiana,* ed. Patrick Madden, September 23, 2006, http://essays.quotidiana.org/montaigne/smells/.

8 Lawless, *Aromatherapy and the Mind,* 83.

9 *Beyond Scents* 1, no. 2 (Spring 1993), 8.

10 Suzanne Fischer-Rizzi, *The Complete Aromatherapy Handbook* (New York: Sterling, 1990), 27.

11 Anonymous, "From the Kaushitaki Upanishad," *The Upanishads,* trans. Juan Mascaró (London: Penguin Books, 1965), 106.

12 Jane Kenyon, "February: Thinking of Flowers," *Otherwise: New and Selected Poems* (Minneapolis, MN: Graywolf Press, 1996), 85.

13 "Nurse Wellness," Vanderbilt University Medical Center, www.mc .vanderbilt.edu/root/vumc.php?site=nurse-wellness&doc=41043.

14 Ibid.

15 "Generally Recognized as Safe (GRAS)," FDA, www.fda.gov/Food /IngredientsPackagingLabeling/GRAS/.

16 Hippocrates, quoted in Samuel L. Metcalfe, *Caloric: Its Mechanical, Chemical, and Vital Agencies in the Phenomena of Nature,* vol. 2 (London: William Pickering, 1843), 1065.

17 David K. Osborn, "The Water Cure," Greek Medicine, www.greekmedicine .net/therapies/The_Water_Cure.html.

18 "Gua Sha Treatment," *Cultural China,* http://kaleidoscope.cultural-china .com/en/207Kaleidoscope742.html.

19 Ibid.

20 James C. Jackson, *How to Treat the Sick without Medicine* (New York: Austin, Jackson, & Company, 1868), 31.

21 Shelton, *The Hygienic System,* 239.

22 Saleeby, *Sunlight and Health,* 140.

23 Sylvia Plath, *The Unabridged Journals of Sylvia Plath* (New York: Anchor, 2000), 75–76.

24 Paavo Airola, *How to Get Well* (Phoenix: Health Plus Publishers, 1974), 239.

25 Sylvia Plath, *The Bell Jar* (New York: Harper Perennial, 2005), 19.

26 Thoreau, *Walden,* 96.

27 Tom Ford, quoted in "My List: Tom Ford in 24 Hours," *Harper's Bazaar*, February 8, 2012, www.harpersbazaar.com/fashion/trends/a856/24-hours-with-tom-ford-0312/.

28 These types of molds are easily found on Amazon or eBay and are handy for making the Tooth Butter Cups in Chapter Eight, the yoni Soothing Suppository in Chapter Ten, and the Botanical-Biotic Suppositories in Chapter Sixteen.

29 Thomas Moore, "Paradise and the Peri," *The Poetical Works of Thomas Moore* (Paris: A. & W. Galignani, 1827), 25.

CHAPTER FOURTEEN

1 The FDA has not defined the term "natural" and has not established a regulatory definition for this term in cosmetic labeling.

2 Take, for example, bottled aloe vera gel that is labeled 100 percent pure. There are likely nonorganic chemicals used in its processing that do not have to be put on the ingredients list. These gels also include preservatives and thickeners . . . or even worse, green coloring. This is not 100 percent pure aloe vera.

3 "Multi-ingredient agricultural products in the 'Made with organic' category must contain at least 70 percent certified organic ingredients (not including salt or water). These products may contain up to 30 percent of allowed non-organic ingredients." USDA, "Organics 101," May 16, 2014, http://blogs.usda.gov/2014/05/16/organic-101-understanding-the-made-with-organic-label/. There is no single standard or protocol for what it means to be "organic." Every organic certifier has its own protocol to determine what percentage of synthetic ingredients can be in a product and still get an "organic" stamp of approval. Some are strict, and some are so ridiculously relaxed that the organic stamp has no meaning or authority.

4 "Therapeutic grade" is a made-up marketing term used by an essential-oils company in the United States. This is all a ploy; there are no standards or grades of essential oils nor are there authentication processes to verify them. There are also no governing bodies to crack down on this type of marketing. Read this very interesting article on "therapeutic grade" in Cropwatch: http://cropwatch.org.uk/Therapeutic%20Grade%20Essential%20Oils%20corrected.pdf.

5 The FDA does not maintain a list of noncomedogenic cosmetic ingredients, and there aren't standardized tests to determine if a product is comedogenic. So, claims by manufacturers that ingredients are or are not comedogenic have limited usefulness.

6 "There are no Federal standards or definitions that govern the use of the term 'hypoallergenic.' The term means whatever a particular company wants it to mean. Manufacturers of cosmetics labeled as hypoallergenic are not required to submit substantiation of their hypoallergenicity claims to FDA." "Labeling," FDA, www.fda.gov/Cosmetics/Labeling/Claims/ucm2005203.htm.

7 Russel M. Walters, Guangru Mao, Euen T. Gunn, and Sidney Hornby, "Cleansing Formulations That Respect Skin Barrier Integrity," *Dermatology Research and Practice,* 2012: 495917, www.ncbi.nlm.nih.gov/pmc/articles/PMC3425021/.

8 Hafiz, *I Heard God Laughing,* 8.

9 For a list of common harmful ingredients found in cosmetics, read "Deciphering Cosmetic Codes" at www.livinglibations.com/default/body-care-articles/body-care-articles/the_whole_being/deciphering_cosmetic_codes.

10 Coleman Barks, "Mathnawi IV," *The Essential Rumi* (San Francisco: HarperOne, 2004), 2683–96.

CHAPTER FIFTEEN

1 Marcus Aurelius, quoted in Julia Cameron and Emma Lively, *It's Never Too Late to Begin Again* (New York: TarcherPerigee, 2016), 76.

2 R. M. Gattefossé, quoted in Jean Valnet, *The Practice of Aromatherapy* (London: Vermillion, 2011), 11–12.

3 *Materia medica* translates from the Latin as "medical matter": a traditional text or treatise that defines the composition and use of botanical substances for medical remedies.

4 D. Hettiarachchi et al., "Western Australia Sandalwood Seed Oil: New Opportunities," *Lipid Technology* 22, no. 2 (February 2010): 27–29.

5 Brigitte Mars, *The Desktop Guide to Herbal Medicine* (Surry Hills, Australia: Accessible Publishing Systems, 2008), 134.

6 Schnaubelt, *Advanced Aromatherapy,* 62.

7 Harvey Grady, "Immunomodulation through Castor Oil Packs," *Journal of Naturopathic Medicine* 7, no. 1 (1999).

8 Nathaniel Altman, *The Honey Prescription* (Rochester, VT: Healing Arts Press, 2010), 123.

9 Jane-Ling Wang, "Jeanne Louise Calment: World's Oldest," Department of Statistics, University of California, Davis, http://anson.ucdavis.edu/~wang/calment.html.

10 Dave Oomah, "Characteristics of Red Raspberry Seed," *Food Chemistry* 69, no. 2 (May 2000): 187–93.

11 Gibran, *The Prophet*, 55.

12 Kurt Schnaubelt, *The Healing Intelligence of Essential Oils* (Rochester, VT: Healing Arts Press, 2011), 52.

13 Schnaubelt, *Medical Aromatherapy*, 205.

14 Ibid., 211.

15 Peter Holmes, *Aromatica: A Clinical Guide to Essential Oil Therapeutics* (Philadelphia: Singing Dragon, 2016), 191.

16 Kathi Keville and Mindy Green, *Aromatherapy: A Complete Guide to the Healing Art* (Freedom, CA: Crossing Press, 2008).

17 Schnaubelt, *The Healing Intelligence of Essential Oils*, 178.

18 Schnaubelt, *Medical Aromatherapy*, 214.

19 Schnaubelt, *The Healing Intelligence of Essential Oils*, 51.

20 Schnaubelt, *Medical Aromatherapy*, 185.

21 Lawless, *Aromatherapy and the Mind*.

22 Schnaubelt, *The Healing Intelligence of Essential Oils*, 179.

23 Schnaubelt, *Medical Aromatherapy*.

24 Schnaubelt, *The Healing Intelligence of Essential Oils*, 129.

25 "Bowles (2003) gives the main constituents of niaouli from Madagascar as 1,8-cineole at 41.8%, viridiflorol (a sesquiterpene alcohol) at 18.1% and limonene at 5% . . . A study conducted by Donoyama and Ichiman (2006) revealed that niaouli was the best oil for 'hygienic massage practice,' in that it showed greater anti-bacterial activity than eucalyptus, lavender, sage, tea tree and thyme linalool in relation to the bacteria found on the therapists' hands and the subjects' skin." Jennifer Peace Rhind, *Essential Oils: A Handbook for Aromatherapy Practice* (Philadelphia: Singing Dragon, 2012), 195.

26 Roberta Wilson, *Aromatherapy: Essential Oils for Vibrant Health and Beauty* (New York: Avery, 1995).

27 Holmes, *Aromatica*, 278.

28 Schnaubelt, *Advanced Aromatherapy,* 118.

29 Kaur, "Skin Cancer Chemopreventive Agent, {Alpha}-Santalol, Induces Apoptotic Death of Human Epidermoid Carcinoma A431 Cells."

30 X. Zhang et al., "Alpha-Santalol, a Chemopreventive Agent against Skin Cancer, Causes G_2/M Cell Cycle Arrest in Both p53-Mutated Human Epidermoid Carcinoma A431 Cells and p53 Wild-Type Human Melanoma UACC-62 Cells," *BMC Research Notes* 3 (2010): 220, https://bmcresnotes .biomedcentral.com/articles/10.1186/1756-0500-3-220.

31 Schnaubelt, *Advanced Aromatherapy,* 93.

32 Holmes, *Aromatica,* 359.

33 Lawless, *Aromatherapy and the Mind,* 133.

34 M. T. Corasaniti, J. Maiuolo, S. Maida, V. Fratto, M. Navarra, R. Russo, D. Amantea, L. A. Morrone, et al., "Cell Signaling Pathways in the Mechanisms of Neuroprotection Afforded by Bergamot Essential Oil against NMDA-Induced Cell Death In Vitro," *British Journal of Pharmacology* 151 (2007): 518–29.

35 M. Borgatti, I. Mancini, N. Bianchi, A. Guerrini, I. Lampronti, D. Rossi, G. Sacchetti, and R. Gambari, "Bergamot (Citrus bergamia Risso) Fruit Extracts and Identified Components Alter Expression of Interleukin 8 Gene in Cystic Fibrosis Bronchial Epithelial Cell Lines," *BMC Biochemistry* 12 (2011): 15.

36 Shaila V. Kothiwale, Vivek Patwardhan, Megha Gandhi, Rahul Sohoni, and Ajay Kumar, "A Comparative Study of Antiplaque and Antigingivitis Effects of Herbal Mouthrinse Containing Tea Tree Oil, Clove, and Basil with Commercially Available Essential Oil Mouthrinse," *Journal of Indian Society Periodontology* 18, no. 3 (May–June 2014): 316–20.

37 Aloe vera is a fascinating plant. Dig deeper into its history and uses: Amar Surjushe, Resham Vasani, and D. G. Saple, "Aloe Vera: A Short Review," *Indian Journal of Dermatology* 53, no. 4 (2008): 163–66.

38 Rumi, *The Essential Rumi,* 222.

39 Len Price and Shirley Price, *Understanding Hydrolats: The Specific Hydrosols for Aromatherapy: A Guide for Health Professionals* (Edinburgh: Churchill Livingstone, 2004), 135.

40 For more information on the Keyes Method, the *Saturday Evening Post* has an interview with Dr. Thomas Rams, the Paul H. Keyes Professor of Periodontology at Temple University School of Dentistry in Philadelphia: www.thefreelibrary.com/ /taking+the+bite+out+of+gum+disease %3a+an+interview+with+thomas+Rams,...-a0160421172.

41 Rudolf Steiner, *Nine Lectures on Bees,* http://wn.rsarchive.org/Lectures /GA351/English/SGP1975/NinBee_index.html.

42 T. Alandejani et al., "Effectiveness of Honey on Staphylococcus aureus and Pseudomonas aeruginosa Biofilms," *Otolaryngology and Head and Neck Surgery* 141, no. 1 (July 2009): 114–18, www.ncbi.nlm.nih.gov /pubmed/19559969.

43 P. C. Molan, "The Evidence Supporting the Use of Honey as a Wound Dressing," *International Journal of Lower Extremity Wounds,* March 1, 2006.

44 Winit Phuapradit, "Topical Application of Honey in Treatment of Abdominal Wound Disruption," *Australian and New Zealand Journal of Obstetrics and Gynaecology* 32, no. 4 (November 1992): 381–84.

45 N. S. Al-Waili, "Mixture of Honey, Beeswax and Olive Oil Inhibits Growth of Staphylococcus aureus and Candida albicans," *Archives of Medical Research* 36, no. 1 (January–February 2005): 10–13.

46 Tullio Simoncini, "Treatment Skin Cancer," Cure Naturali Cancro, www .curenaturalicancro.com/en/simoncini-treatment-skin-cancer/.

47 **Reactive skin:** Audrey Guéniche, Philippe Bastien, Jean Marc Ovigne, Michel Kermici, Guy Courchay, Veronique Chevalier, Lionel Breton, and Isabelle Castiel-Higounenc, "*Bifidobacterium longum* Lysate, a New Ingredient for Reactive Skin," *Experimental Dermatology* 19, no. 8 (August 2010): e1–e8, http://onlinelibrary.wiley.com/doi/10.1111/j.1600-0625.2009.00932.x /full?refreshCitedByCounter=true.

    Acne: Whitney P. Bowe and Alan C. Logan, "Acne Vulgaris, Probiotics and the Gut-Brain-Skin Axis—Back to the Future?" *Gut Pathogens* 3, no. 1 (2011), https://gutpathogens.biomedcentral.com /articles/10.1186/1757-4749-3-1.

    Inflammation: Teruaki Nakatsuji et al., "Dermatological Therapy by Topical Application of Non-Pathogenic Bacteria," *Journal of Investigative Dermatology* 134, no. 1 (January 2014): 11–14, www.jidonline.org/article /S0022-202X(15)36443-5/fulltext.

    Barrier function: Benedetta Cinque, Cristina La Torre, Esterina Melchiorre, Giuseppe Marchesani, Giovanni Zoccali, Paola Palumbo, Luisa Di Marzio, Alessandra Masci, and Luciana Mosca, "Use of Probiotics for Dermal Applications," *Probiotics,* vol. 21 of the series Microbiology Monographs, June 2011: 221–41, https://link.springer.com/chapter/10.1007 /978-3-642-20838-6_9.

Collagen, aging, and the sun: H. M. Kim, D. E. Lee, S. D. Park, Y. T. Kim, Y. J. Kim, J. W. Jeong, S. S. Jang, Y. T. Ahn, J. H. Sim, C. S. Huh, D. K. Chung, and J. H. Lee, "Oral Administration of Lactobacillus plantarum HY7714 Protects Hairless Mouse against Ultraviolet B-Induced Photoaging," *Journal of Microbiology and Biotechnology* 24, no. 11 (November 28, 2014): 1583–91.

CHAPTER SIXTEEN

1. Hafiz, "Now Is the Time," *The Gift,* 160–61.
2. Johann Wolfgang von Goethe, *The Maxims and Reflections of Goethe,* trans. Bailey Saunders (New York: Macmillan, 1906), 171.
3. Toni Morrison, *The Bluest Eye* (New York: Vintage, 2007), 176.
4. Schnaubelt, *The Healing Intelligence of Essential Oils,* 136–37.
5. Easily found on eBay or Amazon.

CHAPTER SEVENTEEN

1. Paracelsus, *Selected Writings,* trans. Norbert Guterman (Princeton, NJ: Princeton University Press, 1995), 50.
2. Beyoncé, 2017 Grammy performance.
3. Phyllis Diller, quoted in Steven Pollack, *Ask the Chiropractor* (New York: iUniverse, 2004), 99.
4. Peggy Freydberg, *Poems from the Pond: 107 Years of Words and Wisdom* (Los Angeles: Hybrid Nation, 2015), 100.
5. J. Kulkarni, "Depression as a Side Effect of the Contraceptive Pill," *Expert Opinion on Drug Safety* 6, no. 4 (July 2007): 371–74.
6. T. Piltonen, "Oral, Transdermal and Vaginal Combined Contraceptives Induce an Increase in Markers of Chronic Inflammation and Impair Insulin Sensitivity in Young Healthy Normal-Weight Women: A Randomized Study," *Human Reproduction* 27, no. 10 (October 2012): 3046–56, doi: 10.1093/humrep/des225.
7. F. Zal, "Effect of Vitamin E and C Supplements on Lipid Peroxidation and GSH-Dependent Antioxidant Enzyme Status in the Blood of Women Consuming Oral Contraceptives," *Contraception* 86, no. 1 (July 2012): 62–66.
8. "Long-Term Oral Contraceptive Users Are Twice as Likely to Have Serious Eye Disease," *American Academy of Ophthalmology,* November 18, 2013.

9 Terry Gordon, professor of environmental medicine, New York University, in Scilla Alecci, "In Online Forums, Women Share Copper IUD Fears," March 30, 2015, http://womensenews.org/2015/03/in-online-forums-women-share -copper-iud-fears.

10 Billings Ovulation Method, www.billingsmethod.com/.

11 The Fertility Awareness Center, www.fertaware.com/faqs/what-is-fertility -awareness/.

12 Jyotsna A. Saonere Suryawanshi, "Neem—Natural Contraceptive for Male and Female—an Overview," *International Journal of Biomolecules and Bio- medicine* 1, no. 2 (2011): 1–6.

13 N. D. Vietmeyer, *Neem: A Tree for Solving Global Problems*, report of an ad hoc panel of the Board on Science and Technology for International Devel- opment, National Research Council (Washington, DC: National Academy Press, 1992), 71–72.

14 S. N. Upadhyay, S. Dhawan, and G. P. Talwar, "Antifertility Effects of Neem Oil in Male Rats by Single Intra-Vas Administration: An Alternate Approach to Vasectomy," *Journal of Andrology* 14, no. 4 (1993): 275–81.

15 Robbins, *Still Life with Woodpecker*, 14.

16 We use Kinesio Tape for making "homemade" bandages.

17 Naomi Wolf, *The Beauty Myth* (New York: Perennial, 2002), 187.

18 Modified excerpt from Meghan Telpner, *UnDiet: Eat Your Way to Vibrant Health* (Toronto: McClelland & Stewart, 2013).

19 W. C. Willett, "The Role of Dietary n-6 Fatty Acids in the Prevention of Car- diovascular Disease," *Journal of Cardiovascular Medicine* 8, Suppl. 1 (Sep- tember 2007): S42–S45.

20 For more information, read Ancel Keys's Seven Countries Study, www .sevencountriesstudy.com/.

21 P. W. Siri-Tarino, Q. Sun, et al., "Meta-analysis of Prospective Cohort Studies Evaluating the Association of Saturated Fat with Cardiovascular Disease," *American Journal of Clinical Nutrition* 91, no. 3 (2010): 535–46.

22 A. J. Arias, K. Steinberg, A. Banga, and R. L. Trestman, "Systematic Review of the Efficacy of Meditation Techniques as Treatments for Medical Illness," *Journal of Alternative and Complementary Medicine* 12, no. 8 (October 2006): 817–32.

23 E. Shonin, W. Van Gordon, and M. D. Griffiths, "Meditation Awareness Train- ing (MAT) for Improved Psychological Well-Being: A Qualitative Examination of Participant Experiences," *Journal of Religion and Health* 53 (2014): 849.

24 Wendy Hasenkamp and Lawrence W. Barsalou, "Effects of Meditation Experience on Functional Connectivity of Distributed Brain Networks," *Frontiers in Human Neuroscience,* March 1, 2012.

25 Britta K. Hölze, "Mindfulness Practice Leads to Increases in Regional Brain Gray Matter Density," *Psychiatry Research and Neuroimaging* 191, no. 1 (January 30, 2011): 36–43.

26 Zeidan Fadel et al., "Mindfulness Meditation Improves Cognition: Evidence of Brief Mental Training," *Consciousness and Cognition* 19, no. 2 (June 2010): 597–605.

27 Ron Alexander, *Wise Mind, Open Mind* (Oakland, CA: New Harbinger, 2009).

28 Lorenza S. Colzato, Ayca Ozturk, and Bernhard Hommel, "Meditate to Create: The Impact of Focused-Attention and Open-Monitoring Training on Convergent and Divergent Thinking," *Frontiers in Psychology,* April 18, 2012.

29 A. D. Cohen et al., "Cherry Angiomas Associated with Exposure to Bromides," *Dermatology* 202, no. 1 (2001): 52–53.

30 I. E. Sadowski, "Methyl Bromide Toxicity: What's on Your Strawberries?" *Mother Earth News,* August–September 2001, www.motherearthnews.com /organic-gardening/methyl-bromide-toxicity-whats-on-your-strawberries -zmaz01aszsel.

31 Animal and *in vitro* tests have demonstrated this: Y. D. Sharma, "Effect of Sodium Fluoride on Collagen Cross-Link Precursors," *Toxicology Letters* 10, no. 1 (January 1982): 97–100; B. Uslu, "Effect of Fluoride on Collagen Synthesis in the Rat," *Research in Experimental Medicine* 182 (1983): 7–12.

32 CDC, "About Antibiotic Use and Resistance," www.cdc.gov/getsmart /community/about/index.html/uri/ear-infection.html.

33 Thomas R. Abrahamsson and Hedvig E. Jakobsson, "Low Diversity of the Gut Microbiota in Infants with Atopic Eczema," *Journal of Allergy and Clinical Immunology* 129, no. 2 (February 2012): 434–40.

34 University of Michigan Health System, "Staph Infections & Eczema: What's the Connection?" *Science Daily,* October 30, 2013, www.sciencedaily.com /releases/2013/10/131030142414.htm.

35 Baoru Yang, "Effects of Dietary Supplementation with Sea Buckthorn (*Hippophaë rhamnoides)* Seed and Pulp Oils on Atopic Dermatitis," *Journal of Nutritional Biochemistry* (Impact Factor: 4.55) 10, no. 11 (November 1999): 622–30.

36 Food Allergy Research & Education, "Food Allergy Facts and Statistics for the U.S.," www.foodallergy.org/file/facts-stats.pdf.

37 Ralph Waldo Emerson, *Journals of Ralph Waldo Emerson: With Annotations,* vol. 6 (Boston: Houghton Mifflin, 1911), 410.

38 John D. McPherson, Brian H. Shilton, and Donald J. Walton, "Role of Fructose in Glycation and Cross-Linking of Proteins," *Biochemistry* 27, no. 6 (1988): 1901–7.

39 There are so many beautiful options straight from Turkey on etsy.com.

40 Young Hye Cho et al., "Effect of Pumpkin Seed Oil on Hair Growth in Men with Androgenetic Alopecia: A Randomized, Double-Blind, Placebo-Controlled Trial," *Evidence-Based Complementary and Alternative Medicine: eCAM* 2014 (2014): 549721.

41 A. D. Katsambas, A. J. Stratigo, T. M. Lotti, et al., "Melasma," *European Handbook of Dermatological Treatments,* 2nd ed. (Berlin: Springer, 2003), 336–41, www.aad.org/skin-conditions/dermatology-a-to-z/melasma/who-gets-causes/melasma-who-gets-and-causes; P. E. Grimes, "Melasma: Etiologic and Therapeutic Considerations," *Archives of Dermatological Research* 131 (1995): 1453–57; Holly Grigg-Spall, *Sweetening the Pill: or How We Got Hooked on Hormonal Birth Control* (Winchester, UK: Zero Books, 2013); Annika Höhn and Tilman Grune, "Lipofuscin: Formation, Effects and Role of Macroautophagy," *Redox Biology* 1, no. 1 (2013): 140–44; Jordan Lite, "Vitamin D Deficiency Soars in the U.S., Study Says," March 23, 2009, www.scientificamerican.com/article.cfm?id=vitamin-d-deficiency-united-states; M. B. Purba, A. Kouris-Blazos, N. Wattanapenpaiboon, et al., "Skin Wrinkling: Can Food Make a Difference?" *Journal of American College of Nutrition* 20 (2001): 71–80; Y. Kohjimoto, T. Ogawa, et al., "Effects of Acetyl-L-Carnitine on the Brain Lipofuscin Content and Emotional Behavior in Aged Rats," *Japanese Journal of Pharmacology* 48, no. 3 (November 1988): 365–71; "Topical Application of EFAs Is Effective at Delivering Skin Healing Oils and Nutrients to the Skin and Body": For more information, read the Linus Pauling Institute's summary of EFAs and skin health, and M. Press, P. J. Hartop, and C. Prottey, "Correction of Essential Fatty-Acid Deficiency in Man by the Cutaneous Application of Sunflower-Seed Oil," *The Lancet* 1 (1974): 597–98; G. S. Jutley, R. Rajaratnam, J. Halpern, A. Salim, and C. Emmett, "Systematic Review of Randomized Controlled Trials on Interventions for Melasma: An Abridged Cochrane Review," *Journal of the American Academy of Dermatology* 70, no. 2 (February 2014): 369–73; B. Yang and H. P. Kallio, "Fatty Acid Composition of Lipids in Sea Buckthorn (Hippophaë rhamnoides L.) Berries of Different Origins," *Journal of Agricultural Food Chemistry* 49, no. 4 (April 2001): 1939–47;

H. Ando, A. Ryu, A. Hashimoto, M. Oka, and M. Ichihashi, "Linoleic Acid and Alpha-Linolenic Acid Lightens Ultraviolet-Induced Hyperpigmentation of the Skin," *Archives of Dermatological Research* 290, no. 7 (July 1998): 375–81; S. W. Hwang et al., "Clinical Efficacy of 25% L-Ascorbic Acid (C'ensil) in the Treatment of Melasma," *Journal of Cutaneous Medicine and Surgery* 13, no. 2 (March–April 2009): 74–81.

42 Sally Fallon Morel, "Skin Deep," Weston A. Price Foundation, September 24, 2010, www.westonaprice.org/health-topics/skin-deep/.

43 William Shakespeare, *Macbeth*, Act 5, Scene 1.

44 Many olive oils are really oil blends, and companies are not required to own up to that on the label. Finding fresh, unadulterated olive oil can be difficult. To discover how to find and select a really real extra-virgin olive oil, check out the website ExtraVirginity.com.

45 Hsin-Yi Peng et al., "Effect of Vetiveria zizanioides Essential Oil on Melano-genesis in Melanoma Cells: Downregulation of Tyrosinase Expression and Suppression of Oxidative Stress," *Scientific World Journal* (2014).

46 Lane, "Aflatoxin, Tobacco, Ammonia and the p53 Tumor-Suppressor Gene."

47 Sandro Drago, "Gliadin, Zonulin and Gut Permeability: Effects on Celiac and Non-celiac Intestinal Mucosa and Intestinal Cell Lines," *Scandinavian Journal of Gastroenterology* 41, no. 4 (April 2006): 408–19.

48 S. Giuliani et al., "Intestinal Epithelial Barrier Dysfunction in Disease and Possible Therapeutical Interventions," *Current Medicinal Chemistry* 18, no. 3 (2011): 398–426.

49 Schnaubelt, *Advanced Aromatherapy*, 75.

50 "Exposures Add Up—Survey Results," EWG, www.ewg.org/skindeep/2004 /06/15/exposures-add-up-survey-results/.

51 Robbins, *Jitterbug Perfume*, 426.

52 Jerry Seinfeld, interview on *Good Morning America*, December 2012, www .youtube.com/watch?v=8T6uAMaRH3g.

53 Headspace.com is a subscription service for guided breathing and mindful-ness meditations.

54 Available on iTunes at https://itunes.apple.com/us/album/being-beauty -guided-meditation-to-feeling-beautiful/id1206139964.

55 Kelly Brogan, "3 Dietary Changes to Make before You Start an Anti-Depressant," January 23, 2014, www.huffingtonpost.com/kelly-brogan-md /diet-mental-health_b_4257003.html.

56 H. Tsao, C. Bevona, W. Goggins, and T. Quinn, "The Transformation Rate of Moles (Melanocytic Nevi) into Cutaneous Melanoma: A Population-Based Estimate," *Archives of Dermatology* 139 (2003): 282–88.

57 G. Argenziano, "Accuracy in Melanoma Detection: A 10-Year Multicenter Survey," *Journal of the American Academy of Dermatology* 67, no. 1 (July 2012): 54-59.

58 Mayo Clinic, "7 Fingernail Problems Not to Ignore," www.mayoclinic.org /healthy-living/adult-health/multimedia/nails/sls-20076131?s=1.

59 E. Mendelsohn, A. Hagopian, et al., "Nail Polish as a Source of Exposure to Triphenyl Phosphate," *Environment International* 86 (January 2016): 45–51.

60 Schnaubelt, *Medical Aromatherapy*, 226–27.

61 American Microbiome Institute, "Understanding the Nasal Microbiome," June 2015, www.microbiomeinstitute.org/blog/2015/6/7/understanding-the -nasal-microbiome.

62 N. A. Abreu, N. A. Nagalingam, et al., "Sinus Microbiome Diversity Depletion and Corynebacterium tuberculostearicum Enrichment Mediates Rhinosinusitis," *Science Translational Medicine* 4, no. 151 (September 12, 2012): 151RA124.

63 G. J. Leyer, S. Li, M. E. Mubasher, C. Reifer, and A. C. Ouwehand, "Probiotic Effects on Cold and Influenza-like Symptom Incidence and Duration in Children," *Pediatrics* 124 (2009): e172-79.

64 Poonam Sood, Aruna Devi, Ridhi Narang, Swathi V, Diljot Kaur Makkar, "Comparative Efficacy of Oil Pulling and Chlorhexidine on Oral Malodor: A Randomized Controlled Trial," *Journal of Clinical and Diagnostic Research* 8, no. 11 (November 2014): ZC18–ZC21.

65 "How Vitamin D Can Help Psoriasis," National Psoriasis Foundation, September 2015, www.psoriasis.org/advance/how-vitamin-d-can-help-psoriasis.

66 Stanisław Jarmuda and Niamh O'Reilly, "Potential Role of *Demodex* Mites and Bacteria in the Induction of Rosacea," *Journal of Medical Microbiology* 61 (November 2012): 1504–10.

67 American Academy of Dermatology, "Could Probiotics Be the Next Big Thing in Acne and Rosacea Treatments?"

68 Mauro Picardo and Monica Ottaviani, "Skin Microbiome and Skin Disease: The Example of Rosacea," *Journal of Clinical Gastroenterology* 48 (November–December 2014): S85–S86.

69 American Academy of Dermatology, "Could Probiotics Be the Next Big Thing in Acne and Rosacea Treatments?"

70 National Rosacea Society, "Rosacea Triggers Survey," www.rosacea.org /patients/materials/triggersgraph.php.

71 National Rosacea Society, "Skin Care & Cosmetics," www.rosacea.org /patients/skincare/index.php.

72 Amanda Chatel, "Will the Full Bush Continue into Summer?" July 2016, www.huffingtonpost.com/bustle/full-bush-trend-_b_5154274.html.

73 R. C. Cordeiro, K. G. Zecchin, and A. M. de Moraes, "Expression of Estrogen, Androgen, and Glucocorticoid Receptors in Recent Striae distensae," *International Journal of Dermatology* 49, no. 1 (January 2010): 30–32.

74 S. Güngör, T. Sayilgan, G. Gökdemir, and D. Ozcan, "Evaluation of an Ablative and Non-ablative Laser Procedure in the Treatment of Striae distensae," *Indian Journal of Dermatology, Venereology and Leprology* 80, no. 5 (September–October 2014): 409–12.

75 Elsaie, Baumann, and Elsaaiee, "Striae distensae (Stretch Marks) and Different Modalities of Therapy."

76 American Thyroid Association, "General Information," www.thyroid.org /media-main/about-hypothyroidism/.

77 Andrew Weil, "Varicose Veins," www.drweil.com/health-wellness/body-mind -spirit/feet/varicose-veins/.

78 Thomas Cleary, *The Flower Ornament Scripture* (Boston: Shambhala, 1993), 1642.

79 "Drinking up to 1L of a silicon-rich mineral water each day for 12 weeks facilitated the removal of aluminum via the urine in both patient and control groups without any concomitant affect upon the urinary excretion of the essential metals, iron and copper. We have provided preliminary evidence that over 12 weeks of silicon-rich mineral water therapy the body burden of aluminum fell in individuals with Alzheimer's disease and, concomitantly, cognitive performance showed clinically relevant improvements in at least 3 out of 15 individuals." S. Davenward et al., "Silicon-Rich Mineral Water as a Non-invasive Test of the 'Aluminum Hypothesis' in Alzheimer's Disease," *Journal of Alzheimer's Disease* 33, no. 2 (January 2013): 423–30.

80 Richard Buckminster Fuller, *I Seem to Be a Verb* (New York: Bantam, 1970), 101.

81 Masaru Emoto, *The Hidden Messages in Water*, trans. David Thayne (Hillsboro, OR: Beyond Words Publishing, 2004), xxii–xxv.

Image Credits

121 Robert Howard/Nadine Artemis
122 Robert Howard/Nadine Artemis
124 Robert Howard/Nadine Artemis
127 Robert Howard/Nadine Artemis
128 Robert Howard/Nadine Artemis
130 Robert Howard/Nadine Artemis
135 Robert Howard/Nadine Artemis
136 1. Nadine by Karen Dawnn
2. Birth of Venus, Sandro Botticelli, Uffizi Gallery
3. Rose by Spring Oz, Adobe Stock
4. 19th c. painting on Cahors theatre in France, Stephane Bidouze/Shutterstock
5. Two Tahitian Women, Gauguin, The Metropolitan Museum of Art
6. Ravana sculpture in the Dumar Lena Cave Temple (Cave 29), Ellora, India, photographer unknown, British Library Online Gallery
7. Deirdre Plomer Sketch
147 Robert Howard/Nadine Artemis
148 Robert Howard
150 Robert Howard/Nadine Artemis
153 Nadine Artemis/Deirdre Plomer
154 Robert Howard/Nadine Artemis
157 David Woodberry Shutterstock
160 Munimara Shutterstock
167 Ron Artemis
177 Nadine Artemis/Purple Flower by Riderfoot Shutterstock
178 Ron Artemis
183 J. Wong
185 J. Wong
192 Lauren Green
198 Lauren Green
205 Lauren Green
206 Lauren Green
209 Stavklem Shutterstock
211 Goldenjack Shutterstock
212 Lauren Green
215 Robert Howard
217 John Lehmann
218 Lauren Green
220 Ron Artemis
229 Robert Howard/Nadine Artemis/Kristy Bourgeois
230 Robert Howard/Nadine Artemis
231 Robert Howard/Nadine Artemis
232 Lauren Green
232 Lauren Green
233 Lauren Green
233 Lauren Green
238 Lauren Green
239 Susan E. Degginger Alamy Stock
239 Scisettialfio Megapixl.com
241 Jeyaprakash Maria Dreamstime
242 Svetlana Ileva Dreamstime
243 Yongkiet Jitwattanatam Shutterstock
245 Johannes Kornelius Shutterstock
246 Mario Adobestock.com
247 Samopauser Adobestock
248 Wikimedia Commons
249 Star Rush Adobe Stock
250 Scisettialfio Megapixl
251 Alexey Stiop Shutterstock
251 Tamara Kulikova Adobe Stock
252 Kubasiak Zbigniew Shutterstock
252 Lazarenko Megapixl
253 Digital Botany Shutterstock
254 Fotografiecor.nl Shutterstock
254 Ollinka Shutterstock
255 Shutterstock
256 1JMueller Shutterstock
257 Jen Petrie Shutterstock
257 Jukree Boonprasit123RF.com
258 Vicuschka Shutterstock
259 Nmsimoes Megapixl
259 Sandra Schwarzwald Shutterstock
260 Spring Oz Adobe Stock
260 DSLucas Shutterstock
261 All-Stock-Photos Shutterstock
262 Swapan Shutterstock
262 Tooykrub Shutterstock
263 Starover Sibiriak Shutterstock
264 Passakorn Umpornmaha Shutterstock
265 IngridHS Shutterstock

Index

G

GABA (gamma-aminobutyric acid), 61
Gattefossé, R. M., 240
geranium, 253
GERD (gastroesophageal reflux disease), 328–29
German chamomile, 254
Gertz, Jami, 13
Gibran, Kahlil, 3, 37, 41, 57, 84, 178, 198, 229
ginger root, 268
gliadin, 343–44
gluten, 83, 335
glycation, 83, 332
glycerin, 77, 164
glyphosates, 53
Goethe, Johann Wolfgang von, 31
Goldbeck, Nikki and David, 17
golden ratio. See phi
grapefruit, 268
    Grapefruit Glow Body Scrub, 289
gua sha, 217, 218
Guroian, Vigen, 30, 44
gut-brain axis, 61

H

Hadler, Nortin, 132
Hafiz, 5, 39, 40, 48, 52, 97, 180, 209, 230
haircare, 185, 301–3, 332–36
    Beach Breeze Hair Spray, 302
    Happy Hair Dry Shampoo, 303
    Happy Hair Rinse, 301
    Sandalwood Scalp Oil, 302
halides, 142
hands
    Tea Tree Hand Sanitizer, 297
    washing, 86
    See also nails
Hanson, Marla, 16
Happy Hair Dry Shampoo, 303
Happy Hair Rinse, 301
Happy Honey Mask, 290
Hatshepsut, Queen, 189

Headache Help, 294
heavy metals, 142
hemorrhoids, 336–37
Herodotus, 90
herpes simplex, 337
herpes zoster. See shingles
Hildegard of Bingen, Saint, 57, 209
hip baths, 221
Hippocrates, 198, 217, 248
Hof, Wim, 222
honey, 276–77
    Happy Honey Mask, 290
hormone replacement therapy, 133
hormones
    balancing, 338
    bone health and, 135
    herbs for, 135
    See also individual hormones
hot-spring baths, 219–20
Huggins, Hal, 117
Human Microbiome Project, 59, 64
Hurston, Zora Neale, 16, 49
hyaluronic acid, 77
hydration, 232, 270–74
hyperpigmentation, 338–42
hypopigmentation, 342

I

illumination, invitation to, 8–9
immortelle, 254–55
Immune-Boosting Spray, 306
infections, 331, 350
inflammation, 150–51
insects
    bites, 316
    Bye-Bye Insect Repellent, 305
intestinal hyperpermeability, 343–44
intuition, 216
inula, 268
iodine, 143–46, 278
Issels, Josef, 118
IUDs, 314
Iyotake, Tatanka, 40

About the Author

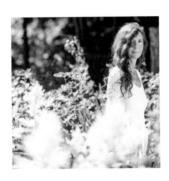

Nadine Artemis is the author of *Holistic Dental Care: The Complete Guide to Healthy Teeth and Gums* and a frequent commentator on health and beauty for media outlets. Alanis Morissette calls her "a true-sense visionary."

Artemis is the creator of Living Libations, a line of botanical health and beauty creations that are among the purest of the pure on the planet. As an innovative aromacologist, Nadine has formulated an elegant collection of rare and exceptional botanical compounds. Her potent dental serums are used worldwide and provide optimal oral care. She and her products have received rave reviews in the *New York Times*, the *National Post*, and the *Hollywood Reporter*.

Her relationship to the cosmos informs her concept of Renegade Beauty, which encourages effortlessness and inspires people to rethink conventional notions of beauty and wellness. This revolutionary vision allows the life force of flowers, dewdrops, plants, sun, and water to be the ingredients of healthy living, and lets everything unessential, contrived, and artificial fall away.

About North Atlantic Books

North Atlantic Books (NAB) is an independent, nonprofit publisher committed to a bold exploration of the relationships between mind, body, spirit, and nature. Founded in 1974, NAB aims to nurture a holistic view of the arts, sciences, humanities, and healing. To make a donation or to learn more about our books, authors, events, and newsletter, please visit www.northatlanticbooks.com.

North Atlantic Books is the publishing arm of the Society for the Study of Native Arts and Sciences, a 501(c)(3) nonprofit educational organization that promotes cross-cultural perspectives linking scientific, social, and artistic fields. To learn how you can support us, please visit our website.